Coronary Artery Disease

Editor

DAVID M. SHAVELLE

CARDIOLOGY CLINICS

www.cardiology.theclinics.com

Consulting Editors
ROSARIO FREEMAN
JORDAN M. PRUTKIN
DAVID M. SHAVELLE
AUDREY H. WU

August 2014 • Volume 32 • Number 3

ELSEVIER

1600 John F. Kennedy Boulevard • Suite 1800 • Philadelphia, Pennsylvania, 19103-2899

http://www.theclinics.com

CARDIOLOGY CLINICS Volume 32, Number 3
August 2014 ISSN 0733-8651, ISBN-13: 978-0-323-32365-9

Editor: Adrianne Brigido
Developmental Editor: Susan Showalter

Cardiology Clinics (ISSN 0733-8651) is published quarterly by Elsevier Inc., 360 Park Avenue South, New York, NY 10010-1710. Months of issue are February, May, August, and November. Business and Editorial Offices: 1600 John F. Kennedy Blvd., Ste. 1800, Philadelphia, PA 19103-2899. Customer Service Office: 3251 Riverport Lane, Maryland Heights, MO 63043. Periodicals post-age paid at New York, NY and additional mailing offices. Subscription prices are $320.00 per year for US individuals, $530.00 per year for US institutions, $155.00 per year for US students and residents, $390.00 per year for Canadian individuals, $665.00 per year for Canadian institutions, $455.00 per year for international individuals, $665.00 per year for international institutions and $220.00 per year for Canadian and international students/residents. To receive student/resident rate, orders must be accompanied by name of affiliated institution, data of term, and the *signature* of program/residency coordinator on institution letterhead. Orders will be billed at individual rate until proof of status is received. Foreign air speed delivery is included in all *Clinics* subscription prices. All prices are subject to change without notice. **POSTMASTER:** Send address changes to *Cardiology Clinics*, Elsevier Health Sciences Division, Subscription Customer Service, 3251 Riverport Lane, Maryland Heights, MO 63043. **Customer Service: 1-800-654-2452 (U.S. and Canada); 314-447-8871 (outside U.S. and Canada). Fax: 314-447-8029. E-mail: journalscustomerservice-usa@ elsevier.com (for print support); journalsonlinesupport-usa@elsevier.com (for online support).**

Reprints. For copies of 100 or more, of articles in this publication, please contact the Commercial Reprints Department, Elsevier Inc., 360 Park Avenue South, New York, NY 10010-1710. Tel.: 212-633-3874; Fax: 212-633-3820; E-mail: reprints@elsevier.com.

Cardiology Clinics is also published in Spanish by McGraw-Hill Interamericana Editores S. A., P.O. Box 5-237, 06500, Mexico D. F., Mexico; in Portuguese by Reichmann and Alfonso Editores Rio de Janeiro, Brazil; and in Greek by Dimitrios P. Lagos, 8 Pondon Street, GR115-28 Ilissia, Greece.

Cardiology Clinics is covered in *MEDLINE/PubMed (Index Medicus), Excerpta Medica, The Cumulative Index to Nursing and Allied Health Literature* (CINAHL).

Contributors

EDITORIAL BOARD

ROSARIO FREEMAN, MD, MS, FACC
Associate Professor of Medicine;
Director, Coronary Care Unit;
Director, Echocardiography Laboratory,
University of Washington Medical Center,
Seattle, Washington

JORDAN M. PRUTKIN, MD, MHS, FHRS
Assistant Professor of Medicine, Division
of Cardiology/Electrophysiology, University
of Washington Medical Center, Seattle,
Washington

DAVID M. SHAVELLE, MD, FACC, FSCAI
Associate Professor, Keck School of Medicine;
Director, General Cardiovascular Fellowship
Program; Director, Cardiac Catheterization
Laboratory, Los Angeles County + USC
Medical Center; Division of Cardiovascular
Medicine, University of Southern California,
Los Angeles, California

AUDREY H. WU, MD
Assistant Professor, Internal Medicine,
University of Michigan, Ann Arbor, Michigan

EDITOR

DAVID M. SHAVELLE, MD, FACC, FSCAI
Associate Professor, Keck School of Medicine;
Director, General Cardiovascular Fellowship
Program; Director, Cardiac Catheterization
Laboratory, Los Angeles County + USC
Medical Center; Division of Cardiovascular
Medicine, University of Southern California,
Los Angeles, California

AUTHORS

SHILPA AGRAWAL, BS
David Geffen School of Medicine, University
of California, Los Angeles, Los Angeles,
California

NANDAN S. ANAVEKAR, MBBCh
Division of Cardiovascular Diseases, Mayo
Clinic, Rochester, Minnesota

DORON ARONSON, MD
Department of Cardiology, Rambam Medical
Center, Technion, Israel Institute of
Technology, Haifa, Israel

J. WELLS ASKEW, MD
Division of Cardiovascular Diseases, Mayo
Clinic, Rochester, Minnesota

C. NOEL BAIREY MERZ, MD, FACC, FAHA
Director, Department of Medicine, Cedars-
Sinai Medical Center, Barbra Streisand
Women's Heart Center; Professor of Medicine,
Cedars-Sinai Heart Institute, Los Angeles,
California

SUKHDEEP S. BASRA, MD, MPH
Division of Cardiology, Baylor College of
Medicine, Houston, Texas

MATTHEW J. BUDOFF, MD
Principal Investigator, Internal Medicine Department, Los Angeles Biomedical Research Institute, Torrance, California

ELAZER R. EDELMAN, MD, PhD
Cardiovascular Division, Department of Medicine, Institute for Medical Science and Engineering, Massachusetts Institute of Technology, Brigham and Women's Hospital, Harvard Medical School, Boston, Massachusetts

WILLIAM J. FRENCH, MD
Professor of Medicine, David Geffen School of Medicine, University of California Los Angeles, Los Angeles, California; Division of Cardiology, Harbor UCLA Medical Center, Torrance, California

AMBARISH GOPAL, MD, FACC, FSCCT
The Heart Hospital Baylor Plano, Plano, Texas

ELLIOTT M. GROVES, MD, MEng
Division of Cardiology, Department of Internal Medicine; Department of Biomedical Engineering, University of California, Irvine, California

STUART J. HEAD, PhD
Department of Cardiothoracic Surgery, Thoraxcenter Erasmus MC, Rotterdam, The Netherlands

HANI JNEID, MD, FACC, FAHA, FSCAI
Division of Cardiology, Baylor College of Medicine, The Michael E. DeBakey VA Medical Center, Houston, Texas

A. PIETER KAPPETEIN, MD, PhD
Department of Cardiothoracic Surgery, Thoraxcenter Erasmus MC, Rotterdam, The Netherlands

BISWAJIT KAR, MD
Division of Cardiology, Baylor College of Medicine, The Michael E. DeBakey VA Medical Center, Houston, Texas

MORTON J. KERN, MD
Division of Cardiology, Department of Internal Medicine, University of California, Irvine, California; Division of Cardiology, Department of Internal Medicine, Long Beach Veterans Administration Hospital, Long Beach, California

RICHARD KONES, MD, FAHA, FESC, FRSM
The Cardiometabolic Research Institute, Houston, Texas

MOLLY MACK, BA
Research Coordinator, Cardiopulmonary Research Science and Technology Institute (CRSTI), Dallas, Texas

PUJA K. MEHTA, MD, FACC
Assistant Professor, Department of Medicine, Cedars-Sinai Medical Center, Barbra Streisand Women's Heart Center, Cedars-Sinai Heart Institute, Los Angeles, California

TODD D. MILLER, MD
Division of Cardiovascular Diseases, Mayo Clinic, Rochester, Minnesota

DAVID PANIAGUA, MD
Division of Cardiology, Baylor College of Medicine, The Michael E. DeBakey VA Medical Center, Houston, Texas

SWAPNESH PARIKH, MD
Internal Medicine Department, Los Angeles Biomedical Research Institute, Torrance, California

UMME RUMANA, MBBS
The Cardiometabolic Research Institute, Houston, Texas

ARNOLD H. SETO, MD, MPH
Division of Cardiology, Department of Internal Medicine, University of California, Irvine, California; Division of Cardiology, Department of Internal Medicine, Long Beach Veterans Administration Hospital, Long Beach, California

OZLEM SORAN, MD, MPH, FACC, FESC
Associate Professor of Medicine; Associate Professor of Epidemiology/Research; Director of EECP Treatment Lab, Heart and Vascular Institute, University of Pittsburgh, Pittsburgh, Pennsylvania

JOSEPH L. THOMAS, MD
Assistant Professor of Medicine, David Geffen School of Medicine, University of California Los Angeles, Los Angeles, California; Division of Cardiology, Harbor UCLA Medical Center, Torrance, California

NICOLAS M. VAN MIEGHEM, MD
Department of Cardiology, Thoraxcenter Erasmus MC, Rotterdam, The Netherlands

SALIM S. VIRANI, MD, PhD
Division of Cardiology, Baylor College of Medicine, The Michael E. DeBakey VA Medical Center, Houston, Texas

Contents

Coronary artery disease (CAD) mortality has been declining in the United States and in regions where health care systems are relatively advanced. Still, CAD remains the number one cause of death in both men and women in the United States, and coronary events have increased in women. Many traditional risk factors for CAD are related to lifestyle, and preventative treatment can be tailored to modifying specific factors. Novel risk factors also may contribute to CAD. Finally, as the risk for CAD is largely understood to be inherited, further genetic testing should play a role in preventative treatment of the disease.

Classical angina refers to typical substernal discomfort triggered by effort or emotions, relieved with rest or nitroglycerin. The well-accepted pathogenesis is an imbalance between oxygen supply and demand. Goals in therapy are improvement in quality of life by limiting the number and severity of attacks, protection against future lethal events, and measures to lower the burden of risk factors to slow disease progression. New pathophysiological data, drugs, as well as conceptual and technological advances have improved patient care over the past decade. Behavioral changes to improve diets, increase physical activity, and encourage adherence to cardiac rehabilitation programs, are difficult to achieve but are effective.

Non–ST elevation acute coronary syndromes (NSTE-ACS) encompass the clinical entities of unstable angina and non–ST elevation myocardial infarction. Several advances have occurred over the past decade, including the emergence of new antiplatelet and antithrombotic therapies and novel treatment strategies, leading to marked improvements in mortality. However, there has also been an increased incidence in NSTE-ACS as a result of the use of high-sensitivity troponins and the increase in cardiovascular risk factors. This article provides a focused update on contemporary management strategies pertaining to antiplatelet, antithrombotic, and anti-ischemic therapies and to revascularization strategies in patients with ACS.

Advances in reperfusion therapy for ST-segment elevation myocardial infarction (STEMI) provide optimal patient outcomes. Reperfusion therapies, including contemporary primary percutaneous coronary intervention, represent decades of clinical evidence development in large clinical trials and national databases. However, rapid identification of STEMI and guideline-directed management of patients across broad populations have been best achieved in advanced systems of care. Current outcomes in STEMI reflect the evolution of both clinical data and idealized health care delivery networks.

Noninvasive Stress Testing for Coronary Artery Disease

Todd D. Miller, J. Wells Askew, and Nandan S. Anavekar

Stress testing remains the cornerstone for noninvasive assessment of patients with possible or known coronary artery disease (CAD). The most important application of stress testing is risk stratification. Most patients who present for evaluation of stable CAD are categorized as low risk by stress testing. These low-risk patients have favorable clinical outcomes and generally do not require coronary angiography. Standard exercise treadmill testing is the initial procedure of choice in patients with a normal or near-normal resting electrocardiogram who are capable of adequate exercise. Stress imaging is recommended for patients with prior revascularization, uninterpretable electrocardiograms, or inability to adequately exercise.

Invasive Testing for Coronary Artery Disease: FFR, IVUS, OCT, NIRS

Elliott M. Groves, Arnold H. Seto, and Morton J. Kern

Coronary angiography is the gold standard for the diagnosis of coronary artery disease and guides revascularization strategies. The emergence of new diagnostic modalities has provided clinicians with adjunctive physiologic and image-based data to help formulate treatment strategies. Fractional flow reserve can predict whether percutaneous intervention will benefit a patient. Intravascular ultrasonography and optical coherence tomography are intracoronary imaging modalities that facilitate the anatomic visualization of the vessel lumen and characterize plaques. Near-infrared spectroscopy can characterize plaque composition and potentially provide valuable prognostic information. This article reviews the indications, basic technology, and supporting clinical studies for these modalities.

Calcium Scoring and Cardiac Computed Tomography in 2014

Swapnesh Parikh and Matthew J. Budoff

Although recent advances in noninvasive imaging technologies have potentially improved diagnostic efficiency and clinical outcomes of patients with acute chest pain, controversy remains regarding much of the accumulated evidence. This article reviews the role of coronary computed tomography (CT) angiography in the assessment of coronary risk, and its usefulness in the emergency department in facilitating appropriate disposition decisions. Also discussed is coronary artery calcification incidentally found on CT scans when done for indications such as evaluation of pulmonary embolism or lung cancer. The evidence base and clinical applications for both techniques are described, together with cost-effectiveness and radiation exposure considerations.

Alternative Therapy for Medically Refractory Angina: Enhanced External Counterpulsation and Transmyocardial Laser Revascularization

Ozlem Soran

Medically refractory angina pectoris (RAP) is defined by presence of severe angina with objective evidence of ischemia and failure to relieve symptoms with coronary revascularization. Medication and invasive revascularization are the most common approaches for treating coronary artery disease (CAD). Although symptoms are eliminated or alleviated by these invasive approaches, the disease and its causes are present after treatment. New treatment approaches are needed to prevent the disease from progressing and symptoms from recurring. External enhanced counterpulsation therapy provides a treatment modality in the management of CAD and can complement invasive revascularization procedures. Data support that it should be considered as a first-line treatment of RAP.

Diabetes mellitus (DM) is a major risk factor for cardiovascular disease. Near-normal glycemic control does not reduce cardiovascular events. For many patients with 1- or 2-vessel coronary artery disease, there is little benefit from any revascularization procedure over optimal medical therapy. For multivessel coronary disease, randomized trials demonstrated the superiority of coronary artery bypass grafting over multivessel percutaneous coronary intervention in patients with treated DM. However, selection of the optimal myocardial revascularization strategy requires a multidisciplinary team approach ('heart team'). This review summarizes the current evidence regarding the effectiveness of various medical therapies and revascularization strategies in patients with DM.

Coronary artery bypass grafting (CAGB) is superior to percutaneous coronary intervention (PCI) in reducing mortality in certain patients and improving the composite end points of angina, recurrent myocardial infarction, and repeat revascularization procedures. However, CABG is associated with a higher perioperative stroke risk. For patients with less complex disease or left main coronary disease, PCI is an acceptable alternative to CABG. Lesion complexity is an essential consideration for stenting, whereas patient comorbidity is an essential consideration for CABG. All patients with complex multivessel coronary artery disease should be reviewed by a heart team including a cardiac surgeon and interventional cardiologist.

Cardiac Syndrome X (CSX), characterized by angina-like chest discomfort, ST segment depression during exercise, and normal epicardial coronary arteries at angiography, is highly prevalent in women. CSX is not benign, and linked to adverse cardiovascular outcomes and a poor quality of life. Coronary microvascular and endothelial dysfunction and abnormal cardiac nociception have been implicated in the pathogenesis of CSX. Treatment includes life-style modification, anti-anginal, anti-atherosclerotic, and anti-ischemic medications. Non-pharmacological options include cognitive behavioral therapy, enhanced external counterpulsation, neurostimulation, and stellate ganglionectomy. Studies have shown the efficacy of individual treatments but guidelines outlining the best course of therapy are lacking.

CARDIOLOGY CLINICS

DOWNLOAD
Free App!

Review Articles
THE CLINICS

NOW AVAILABLE FOR YOUR iPhone and iPad

Preface
Coronary Artery Disease

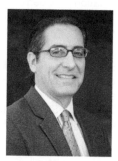

David M. Shavelle, MD, FACC, FSCAI
Editor

Coronary artery disease continues to be a major cause of morbidity and mortality in the United States and throughout the world. Multiple recent, randomized clinical trials have influenced society-based practice guidelines (American College of Cardiology, American Heart Association, and the European Society of Cardiology), altered clinical practice, and improved the care of cardiovascular patients. Our aim in the current issue of *Cardiology Clinics* is to provide a contemporary and concise, yet extensive, review on all aspects of the management of patients with coronary artery disease. To achieve this, we have organized a group of highly accomplished clinicians and research scientists. All authors have sought to provide evidence-based recommendations incorporating the most recent society-based practice guidelines and pivotal clinical trials.

Drs Mack and Gopal begin the issue with an overview of the epidemiology of coronary artery disease, the basis for risk factor equivalents, and a summary of the traditional and emerging cardiovascular risk factors. Drs Kones and Rumana discuss the management of patients with stable ischemic heart disease with a focus on the evidence base to support established medical therapy, including a discussion of silent ischemia and the promise of future medical therapy. Drs Basra, Virani, Kar, Deswal, and Jneid discuss the acute coronary syndromes of unstable angina and non-ST segment elevation myocardial infarction, including the pathophysiology, risk stratification, and the various medical therapies used, with a concise summary of the newest iteration of antiplatelet therapy (Prasugrel, Ticangrelor, and Cangrelor). Drs French and

Thomas contribute an article on the acute coronary syndrome of ST segment elevation myocardial infarction (STEMI) with a focus on evidence-based therapies and the use of advanced systems of care (ie, STEMI receiving systems).

Drs Miller, Askew, and Anavekar provide an article on noninvasive testing, including information on exercise treadmill, exercise and pharmacologic echocardiography, and exercise and pharmacologic nuclear stress testing. At the conclusion of the article, the authors summarize two recent randomized studies comparing several of these imaging methods and also review pertinent data on the use of stress testing from several recently published clinical trials: Clinical Outcomes Using Revascularization and Aggressive Drug Evaluation (COURAGE); Bypass Angioplasty Revascularization Investigation 2 Diabetes (BARI 2D); and Surgical Treatment for Ischemic Heart Failure (STICH). Drs Groves, Seto, and Kern discuss the basis for invasive testing for ischemia and the evaluation of plaque morphology in the cardiac catheterization laboratory using fractional flow reserve, coronary flow reserve, optimal coherence tomography, and near-infrared spectroscopy. Drs Parikh and Budoff focus on the use of coronary calcium scanning for risk stratification and the role of cardiac computed tomography in evaluating patients with chest pain. Dr Soran presents the current status on patients with medical refractory angina and discusses the evidence to support the use of external enhanced counterpulsation and transmyocardial laser revascularization.

A substantial number of patients with coronary artery disease also have diabetes mellitus, and

Cardiol Clin 32 (2014) xi–xii
http://dx.doi.org/10.1016/j.ccl.2014.06.001
0733-8651/14/$ – see front matter

Drs Aronson and Edelman present an article on the contemporary management of these patients, including information from the recently completed BARI-2D, SYNergy Between PCI With TAXus and Cardiac Surgery (SYNTAX), and the Future Revascularization Evaluation in Patients with Diabetes Mellitus: Optimal Management of Multivessel Disease (FREEDOM) trials. Drs Kappetien, van Mieghem, and Head discuss the respective roles of coronary artery bypass surgery and percutaneous coronary intervention for patients with multivessel and left main coronary artery disease. Drs Agrawal, Mehta, and Bairey Merz conclude the issue with a summary of Cardiac Syndrome X, including the role of diagnostic testing and coronary microvascular dysfunction, the natural history, options for pharmacologic and nonpharmacologic treatment, and the use of lifestyle modifications.

We hope you enjoy this issue of *Cardiology Clinics* and that the information provided enhances your medical knowledge and further improves the care of your patients with coronary artery disease.

David M. Shavelle, MD, FACC, FSCAI
Division of Cardiovascular Medicine
University of Southern California
1510 San Pablo Street, Suite 322
Los Angeles, CA 90033, USA

E-mail address:
shavelle@usc.edu

Epidemiology, Traditional and Novel Risk Factors in Coronary Artery Disease

Molly Mack, BA[a], Ambarish Gopal, MD, FSCCT[b],*

KEYWORDS

- Coronary artery disease • Epidemiology • Risk factors

KEY POINTS

- The top risk factors related to coronary artery disease (CAD) include suboptimal diet, tobacco use, high body mass index, high blood pressure, high fasting plasma glucose, and physical inactivity.
- Various lifestyle factors, including tobacco use, diet, exercise, alcohol intake, and obesity, significantly impact the risk of developing CAD.
- Many risk factors for CAD are modifiable by specific, preventable measures.
- All patients with a CAD risk equivalent (noncoronary atherosclerotic arterial disease, diabetes mellitus, or chronic kidney disease) should be managed as aggressively as those with prior CAD.
- Emerging risk factors for CAD, including C-reactive protein, Interleukin-6, myeloperoxidase, radiation, metabolic syndrome, and microalbuminuria warrant further analysis.

EPIDEMIOLOGY OF CORONARY ARTERY DISEASE

Introduction

By analyzing the patterns, causes and effects of coronary artery disease (CAD) in different populations, the field of epidemiology has helped identify risk factors for CAD and directs specific therapy for the primary and secondary prevention of cardiovascular disease.

In developed nations, CAD is a major cause of death and disability.[1,2] CAD remains the number one cause of death in both men and women in the United States.[1,2] Although mortality rates related to CAD have continued to decline over past years, CAD remains accountable for about one-third of all deaths over the age of 35 years.[1,2] Additionally, about a half of all middle-aged men and a third of middle-aged women in the United States will have some form of CAD.[3]

CAD is typically a chronic disease with progression over a period of years or decades. It remains a large public health burden. In 2010, 1 in 6 deaths in the United States was caused by CAD (379,599 Americans died of the disease).[4] In the same year, the American Heart Association (AHA) reported cardiovascular-related health costs at an estimated $315.4 billion.[1,4] According to the AHA, the 2010 overall death rate related to CAD was 235.5 deaths per 100,000 population.[1] Every 31 seconds, an American has a coronary event, and every 1 minute and 23 seconds, an American dies of CAD.[1] Although women have historically been at lower risk for CAD, current data indicate that the prevalence of cardiac events in men is decreasing, while women are experiencing an increase in cardiac events, including myocardial infarction.[5]

Prevalence

According to data from the National Heart, Lung, and Blood Institute's National Health and Nutrition Examination Survey (NHANES) 2007 to 2010, an

[a] Cardiopulmonary Research Science and Technology Institute (CRSTI), 7777 Forest Lane, C-742, Dallas, TX 75230, USA; [b] The Heart Hospital Baylor Plano, 1100 Allied Drive, Plano, TX 75093, USA
* Corresponding author.
E-mail address: Ambarish.gopal@baylorhealth.edu

Cardiol Clin 32 (2014) 323–332
http://dx.doi.org/10.1016/j.ccl.2014.04.003
0733-8651/14/$ – see front matter © 2014 Elsevier Inc. All rights reserved.

estimated 15.4 million Americans at least 20 years of age have CAD.[1] The reported prevalence increases with age for both women and men.[1] Myocardial infarction (MI) prevalence was compared by gender in middle-aged individuals (age 35–54 years) during the 1988 to 1994 and 1999 to 2004 time periods.[5] Despite MI prevalence being significantly greater in men than women during both time periods, there were trends showing a decrease in men and an increase in women, repectively.[5]

Data that rely on self-reported MI and angina probably underestimate the actual prevalence of advanced CAD (advanced obstructive CAD can commonly exist with few symptoms or no obvious clinical findings, as silent ischemia can account for about 75% of all ischemic episodes).[6]

Incidence

The incidence of initial coronary events (identified and unidentified MI, angina pectoris, unstable coronary syndromes and coronary deaths) can be summarized as follows[7–9]:

- Lifetime risk of developing CAD is 49% in men and 32% in women for individuals aged 40 years. The lifetime risk is 35% in men and 24% in women for individuals aged 70 years.
- Incidence of all coronary events rises with age (females lagging behind males by about 10 years). For MI and sudden death, women lag behind men in incidence by about 20 years (the sex ratio for incidence narrows progressively with advancing age).[2] The incidence at ages 65 to 94 years compared with ages 35 to 64 years approximately more than doubles in men and triples in women.
- In premenopausal women, MI and sudden death are relatively rare. After menopause, the incidence and severity of CAD increases abruptly, with rates about 3 times those of women the same age who are premenopausal.[7]
- Initial presentation of coronary disease in women less than 75 years is more likely to be angina pectoris than MI.[8] Angina in women is more likely to be uncomplicated, while angina in men often occurs after an MI.[8,9]
- Incidence of CAD has decreased over time in developed countries.[10,11]
- Although in developed countries heart disease mortality has been declining, the experience is often quite different around the world.[12] CAD is the number one cause of death in adults from both low- and middle-income countries, as well as from those high-income countries.[13]

- In India, CAD may not mostly be explained by traditional CAD risk factors.[14] In China, risk factor trends complement tracking of event rates (for example, higher cholesterol levels correlate with increased CAD mortality).[15] In Latin America, declines in vascular event rates have not been as favorable as in the United States (unfavorable patterns in physical activity, obesity, and smoking may explain this).[16]

Clinical Presentation of CAD

Myocardial infarction

Despite the reported declining incidence of CAD over the past years and decades in the United States, most observational studies have not documented a reduction in the incidence of MI in different time periods ranging from 1971 to 2006.[10,17–21] This conflict may possibly be explained by the use of the more sensitive troponin assays, which began around 2000. These sensitive assays diagnose MI even when less of the myocardium is infarcted, an effect that could possibly mask a reduction in MI incidence over time.[22] However, another study did not show this to be the case, even when including all infarctions irrespective of biomarker used for diagnosis.[21] There has been a relative increase in the presentation of non-ST segment elevation MI (NSTEMI) in relation to ST segment elevation MI (STEMI) over the past.[17,18,21]

CAD is the leading cause of death in adults in the United States, accounting for about one-third of all deaths in subjects over the age of 35 years.[3] The death rate is higher in men than in women (3 times higher at ages 25–34 years and decreasing to 1.6 times at ages 75–84 years), and in blacks compared with whites, an excess difference that resolves by age 75 years.[3] Among the Hispanic population, coronary mortality is not as high as it is among blacks and whites.[3]

Mortality rates for CAD in men and women, and in blacks and whites, have decreased in most developed countries by about 24% to 50% since 1975, although this decrease has slowed down since 1990.[3,10,23–32] From 1996 to 2006, death rates from CAD were reported to have come down by about 29%.[3] In the United States, from 1980 to 2000, the factors responsible for the reduction in CAD mortality were evaluated in adults between the ages of 25 and 84 years.[30] Approximately 50% of this effect was due to improvements in therapy, including secondary preventive measures after MI or revascularization, initial management for acute coronary syndromes, management of heart failure, and revascularization for chronic angina. The other half of this effect was due to risk factor modification, including reductions in total cholesterol, systolic blood pressure, smoking prevalence, and physical inactivity. These were counterbalanced by increases in body mass index and diabetes mellitus, which together contributed to an 18% increase in the number of deaths.[33]

Silent myocardial ischemia and infarction

In silent myocardial ischemia, the development of a Q wave MI in the absence of typical symptoms is considered a specific finding with electrocardiogram (ECG).[34] MI was silent in about 26% to 33% of the men and about 33% to 54% of the women.[35–38] This was higher in diabetic men than in nondiabetic men.[39] Silent MI is strongly age dependent, with incidence being almost zero before age 40 years with increases to about 3 cases per 1000 population per year at age 60.[38] A similar pattern was noted in almost 13,000 women with another study.[37] With ECGs, approximately 10% of anterior MIs and 25% of inferior MIs revert to a nondiagnostic pattern within 2 years after the MI, and some unidentified MIs may result in sudden death before they can be discovered.[40,41] Both hypertension and diabetes mellitus are associated with silent MIs. Among individuals with blood pressure greater than 160/95 mm Hg who had MIs, the MI was silent in about 48% of the women and about 32% of the men.[42]

Silent MIs were more than twice as prevalent in men with diabetes mellitus than in those without (about 39 vs 18%). In contrast, women with diabetes mellitus were less likely to have unrecognized MIs.[39,43]

About 2% to 4% of the general population has CAD that is asymptomatic but detectable by an exercise ECG or an ambulatory ECG monitoring.[44,45] Prevalence of silent ischemia may be as high as 10% in asymptomatic men with 2 or more major coronary risk factors.[44,45] Silent ischemia is even more common in those with known CAD.[44,45] In patients with stable angina who undergo exercise testing and ambulatory monitoring, the prevalence of silent ischemia is estimated to range from 25% to 50%, and about 70% to 80% of ischemic episodes are silent.[44,45]

Sudden cardiac death

Sudden cardiac death (SCD) is the initial clinical coronary event in about 15% of individuals with CAD.[46] SCD is also the most frequent mode of death in patients with CAD (about 30%–50%).[47,48] The occurrence of SCD after acute MI is the same with STEMI and NSTEMI, and with symptomatic and silent infarctions.[49,50] Women have been found to be significantly less likely to have severe left ventricular dysfunction or a

diagnosis of CAD.[51] Women were also less likely than men to have ventricular fibrillation as an initial presenting rhythm and were more likely to have pulseless electrical activity/asystole.[52] After adjusting for the presence of ventricular fibrillation and other factors, women had a similar comparable rate of survival to hospital discharge.[50]

Risk Factors

CAD risk equivalents

Some individuals without known CAD have a risk of major cardiovascular events that is equivalent to that of patients with established CAD (**Table 1**). All patients with a CAD risk equivalent should be managed as aggressively as those with prior, established CAD.

The following are established CAD risk equivalents:

- Noncoronary atherosclerotic disease process that includes carotid artery disease, peripheral artery disease or abdominal aortic aneurysm. The 10-year risk of developing CAD exceeds 20% in these patient groups.
- Diabetes mellitus (insulin resistance, hyperinsulinemia, and elevated blood glucose) are associated with atherosclerotic cardiovascular disease.[53–60] The all-cause mortality risk associated with diabetes mellitus is

Table 1
Traditional and novel risk factors of coronary artery disease

Traditional Risk Factors	Suboptimal diet
	Tobacco smoking
	High BMI
	High blood pressure (>140/90 mm Hg, or use of antihypertensive medication)
	High fasting plasma glucose
	Physical inactivity
	Age (male >45 y, female >55 y)
	Family history of premature CAD
	HDL cholesterol (<40 mg/dL)
Novel Risk Factors	Plasma concentration of C-reactive protein
	IL-6 and membrane-bound IL-6 receptors
	Increased levels of the leukocyte enzyme myeloperoxidase
	HIV-positive status
	Mediastinal or chest wall radiation
	Metabolic syndrome
	Microalbuminuria
	Remnant lipoproteins

comparable to the all-cause mortality risk associated with a prior MI.[61]

- Hyperglycemia without overt diabetes mellitus correlates with cardiovascular risk in patients with and without diabetes at baseline.
- Chronic kidney disease with even mild-to-moderate renal dysfunction is associated with a substantial increase in CAD risk.[62]

Risk factors of CAD

Over 90% of CAD events occur in individuals with at least 1 risk factor.[63,64] The absence of major risk factors predicts a much lower risk of CAD.[61] The frequency and predictive value of 5 major risk factors (blood pressure, low-density lipoprotein [LDL] and high-density lipoprotein [HDL] cholesterol, glucose intolerance, and smoking) were evaluated in 35- to 74-year-old white non-Hispanic individuals without coronary heart disease (CHD) in the Framingham Heart Study and the Third National Health and Nutrition Examination Survey (NHANES III).[62] The frequency of borderline risk factors (defined as systolic pressure 120–139 mm Hg, diastolic pressure 80–89 mm Hg, LDL cholesterol 100–159 mg/dL [2.6–4.1 mmol/L], HDL cholesterol 40–59 mg/dL [1.0–1.5 mmol/L], impaired fasting glucose without overt diabetes, and a past history of smoking) was also assessed in the same cohorts.[62] In NHANES III, about 60% of men and about 50% of women had 1 to 2 elevated risk factors, and about 26% of men and about 41% of women had at least 1 borderline risk factor.[62]

Recent analyses from the US Burden of Disease Collaborators demonstrated that each of the 7 health factors and behaviors causes substantial mortality and morbidity in the United States. The top risk factors related to overall disease burden were suboptimal diet, followed by tobacco smoking, high body mass index (BMI), high blood pressure, high fasting plasma glucose, and physical inactivity.[1]

Factors that may synergistically increase the risk of CAD are[65]

- Age: men at least 45 years of age, women at least 55 years of age or premature menopause without estrogen replacement therapy
- Family history of premature CAD: definite myocardial infarction or sudden death before age 55 years in male first-degree relative and before age 65 in female first-degree relative
- Current cigarette smoking
- Hypertension: blood pressure greater than 140/90 mm Hg, or use of an antihypertensive medication
- HDL cholesterol less than 40 mg/dL (1.03 mmol/L)

Factors that may reduce the risk of CAD are

- HDL cholesterol of at least 60 mg/dL (1.55 mmol/L)

The presence of the previously mentioned established risk factors is associated with CAD, and the AHA therefore promotes 7 ideal cardiovascular health metrics.[66]

- Not smoking
- Being physically active
- Having a normal blood pressure
- Having a normal blood glucose level
- Having a normal total cholesterol level
- Being normal weight
- Eating a healthy diet

The following specific lipid and lipoprotein abnormalities are associated with an increased risk of CAD:

- Elevated total cholesterol and elevated LDL cholesterol
- Low HDL cholesterol
- Hypertriglyceridemia
- Increased non-HDL cholesterol
- Increased Lipoprotein(a)
- Increased apolipoprotein C-III
- Small, dense LDL particles
- Different genotypes of apolipoprotein E (apoE) influence cholesterol and triglyceride levels as well as the risk of CAD

There is growing evidence showing fruit and vegetable consumption is inversely related to the risk of CAD and stroke.[65,67–73] Higher intake of red meat and high-fat dairy products has been associated with increased risk of CAD.[74,75] High fiber intake is also associated with decrease in the risk of CAD and stroke compared with low fiber intake.[65,66] High serum concentrations of enterolactone (biomarker of a diet high in fiber and vegetable) inversely correlates with the risk of acute coronary events and with CAD mortality.[68,69]

Exercise may have a variety of beneficial effects as follows[74,76–85]:

- Exercise of even moderate degree renders protection against CAD and all-cause mortality.
- An elevation in serum HDL cholesterol, a reduction in blood pressure, and a reduction of insulin resistance promotes weight loss.
- The degree of cardiovascular fitness (a measure of physical activity) is associated with a reduction in CAD risk and overall cardiovascular mortality. This is determined by duration of exercise and maximal oxygen uptake on a treadmill.

Obesity is associated with several risk factors for atherosclerosis, CAD, and cardiovascular mortality, including hypertension, insulin resistance and glucose intolerance, hypertriglyceridemia, reduced HDL cholesterol, and decreased levels of adiponectin.[86–89]

Psychosocial factors may contribute to the early development of CAD as well as to the acute precipitation of MI and sudden cardiac death (damage of the endothelium and aggravation of traditional risk factors such as smoking, hypertension, and lipid metabolism).[90–93] Depression, anger, stress, and other factors have been associated with negative cardiovascular outcomes.[88–91]

NOVEL AND EMERGING RISK FACTORS

A person's baseline level of inflammation, as evaluated by the plasma concentration of c-reactive protein (CRP), predicts the long-term risk of a first MI, ischemic stroke, or peripheral artery disease.[94–96] It improves risk stratification of a patient for CAD[97,98] and may help direct further evaluation and therapy for primary prevention.[99–101]

Interleukin-6 (IL-6) and membrane-bound IL-6 receptors (IL-6Rs) appear to have a role in the development of CAD and may be a future target for therapeutic interventions to help prevent CAD.[102–104] The presence of Asp358Ala (rs2228145, formerly rs8192284), a variant allele of the *IL6R* gene encoding IL-6R, has been associated with decreased membrane-bound IL-6R, resulting in reduced IL-6R signaling and thus less inflammation.[96–98] Elevated soluble circulating IL-6R levels have led to decreased membrane-bound IL-6R, thereby decreasing signaling and downstream inflammation (reduced CRP levels).[96–98]

Increased levels of the leukocyte enzyme myeloperoxidase, which is secreted during acute inflammation and promotes oxidation of lipoproteins, are associated with the presence of coronary disease and may be predictive of the presence of acute coronary syndrome in patients with chest pain.[105–108] Among patients with chronic systolic heart failure, elevated plasma myeloperoxidase levels have been associated with an increased likelihood of more advanced heart failure and may be predictive of a higher rate of adverse clinical outcomes.[109]

The risk of CAD in human immunodeficiency virus (HIV)-positive patients is predominantly driven by traditional CAD risk factors.[110–114] However, studies correcting for traditional CAD risk factors have shown higher rates of CAD and MI in HIV-positive patients when compared with HIV-negative controls.[104–108]

Mediastinal or chest wall radiation during treatment for malignancy (eg, Hodgkin lymphoma or breast cancer) has been linked to CAD, pericardial disease, valvular disease, and cardiomyopathy.[115,116] Radiation CAD tends to involve the ostia of the left main and right coronary arteries, and may present as either angina or acute MI, potentially requiring revascularization.[104,105]

Individuals with metabolic syndrome (abdominal obesity, hypertension, diabetes, and dyslipidemia) have a markedly increased risk of CAD.[117–119] This is also called the insulin resistance syndrome or syndrome X. Remnant lipoproteins (RLPs) are precursors to LDLs. In people with metabolic syndrome and diabetes, poor triglyceride lipolysis can increase these remnants, including very low-density lipoproteins (VLDL3) and intermediate-density lipoproteins (IDLs), which are correlated with risk for CAD.

Microalbuminuria is associated with vascular damage and appears to be a marker of early CAD. While microalbuminuria is considered an important risk factor for CAD and early cardiovascular mortality, the mechanism by which microalbuminuria is associated with CAD remains unclear.[120,121]

GENETIC TESTING

As up to 40% to 60% of susceptibility to CAD is said to be inherited, genetic testing should continue to play a larger role in identifying risk factors and determining preventative treatment. Currently, genome-wide association studies (GWAS) have identified 33 genetic variants that increase a person's risk for CAD. As many of the variants mediate risk through loci independent of the known risk factors (only 10 of the variants mediate through hypertension or lipids), further genetic analysis is necessary.[122]

SUMMARY

CAD mortality has been declining in the United States and in regions where health care systems are relatively advanced. Although prevalence has decreased, CAD remains the number one cause of death in both men and women in the United States, and coronary events have increased in women. Many traditional risk factors for CAD are related to lifestyle, and preventative treatment can be tailored to modifying specific factors. These top risk factors include suboptimal diet, tobacco use, high BMI, high blood pressure, high plasma glucose, and physical inactivity. Novel risk factors, including plasma concentration of C-reactive protein, IL-6, myeloperoxidase, radiation, metabolic syndrome, and microalbuminuria may contribute to CAD as well. Finally, as the risk for CAD is largely understood to be inherited, further genetic testing should play a role in preventative treatment of the disease.

REFERENCES

1. Go AS, Mozaffarian D, Roger VL, et al. Heart disease and stroke statistics—2014 update: a report from the American Heart Association. Circulation 2014;129:e28–292.
2. Go AS, Mozaffarian D, Roger VL, et al. Executive summary: heart disease and stroke statistics—2014 update: a report from the American Heart Association. Circulation 2014;129:399–410.
3. Lloyd-Jones DM, Larson MG, Beiser A, et al. Lifetime risk of developing coronary heart disease. Lancet 1999;353:89.
4. Murphy SL, Xu J, Kochanek KD. Deaths: final data for 2010. Natl Vital Stat Rep 2013;61(4).
5. Towfighi A, Zheng L, Ovbiagele B. Sex-specific trends in midlife coronary heart disease risk and prevalence. Arch Intern Med 2009;169:1762–6.
6. Deedwania PC, Carbajal EV. Silent myocardial ischemia. A clinical perspective. Arch Intern Med 1991;151:2373.
7. Gordon T, Kannel WB, Hjortland MC, et al. Menopause and coronary heart disease. The Framingham Study. Ann Intern Med 1978;89:157.
8. Lerner DJ, Kannel WB. Patterns of coronary heart disease morbidity and mortality in the sexes: a 26-year follow-up of the Framingham population. Am Heart J 1986;111:383.
9. Kannel WB. Prevalence and clinical aspects of unrecognized myocardial infarction and sudden unexpected death. Circulation 1987;75:II4.
10. Ergin A, Muntner P, Sherwin R, et al. Secular trends in cardiovascular disease mortality, incidence, and case fatality rates in adults in the United States. Am J Med 2004;117:219.
11. Arciero TJ, Jacobsen SJ, Reeder GS, et al. Temporal trends in the incidence of coronary disease. Am J Med 2004;117:228.
12. Yusuf S, Reddy S, Ounpuu S, et al. Global burden of cardiovascular diseases: part II: variations in cardiovascular disease by specific ethnic groups and geographic regions and prevention strategies. Circulation 2001;104:2855.
13. Lopez AD, Mathers CD, Ezzati M, et al. Global and regional burden of disease and risk factors, 2001: systematic analysis of population health data. Lancet 2006;367:1747.
14. Goyal A, Yusuf S. The burden of cardiovascular disease in the Indian subcontinent. Indian J Med Res 2006;124:235.
15. Critchley J, Liu J, Zhao D, et al. Explaining the increase in coronary heart disease mortality in Beijing between 1984 and 1999. Circulation 2004;110:1236.
16. Rodríguez T, Malvezzi M, Chatenoud L, et al. Trends in mortality from coronary heart and cerebrovascular diseases in the Americas: 1970-2000. Heart 2006;92:453.
17. Furman MI, Dauerman HL, Goldberg RJ, et al. Twenty-two year (1975 to 1997) trends in the incidence, in-hospital and long-term case fatality rates from initial Q-wave and non-Q-wave myocardial infarction: a multi-hospital, community-wide perspective. J Am Coll Cardiol 2001;37:1571.
18. Rogers WJ, Frederick PD, Stoehr E, et al. Trends in presenting characteristics and hospital mortality among patients with ST elevation and non-ST elevation myocardial infarction in the National Registry of Myocardial Infarction from 1990 to 2006. Am Heart J 2008;156:1026.
19. Chen J, Normand SL, Wang Y, et al. Recent declines in hospitalizations for acute myocardial infarction for Medicare fee-for-service beneficiaries: progress and continuing challenges. Circulation 2010;121:1322.
20. Hardoon SL, Whincup PH, Lennon LT, et al. How much of the recent decline in the incidence of myocardial infarction in British men can be explained by changes in cardiovascular risk factors? Evidence from a prospective population-based study. Circulation 2008;117:598.
21. Roger VL, Weston SA, Gerber Y, et al. Trends in incidence, severity, and outcome of hospitalized myocardial infarction. Circulation 2010;121:863.
22. Parikh NI, Gona P, Larson MG, et al. Long-term trends in myocardial infarction incidence and case fatality in the National Heart, Lung, and Blood Institute's Framingham Heart study. Circulation 2009;119:1203.
23. Kuulasmaa K, Tunstall-Pedoe H, Dobson A, et al. Estimation of contribution of changes in classic risk factors to trends in coronary-event rates across the WHO MONICA Project populations. Lancet 2000;355:675.
24. McGovern PG, Pankow JS, Shahar E, et al. Recent trends in acute coronary heart disease—mortality, morbidity, medical care, and risk factors. The Minnesota Heart Survey Investigators. N Engl J Med 1996;334:884.
25. Capewell S, Morrison CE, McMurray JJ. Contribution of modern cardiovascular treatment and risk factor changes to the decline in coronary heart disease mortality in Scotland between 1975 and 1994. Heart 1999;81:380.
26. Capewell S, Beaglehole R, Seddon M, et al. Explanation for the decline in coronary heart disease

mortality rates in Auckland, New Zealand, between 1982 and 1993. Circulation 2000;102:1511.

27. Cooper R, Cutler J, Desvigne-Nickens P, et al. Trends and disparities in coronary heart disease, stroke, and other cardiovascular diseases in the United States: findings of the national conference on cardiovascular disease prevention. Circulation 2000;102:3137.

28. McGovern PG, Jacobs DR Jr, Shahar E, et al. Trends in acute coronary heart disease mortality, morbidity, and medical care from 1985 through 1997: the Minnesota heart survey. Circulation 2001;104:19.

29. Rosamond WD, Chambless LE, Folsom AR, et al. Trends in the incidence of myocardial infarction and in mortality due to coronary heart disease, 1987 to 1994. N Engl J Med 1998;339:861.

30. Ford ES, Ajani UA, Croft JB, et al. Explaining the decrease in U.S. deaths from coronary disease, 1980-2000. N Engl J Med 2007;356:2388.

31. Tu JV, Nardi L, Fang J, et al. National trends in rates of death and hospital admissions related to acute myocardial infarction, heart failure and stroke 1994-2004. CMAJ 2009;180:1304.

32. Preis SR, Hwang SJ, Coady S, et al. Trends in all-cause and cardiovascular disease mortality among women and men with and without diabetes mellitus in the Framingham Heart Study, 1950 to 2005. Circulation 2009;119:1728.

33. Fox CS, Coady S, Sorlie PD, et al. Increasing cardiovascular disease burden due to diabetes mellitus: the Framingham Heart Study. Circulation 2007; 115:1544.

34. Sheifer SE, Manolio TA, Gersh BJ. Unrecognized myocardial infarction. Ann Intern Med 2001;135:801.

35. Kannel WB, Cupples LA, Gagnon DR. Incidence, precursors and prognosis of unrecognized myocardial infarction. Adv Cardiol 1990;37:202.

36. de Torbal A, Boersma E, Kors JA, et al. Incidence of recognized and unrecognized myocardial infarction in men and women aged 55 and older: the Rotterdam Study. Eur Heart J 2006;27:729.

37. Jónsdóttir LS, Sigfusson N, Sigvaldason H, et al. Incidence and prevalence of recognised and unrecognised myocardial infarction in women. The Reykjavik Study. Eur Heart J 1998;19:1011.

38. Sigurdsson E, Thorgeirsson G, Sigvaldason H, et al. Unrecognized myocardial infarction: epidemiology, clinical characteristics, and the prognostic role of angina pectoris. The Reykjavik Study. Ann Intern Med 1995;122:96.

39. Kannel WB. Lipids, diabetes, and coronary heart disease: insights from the Framingham Study. Am Heart J 1985;110:1100.

40. Davidoff R, Goldman AP, Diamond TH, et al. The natural history of the Q wave in inferoposterior myocardial infarction. S Afr Med J 1982;61:611.

41. Richter A, Herlitz J, Hjalmarson A. QRS complex recovery during one year after acute myocardial infarction. Clin Cardiol 1987;10:16.

42. Kannel WB, Dannenberg AL, Abbott RD. Unrecognized myocardial infarction and hypertension: the Framingham Study. Am Heart J 1985;109:581.

43. Shlipak MG, Elmouchi DA, Herrington DM, et al. The incidence of unrecognized myocardial infarction in women with coronary heart disease. Ann Intern Med 2001;134:1043.

44. Deedwania PC. Should asymptomatic subjects with silent ischemia undergo further evaluation and follow-up? Int J Cardiol 1994;44:101.

45. Deedwania PC. The need for a cost-effective strategy to detect ambulatory silent ischemia. Am J Cardiol 1994;74:1061.

46. Kannel WB, Doyle JT, McNamara PM, et al. Precursors of sudden coronary death. Factors related to the incidence of sudden death. Circulation 1975; 51:606.

47. Kannel WB, Wilson PW, D'Agostino RB, et al. Sudden coronary death in women. Am Heart J 1998; 136:205.

48. Gillum RF. Sudden coronary death in the United States: 1980-1985. Circulation 1989;79:756.

49. Kannel WB, Cupples LA, D'Agostino RB. Sudden death risk in overt coronary heart disease: the Framingham Study. Am Heart J 1987;113:799.

50. Berger CJ, Murabito JM, Evans JC, et al. Prognosis after first myocardial infarction. Comparison of Q-wave and non-Q-wave myocardial infarction in the Framingham Heart Study. JAMA 1992; 268:1545.

51. Chugh SS, Uy-Evanado A, Teodorescu C, et al. Women have a lower prevalence of structural heart disease as a precursor to sudden cardiac arrest: The Ore-SUDS (Oregon Sudden Unexpected Death Study). J Am Coll Cardiol 2009;54:2006.

52. Kim C, Fahrenbruch CE, Cobb LA, et al. Out-of-hospital cardiac arrest in men and women. Circulation 2001;104:2699.

53. Kannel WB, McGee DL. Diabetes and cardiovascular risk factors: the Framingham study. Circulation 1979;59:8.

54. Kannel WB, McGee DL. Diabetes and glucose tolerance as risk factors for cardiovascular disease: the Framingham study. Diabetes Care 1979;2:120.

55. Almdal T, Scharling H, Jensen JS, et al. The independent effect of type 2 diabetes mellitus on ischemic heart disease, stroke, and death: a population-based study of 13,000 men and women with 20 years of follow-up. Arch Intern Med 2004; 164:1422.

56. Reaven GM. Banting lecture 1988. Role of insulin resistance in human disease. Diabetes 1988;37: 1595.

57. Zavaroni I, Bonora E, Pagliara M, et al. Risk factors for coronary artery disease in healthy persons with hyperinsulinemia and normal glucose tolerance. N Engl J Med 1989;320:702.

58. Al-Delaimy WK, Merchant AT, Rimm EB, et al. Effect of type 2 diabetes and its duration on the risk of peripheral arterial disease among men. Am J Med 2004;116:236.

59. Gerstein HC, Pais P, Pogue J, et al. Relationship of glucose and insulin levels to the risk of myocardial infarction: a case-control study. J Am Coll Cardiol 1999;33:612.

60. Singer DE, Nathan DM, Anderson KM, et al. Association of HbA1c with prevalent cardiovascular disease in the original cohort of the Framingham Heart Study. Diabetes 1992;41:202.

61. Vaccaro O, Eberly LE, Neaton JD, et al. Impact of diabetes and previous myocardial infarction on long-term survival: 25-year mortality follow-up of primary screenees of the Multiple Risk Factor Intervention Trial. Arch Intern Med 2004;164:1438.

62. Gansevoort RT, Correa-Rotter R, Hemmelgarn BR, et al. Chronic kidney disease and cardiovascular risk: epidemiology, mechanisms, and prevention. Lancet 2013;382:339.

63. Stamler J, Stamler R, Neaton JD, et al. Low risk-factor profile and long-term cardiovascular and noncardiovascular mortality and life expectancy: findings for 5 large cohorts of young adult and middle-aged men and women. JAMA 1999;282: 2012.

64. Vasan RS, Sullivan LM, Wilson PW, et al. Relative importance of borderline and elevated levels of coronary heart disease risk factors. Ann Intern Med 2005;142:393.

65. Wilson PW. Established risk factors and coronary artery disease: the Framingham Study. Am J Hypertens 1994;7:7S.

66. Lloyd-Jones DM, Hong Y, Labarthe D, et al. Defining and setting national goals for cardiovascular health promotion and disease reduction: the American Heart Association's strategic Impact Goal through 2020 and beyond. Circulation 2010; 121:586.

67. Rimm EB, Ascherio A, Giovannucci E, et al. Vegetable, fruit, and cereal fiber intake and risk of coronary heart disease among men. JAMA 1996; 275:447.

68. Wolk A, Manson JE, Stampfer MJ, et al. Long-term intake of dietary fiber and decreased risk of coronary heart disease among women. JAMA 1999; 281:1998.

69. Law MR, Morris JK. By how much does fruit and vegetable consumption reduce the risk of ischaemic heart disease? Eur J Clin Nutr 1998;52:549.

70. Vanharanta M, Voutilainen S, Lakka TA, et al. Risk of acute coronary events according to serum concentrations of enterolactone: a prospective population-based case-control study. Lancet 1999;354:2112.

71. Vanharanta M, Voutilainen S, Rissanen TH, et al. Risk of cardiovascular disease-related and all-cause death according to serum concentrations of enterolactone: Kuopio Ischaemic Heart Disease Risk Factor Study. Arch Intern Med 2003;163:1099.

72. Dauchet L, Amouyel P, Dallongeville J. Fruit and vegetable consumption and risk of stroke: a meta-analysis of cohort studies. Neurology 2005;65:1193.

73. Dehghan M, Mente A, Teo KK, et al. Relationship between healthy diet and risk of cardiovascular disease among patients on drug therapies for secondary prevention: a prospective cohort study of 31 546 high-risk individuals from 40 countries. Circulation 2012;126:2705.

74. Bernstein AM, Sun Q, Hu FB, et al. Major dietary protein sources and risk of coronary heart disease in women. Circulation 2010;122:876.

75. Pan A, Sun Q, Bernstein AM, et al. Red meat consumption and mortality: results from 2 prospective cohort studies. Arch Intern Med 2012;172:555.

76. Powell KE, Thompson PD, Caspersen CJ, et al. Physical activity and the incidence of coronary heart disease. Annu Rev Public Health 1987;8:253.

77. Paffenbarger RS Jr, Hyde RT, Wing AL, et al. The association of changes in physical-activity level and other lifestyle characteristics with mortality among men. N Engl J Med 1993;328:538.

78. Leon AS, Connett J, Jacobs DR Jr, et al. Leisure-time physical activity levels and risk of coronary heart disease and death. The Multiple Risk Factor Intervention Trial. JAMA 1987;258:2388.

79. Lee DC, Sui X, Artero EG, et al. Long-term effects of changes in cardiorespiratory fitness and body mass index on all-cause and cardiovascular disease mortality in men: the Aerobics Center Longitudinal Study. Circulation 2011;124:2483.

80. Sandvik L, Erikssen J, Thaulow E, et al. Physical fitness as a predictor of mortality among healthy, middle-aged Norwegian men. N Engl J Med 1993;328:533.

81. Blair SN, Kohl HW 3rd, Paffenbarger RS Jr, et al. Physical fitness and all-cause mortality. A prospective study of healthy men and women. JAMA 1989; 262:2395.

82. LaMonte MJ, Eisenman PA, Adams TD, et al. Cardiorespiratory fitness and coronary heart disease risk factors: the LDS Hospital Fitness Institute cohort. Circulation 2000;102:1623.

83. Laukkanen JA, Lakka TA, Rauramaa R, et al. Cardiovascular fitness as a predictor of mortality in men. Arch Intern Med 2001;161:825.

84. Myers J, Prakash M, Froelicher V, et al. Exercise capacity and mortality among men referred for exercise testing. N Engl J Med 2002;346:793.

85. Barlow CE, Defina LF, Radford NB, et al. Cardiorespiratory fitness and long-term survival in "low-risk" adults. J Am Heart Assoc 2012;1: e001354.

86. Eckel RH, York DA, Rössner S, et al. Prevention Conference VII: obesity, a worldwide epidemic related to heart disease and stroke: executive summary. Circulation 2004;110:2968.

87. Calle EE, Thun MJ, Petrelli JM, et al. Body-mass index and mortality in a prospective cohort of U.S. adults. N Engl J Med 1999;341:1097.

88. Wolk R, Berger P, Lennon RJ, et al. Association between plasma adiponectin levels and unstable coronary syndromes. Eur Heart J 2007;28:292.

89. Tirosh A, Shai I, Afek A, et al. Adolescent BMI trajectory and risk of diabetes versus coronary disease. N Engl J Med 2011;364:1315.

90. Januzzi JL Jr, Stern TA, Pasternak RC, et al. The influence of anxiety and depression on outcomes of patients with coronary artery disease. Arch Intern Med 2000;160:1913.

91. Siegman AW, Kubzansky LD, Kawachi I, et al. A prospective study of dominance and coronary heart disease in the Normative Aging Study. Am J Cardiol 2000;86:145.

92. Kawachi I, Sparrow D, Spiro A 3rd, et al. A prospective study of anger and coronary heart disease. The Normative Aging Study. Circulation 1996;94:2090.

93. Sesso HD, Kawachi I, Vokonas PS, et al. Depression and the risk of coronary heart disease in the Normative Aging Study. Am J Cardiol 1998; 82:851.

94. Ridker PM, Glynn RJ, Hennekens CH. C-reactive protein adds to the predictive value of total and HDL cholesterol in determining risk of first myocardial infarction. Circulation 1998;97:2007.

95. Koenig W, Sund M, Fröhlich M, et al. C-Reactive protein, a sensitive marker of inflammation, predicts future risk of coronary heart disease in initially healthy middle-aged men: results from the MONICA (Monitoring Trends and Determinants in Cardiovascular Disease) Augsburg Cohort Study, 1984 to 1992. Circulation 1999;99:237.

96. Ridker PM, Buring JE, Shih J, et al. Prospective study of C-reactive protein and the risk of future cardiovascular events among apparently healthy women. Circulation 1998;98:731.

97. Ridker PM, Buring JE, Rifai N, et al. Development and validation of improved algorithms for the assessment of global cardiovascular risk in women: the Reynolds Risk Score. JAMA 2007; 297:611.

98. Wilson PW, Pencina M, Jacques P, et al. C-reactive protein and reclassification of cardiovascular risk in the Framingham Heart Study. Circ Cardiovasc Qual Outcomes 2008;1:92.

99. Pearson TA, Mensah GA, Alexander RW, et al. Markers of inflammation and cardiovascular disease: application to clinical and public health practice: a statement for healthcare professionals from the Centers for Disease Control and Prevention and the American Heart Association. Circulation 2003;107:499.

100. Genest J, McPherson R, Frohlich J, et al. 2009 Canadian Cardiovascular Society/Canadian guidelines for the diagnosis and treatment of dyslipidemia and prevention of cardiovascular disease in the adult—2009 recommendations. Can J Cardiol 2009;25:567.

101. U.S. Preventive Services Task Force. Using nontraditional risk factors in coronary heart disease risk assessment: U.S. Preventive Services Task Force recommendation statement. Ann Intern Med 2009;151:474.

102. IL6R Genetics Consortium Emerging Risk Factors Collaboration, Sarwar N, Butterworth AS, Freitag DF, et al. Interleukin-6 receptor pathways in coronary heart disease: a collaborative meta-analysis of 82 studies. Lancet 2012;379:1205.

103. Interleukin-6 Receptor Mendelian Randomisation Analysis (IL6R MR) Consortium, Hingorani AD, Casas JP. The interleukin-6 receptor as a target for prevention of coronary heart disease: a mendelian randomisation analysis. Lancet 2012;379:1214.

104. Reich D, Patterson N, Ramesh V, et al. Admixture mapping of an allele affecting interleukin 6 soluble receptor and interleukin 6 levels. Am J Hum Genet 2007;80:716.

105. Brennan ML, Penn MS, Van Lente F, et al. Prognostic value of myeloperoxidase in patients with chest pain. N Engl J Med 2003;349:1595.

106. Zheng L, Nukuna B, Brennan ML, et al. Apolipoprotein A-I is a selective target for myeloperoxidase-catalyzed oxidation and functional impairment in subjects with cardiovascular disease. J Clin Invest 2004;114:529.

107. Zhang R, Brennan ML, Fu X, et al. Association between myeloperoxidase levels and risk of coronary artery disease. JAMA 2001;286:2136.

108. Karakas M, Koenig W, Zierer A, et al. Myeloperoxidase is associated with incident coronary heart disease independently of traditional risk factors: results from the MONICA/KORA Augsburg study. J Intern Med 2012;271:43.

109. Tang WH, Tong W, Troughton RW, et al. Prognostic value and echocardiographic determinants of plasma myeloperoxidase levels in chronic heart failure. J Am Coll Cardiol 2007;49:2364.

110. Grover SA, Coupal L, Gilmore N, et al. Impact of dyslipidemia associated with highly active antiretroviral therapy (HAART) on cardiovascular risk and life expectancy. Am J Cardiol 2005; 95:586.

111. Kamin DS, Grinspoon SK. Cardiovascular disease in HIV-positive patients. AIDS 2005;19:641.

112. Currier JS, Lundgren JD, Carr A, et al. Epidemiological evidence for cardiovascular disease in HIV-infected patients and relationship to highly active antiretroviral therapy. Circulation 2008;118:e29.

113. Grinspoon SK, Grunfeld C, Kotler DP, et al. State of the science conference: initiative to decrease cardiovascular risk and increase quality of care for patients living with HIV/AIDS: executive summary. Circulation 2008;118:198.

114. Tseng ZH, Secemsky EA, Dowdy D, et al. Sudden cardiac death in patients with human immunodeficiency virus infection. J Am Coll Cardiol 2012;59:1891.

115. Moslehi J. The cardiovascular perils of cancer survivorship. N Engl J Med 2013;368:1055.

116. Darby SC, Ewertz M, McGale P, et al. Risk of ischemic heart disease in women after radiotherapy for breast cancer. N Engl J Med 2013;368:987.

117. Ford ES. Risks for all-cause mortality, cardiovascular disease, and diabetes associated with the metabolic syndrome: a summary of the evidence. Diabetes Care 2005;28:1769.

118. Gami AS, Witt BJ, Howard DE, et al. Metabolic syndrome and risk of incident cardiovascular events and death: a systematic review and meta-analysis of longitudinal studies. J Am Coll Cardiol 2007;49:403.

119. Galassi A, Reynolds K, He J. Metabolic syndrome and risk of cardiovascular disease: a meta-analysis. Am J Med 2006;119:812.

120. Toth PP, Massaro J, Jones S, et al. Quantitative impact of remnant lipoproteins on risk for hard CHD events: a meta-analysis of the Framinham Offspring and Jackson Heart Studies. J Am Coll Cardiol 2014;63(12_S). http://dx.doi.org/10.1016/S0735-1097(14)61317-6.

121. Mann JF, Gerstein HC, Yi QL, et al. Development of renal disease in people at high cardiovascular risk: results of the HOPE randomized study. J Am Soc Nephrol 2003;14:641.

122. Roberts R, Steward AF. Genes and coronary artery disease: where are we? J Am Coll Cardiol 2012;18:1715–21.

Stable Ischemic Heart Disease

Richard Kones, MD, FAHA, FESC, FRSM*, Umme Rumana, MBBS

KEYWORDS

- Angina • Stable ischemic heart disease • Coronary artery disease • Myocardial oxygen balance
- Cardiovascular risk assessment • Silent ischemia • Nitrates • β-Blockers
- Calcium channel blockers

KEY POINTS

- Because angina is the most common presentation of stable ischemic heart disease (SIHD), a patient's first visit is frequently the gateway into the cardiac health system and is critical to the patient's successful journey.
- The pretest probability of ischemic heart disease (IHD) should be estimated and guideline-based therapies begun if appropriate; further investigation proceeds according to a patient's current condition or response to therapies.
- A patient's post-test risk and options should be evaluated, if necessary, with an invasive cardiologist or surgeon.
- A patient discussion concerning choices, risks, and benefits allows personalization of therapy and enlists the patient as a partner in therapy.
- Assessment of clinical and functional status, adherence to medications, and reinforcement for overall management continues on an outpatient basis.

DEFINITION AND CLINICAL DIAGNOSIS

Typical angina is commonly triggered by exertion, emotional stress, cold, wind, or fever. Exertional angina is relieved within 1 to 5 minutes through rest or sooner using sublingual nitroglycerin (NGN); otherwise, episodes may last 2 to 10 minutes. There is heaviness or pressure in the precordium, retrosternum, or epigastrium, with possible radiation to the outer aspects of both arms, neck, jaw, shoulders, or midabdomen. Quality is described as crushing, tightness, pressure, or gripping, with or without numbness. The average frequency of attacks in patients under medical care is approximately 2 per week, and many patients limit activities to avoid attacks.

In some patients, in particular diabetics and the elderly, myocardial ischemia may cause symptoms other than precordial discomfort, including dyspnea, diaphoresis, nausea and emesis, fatigue, weakness, altered sensorium, lightheadedness, and fainting as "equivalents" of angina. Often chest pain and restricted breathing occur together. Diminished pain perception of afferent signals or presence of dysautonomia in diabetes may modulate symptom expression and prolong anginal perceptual threshold. The insensitivity of chest pain as an index of heart disease or its severity and burden pose special difficulty, because cardiovascular mortality is 3-fold higher in diabetic men and between 2- and 5-fold higher among diabetic women compared with nondiabetic counterparts.

During classical angina, discomfort does not usually vary with position, the respiratory cycle, or cough. Angina or any "equivalent" may be accompanied by dyspnea, nausea, diaphoresis, weakness/fatigue, and apprehension. Pain of

The Cardiometabolic Research Institute, 8181 Fannin Street, Unit 314, Houston, TX 77054, USA
* Corresponding author.
E-mail address: cardiacresearchinstitute@gmail.com

Cardiol Clin 32 (2014) 333–351
http://dx.doi.org/10.1016/j.ccl.2014.04.004
0733-8651/14/$ – see front matter © 2014 Elsevier Inc. All rights reserved.

cardiology.theclinics.com

longer duration (>15 minutes), radiating to both arms, or accompanied by diaphoresis, a third heart sound, or hypotension suggests a myocardial infarction (MI).

Approximately 77% of individuals with chest pain do not seek medical care, often mistakenly attributing it to benign causes. Approximately 12% of patients presenting with chest pain are found to have IHD. Of those seen in emergency departments (EDs), 45% to 50% have a cardiac cause.[1,2] In primary care, the most common conditions encountered are musculoskeletal (including costochondritis), 36%; gastrointestinal conditions, including gastroesophageal reflux disease (GERD), 19%; panic disorder and psychiatric, 8%; pulmonary disease, 5%; stable angina, 10.5%; other cardiac conditions, 5.3%; and other/unknown, 16%.[3] Diagnoses that could produce sudden death should be efficiently eliminated: acute coronary syndrome (ACS)/MI, pulmonary embolus, aortic dissection, and tension pneumothorax (**Table 1**).

Silent Ischemia and Infarction Is Frequent

Data relying on clinical reports of anginal pain leave SIHD prevalence vastly underestimated, because silent (asymptomatic) ischemia is the most common manifestation of SIHD; 17% to 59% of diabetics have silent ischemia. During continuous monitoring or testing in high-risk patients, evidence of silent ischemia is apparent in many clinical situations. Perhaps 75% of ischemic episodes may occur without pain, especially in the early morning hours. When patients with SIHD are considered to be controlled clinically, at least 40% of patients show ischemia when monitored.[4,5] Silent MIs account for 33% of those identified by ECG retrospectively.[6] Such patients have a poorer prognosis than counterparts with chest pain,[7,8] in part because they may be incorrectly diagnosed and are less likely to receive appropriate treatment, resulting in poorer outcomes. In patients with unstable angina, one or more instances of

Table 1
Some noncoronary causes of chest pain

System	Diagnoses
Gastrointestinal	Peptic ulcer, gastritis, GERD, cholecystitis, cholelithiasis, choledocholithiasis, esophageal spasm/motility disorders, esophagitis, esophageal perforation, pancreatic diseases, some causes of acute abdomen, such as perforations, volvulus, mesenteric adenitis, etc. GERD accounts for up to 60% of noncardiac cases.
Musculoskeletal	Chest wall trauma/rib fracture, costochondritis, muscle/ligament/tendon strains, myositis, chronic overuse injuries, sternoclavicular arthritis, cervical radiculitis, brachial plexus compression, left shoulder bursitis
Pulmonary	Pulmonary embolism, severe pulmonary hypertension, pleuritis, pneumonia, pneumothorax, bronchiectasis
Other cardiovascular	Pericarditis, acute aortic dissection, aortic stenosis, mitral valve prolapse, idiopathic hypertrophic subaortic stenosis, cardiac contusion, acute stress cardiomyopathy (Takotsubo disease), uncontrolled hypertension, coronary anomalies, Kawasaki disease, polyarteritis nodosa, Takayasu arteritis (aortic arch syndrome)
Related processes that modulate oxygen supply and demand	Angina may be intensified or caused by hypotension; hypoxia; anemia; bradycardia; fever; thyrotoxicosis; high-output states, such as AV shunts; systemic and inflammatory diseases, especially sepsis, an example of demand ischemia. A hemoglobinopathy or carbon monoxide poisoning may interfere with oxygen delivery.
Nervous	Cervical radiculopathy, peripheral neuropathy, brachial plexus impingement, brachial neuritis
Psychiatric	Generalized anxiety disorder, panic disorder, hyperventilation, affective disorders (eg, depression), somatoform disorders, fixed delusions in thought disorders
Infectious	Herpes zoster prior to rash, acute lymphadenopathy, Pott disease (tuberculous spondylitis)
Metabolic	Hyperviscosity syndrome, acute thyrotoxicosis

ST depression on 24-hour monitoring is associated with a 7.43-fold increase in risk of MI or death.[8,9] Even with clear objective findings, such as subsequent ST-segment elevation, the absence of chest pain during the initial presentation still decreases utilization of both fibrinolysis and percutaneous coronary intervention (PCI).

SIHD and CHD in women, with a lower incidence of IHD than men until later ages, present a unique challenge in both diagnosis and management. Even though angina is the most common initial manifestation of IHD in women, they present with more atypical features, such as variable pain thresholds, palpitation, or even sharp lancinating pain, and more "equivalents." Young women also have a higher incidence of microvascular than macrovascular disease, yet when older, present with SIHD rather than acute MI or SCD as seen in men. Younger women have a higher false-positive rate on exercise and nuclear stress tests, poorer outcomes than men after MI, and higher inpatient mortality post-PCI. Nonetheless, guideline-directed medical care (discussed later) applies fully to women, independent of other differences and persisting disparities.

SIHD in the elderly is associated with more diffuse and severe disease, because age is a strong determinant of CHD risk. Clinical presentations may be confounded by comorbidities, and their effects on pathophysiological limitations must be teased apart. Pharmacologic stress testing is informative, and response to guideline-directed therapies prolongs survival after acute events.[10] Due to greater triple-vessel and left main disease and frequency of left ventricular (LV) dysfunction and other comorbidities, revascularization decisions are made on an individual basis.

GOALS OF THERAPY, FUNCTIONAL CLASSIFICATION, AND SEVERITY

The goals of treatment of SIHD are to (1) limit the number and severity of anginal attacks and improve quality of life, (2) protect against lethal events, and (3) lower the burden of risk factors to slow disease progression. Strategies to achieve these goals are patient education and counseling, lifestyle improvement, optimum medical therapy, and revascularization.

Angina is classified according to severity by the Canadian Cardiovascular Society or functional capacity—ability to perform specific activities (**Table 2**). The Canadian Cardiovascular Society classes correspond to the exercise tolerances given in metabolic equivalents (METs) in **Table 2** (1 MET = V_{O_2} of 3.5 mL O_2 per [kg • min], equal

to the energy produced per unit surface area of an average person seated at rest).[13]

Myocardial Energy (Oxygen) Imbalance and Ischemic Pain

Myocardial ischemia results from an imbalance between myocardial energy supply and myocardial oxygen demand (**Fig. 1**).[14,15]

Pretest Probability of Ischemia Graded According to Gender, Age, and Symptoms

The 3 elements of typical angina include (1) substernal discomfort with location, characteristics, and duration, as discussed previously; (2) provocation by effort or emotional stress; and (3) relief by rest or NGN. The likelihood that a patient has IHD may be estimated from the character of chest pain, age, and gender (**Table 3**). Estimating probability assists in choosing which next tests would be most productive. Details influencing this decision include what degree of uncertainty is tolerable to the physician and patient; probability of a different diagnosis, accuracy (specificity and sensitivity), and reliability of the diagnostic procedure contemplated; probability of an alternative diagnosis; and the risk/benefit ratio of additional testing versus no further testing.

For example, at age 45, if the chest pain were classic ("yes" to 3 questions top panel, **Table 3**), 87% of men would have IHD (high) but only 55% of women (intermediate).[16] If the chest pain satisfied 2 elements (atypical), these figures would be 51% and 22%, respectively, both intermediate. If the chest discomfort described had none of the 3 elements (noncardiac), 13% of men and 3% of women would have IHD.

At age 65, if all 3 elements of typical angina were present, 94% of men and 86% of women would have IHD. If no elements are present, 27% of men and 14% of women would have IHD. As age increases, the relationship between the number of typical symptoms and diagnosis tightens.[17,18]

Classifications that Include Additional Clinical and Baseline ECG Findings

Califf and colleagues[19] proposed another classification with predictive value, rating risk probability as low, intermediate, and high (**Table 4**). It is also possible to describe a general continuum of severity of ischemia from low to intermediate to high using history, type of pain, clinical findings, and biomarkers.[17]

A high probability does not mean certainty, and diagnostic errors in the absence of coronary angiograms persist; up to 12% of patients

Table 2
Comparison of two classifications of impaired functional capacity and severity in angina patients

Canadian Cardiovascular Society Class (Severity and Limitation of Activity)	Canadian Cardiovascular Society Severity Classification[11]	Specific Activity Scale (Quantitated in METs)[12]
Class I (minimal/no limitation)	Ordinary physical activity does not cause symptoms. Strenuous rapid or prolonged exertion at work or recreation may produce angina. Equivalent >7 METs, strenuous activity[13]	Patients can perform tasks involving >7 METs: carry 24 lb up 8 steps; carry a weight of 80-lb level; do outdoor work (shovel snow, spade soil), recreation (basketball, squash, handball, ski, walk or jog 5 mph).
Class II (mild/slight limitation)	Slight limitation of physical activity, not at rest, but only during vigorous activity: Angina may occur with • Walking straight or uphill or climbing stairs rapidly • Walking or stair climbing after meals or in the cold, wind, or during emotional stress • Walking level ≥2 blocks, normal pace under normal conditions • Climbing >1 flight of ordinary stairs, normal pace and normal conditions	Patients can perform tasks using >5 METs: walk at 4 mph on level ground, sexual intercourse to completion, roller skate, dance fox trot, garden, rake, weed but cannot perform those that involve ≥7 METs.
Class III (severe/marked limitation)	Symptoms with everyday living activities, but not at rest (ie, appreciable limitation): Angina may occur after • Walking 1–2 blocks on the level or • Climbing 1 flight of stairs, normal conditions, normal pace	Patients can perform tasks using >2 METs: walk 2.5 mph, clean windows, play golf, dress completely, clean windows, strip and make bed, but not those involving ≥5 METs.
Class IV (extreme/ unable)	Inability to perform any activity without angina, or angina at rest; severe limitation. May be self-confined to bed or a chair. Equivalent ≈1–2 METs, slowest walk[13]	Patients are severely limited and cannot perform tasks requiring 1–2 METs, including any of the above activities.

discharged from EDs may have MIs, although the use of high-sensitivity cardiac troponin assays and coronary CT angiography minimizes such pitfalls.

ANTI-ISCHEMIC THERAPY

Three traditional antianginal agents—nitrates, β-blockers, and calcium channel blockers (CCBs)—decrease the severity, duration, or frequency of angina, usually increasing exercise performance and time to ST-segment depression. They improve myocardial oxygen balance by reducing demand (heart rate, contractility, afterload, and preload), and increase supply through a rise in coronary blood flow (CBF), distancing

the threshold producing anginal symptoms. Frequently a combination of these drugs is necessary for symptom control. Discontinuance of some agents, if possible, is left to the clinician.[21]

Organic Nitrates

NGN causes dilatation of epicardial coronary arteries by relaxing arterial smooth muscle and also of other arteries and venous conduits, with less effect on small arterioles. The short-acting organic nitrates react with intracellular sulfhydryl groups (from methionine or cysteine) and mitochondrial aldehyde dehydrogenase to form S-nitrosothiol, which is reduced to nitric oxide (NO). NO then activates smooth muscle guanylyl

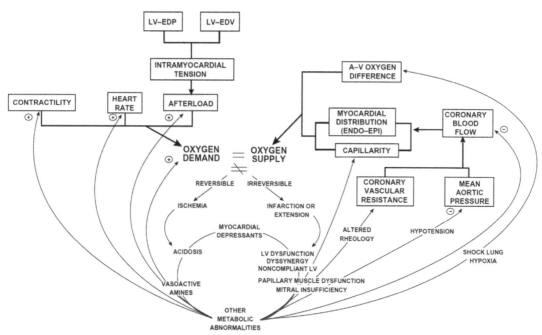

Fig. 1. Energy for myocardial work as ATP is a function of oxidative phosphorylation and nutrient supply. Myocardial oxygen demand is determined by heart rate, blood pressure, and myocardial wall tension, the latter dependent on preload, afterload, and contractility. When oxygen demand is increased due to effort, it cannot be supplied by higher oxygen extraction. In the presence of coronary obstruction, CBF is also compromised, resulting in an imbalance between oxygen need and supply and clinical chest pain. ENDO, endocardium; EPI, epicardium; LV-EDP, LV end-diastolic pressure; LV-EDV, LV end-diastolic volume. (*From* Kones R. Pathogenesis of cardiogenic shock II. N Y State J Med 1973;73:1662–70; with permission.)

cyclase, raising cyclic guanosine monophosphate (cGMP) levels to inhibit calcium entry into the muscle, producing relaxation.[22] NO also inhibits potassium channels to hyperpolarize muscle membranes and activates light chain phosphatase, both effecting relaxation, accounting for more vasodilatation. NO increases cGMP in platelets to reduce calcium and suppress platelet

Table 3 Variables that determine pretest probability of IHD: symptoms, gender, and age	
Variables	**Categories**
Characteristics of pain	How typical are the clinical characteristics (elements) of the chest pain? 1. Pain or discomfort substernal? 2. Pain triggered by exertion? 3. Pain relieved by rest of NGN within 10 min?
Character of pain (probability rises with number of elements)	1. Typical (classical) angina features all 3 criteria above. 2. Atypical angina satisfies 2 of the 3 features above. 3. Nonanginal chest pain satisfies 0–1 of the features above.
Probability when adding age, gender, and above together (probability rises with male gender and age)	High probability • Men ≥40 y with typical angina • Women ≥65 y with typical angina Intermediate probability—10%–90% • Men, all ages, with atypical angina • Women ≥50 y with atypical angina • Women 30–50 y with typical angina Low probability—less than 10% • Asymptomatic men and women of all ages • Women <50 y with atypical chest pain

Table 4
Classification using clinical and ECG findings

Probability of IHD	Clinical Findings	ECG Changes
High	Pain >20 min at rest, similar prior pain diagnosed as angina, and/or hypotension, diaphoresis, rales, transient mitral regurgitation	New ST-segment depression ≥0.5 mm, T-wave inversion ≥2 mm, recent left bundle branch block or life-threatening ventricular arrhythmia, and/or diagnostic elevations in biomarkers
Intermediate	Pain >20 min relieved by rest or NGN, male, age ≥70 y, coexistence of diabetes/extracardiac disease	Fixed Q waves and resting ST depression ≤1 mm in multiple lead groups, LV hypertrophy and/or traditional risk factors suggestive but not necessary for the diagnosis.
Low	Absence of above, history of panic attacks, hyperventilation or cocaine use; chest wall tenderness	ECG normal or unchanged, T-wave inversions in leads with dominant R waves, or T-wave flattening[20]

Data from Califf RM, Harrell FE, Lee KL, et al. The evolution of medical and surgical therapy for coronary artery disease. JAMA 1989;261:2077–86.

activation.[23] In modest doses, nitrates reduce preload; in higher doses, they lower afterload. Myocardial oxygen consumption falls, increasing exercise capacity. NO improves endothelial function, optimizing vasodilation,[24] whereas CBF may redistribute to ischemic zones.

Long-acting nitrates in use include an ointment, patches, isosorbide dinitrate, and isosorbide mononitrate (**Table 5**). Higher doses of oral forms are necessary because of metabolism by the liver, except for isosorbide mononitrate. None provides full 24-hour protection—tolerance develops within 12 to 24 hours, which may be prevented with a nitrate-free 6- to 12-hour period daily. Tolerance develops via oxidation of tetrahydrobiopterin (BH4), a cofactor for endothelial NO synthase.[25] When BH4 is deficient, NO synthesis is uncoupled from energy sources, and endothelial NO synthase action actually reverses to produce atherogenic superoxide. Recoupling is promoted by angiotensin-converting enzyme inhibitors (ACEIs), AT1-receptor blockers, statins, nebivolol, and resveratrol.

β-Blockers

All β-blockers lower heart rate at rest and limit rate rises during exercise, keeping myocardial oxygen demand below the angina-producing threshold; in so doing, diastole is prolonged, increasing CBF. Used alone, β-blockers may be more effective than long-acting nitrates or CCBs in reducing mild ischemic episodes.[26] Specific β_1 effects include raising heart rate and contractility, enhanced automaticity and conduction velocity, release of renin from juxtaglomerular cells, ghrelin from the stomach, and lipolysis. β_2-Adrenergic receptor stimulation relaxes smooth muscle in the bronchi and uterus; dilates coronary, carotid, and peripheral arteries; and promotes gluconeogenesis and glycogenolysis, in part though insulin release.

β-Blocker dosages are titrated to a resting heart rate of 55 to 60 beats per minute and an exercise heart rate response less than 75% of the rate that precipitates ischemia. As far as anti-ischemic efficacy is concerned, equipotent doses produce similar effects; in larger doses, β_1 blockers may lose some selectivity and inhibit β_2 receptors. Pertinent clinical information is summarized in **Table 6**.

Calcium Channel Blockers

CCBs bind to and inhibit L-type calcium channels, reducing calcium influx into cells to bring about smooth muscle relaxation. The dihydropyridine class mainly affects arteries, causing vasodilation in the peripheral and coronary beds and increased CBF; reflex tachycardia is more likely. The phenylalkylamine class of CCBs, such as verapamil, reduces myocardial oxygen demand chiefly through a negative inotropic action. The benzothiazepine class of CCBs, such as diltiazem, combines the effects of the other 2 classes. Both nondihydropyridine CCBs, verapamil and diltiazem, lower myocardial oxygen need by slowing sinoatrial nodal (SAN) and atrioventricular (AV) nodal conduction to lower heart rate and depress contractility under physiologic conditions, and all the CCBs are effective coronary vasodilators.

CCBs find clinical use in patients who cannot tolerate β-blockers, when they are ineffective, and in combination for additional anti-ischemic

Table 5
Common forms of nitrates used for SIHD

Compound	Route	Usual Dose (Daily Unless Mentioned)	Onset of Action (min)	Duration	Notes
NGN	Sublingual	Offer to all eligible candidates. 0.3–0.6 mg, up to 1.5 mg as needed, or up to 3 tablets, not to exceed 1.2 mg within 15 min. If pain persists, have patient go to ED. Use prophylactically 5–10 min prior to activities that may trigger angina.	1–3	10–30 min	Underutilized frequently. Potency lost over time so replace regularly.
NGN	Spray/mist/aerosol	0.4 mg, 1–2 sprays prn as needed, up to 3 doses, 5 min apart, not to exceed 1.2 mg within 15 min	2–5	10–30 min	
NGN	Transdermal patch	0.2–0.8 mg/h q24h; remove at night for 12 h	60–100	8–12 h	Need 8–10 h NGN-free recovery to avoid tolerance
NGN	Intravenous	5–200 µg/min (ACS) titrated to symptom relief, headache, or hypotension	1–2 min	While infusing	Tolerance possible in 7–8 h
Isosorbide dinitrate	Oral	5–80 mg, 2–3 times daily	30–60	8 h	Need 8–12 h NGN-free recovery to avoid tolerance
Isosorbide mononitrate	Oral	20 mg twice daily, 7–8 h apart	30–60	6–8 h	Metabolite of isosorbide dinitrate
Isosorbide mononitrate SR	Oral	30–240 mg daily, given once daily	30–60	12–18 h	

Side effects of immediate nitrates include cerebral vasodilation and headache, postural hypotension, dizziness, and syncope.

Contraindications include caution with cGMP-dependent phosphodiesterase inhibitors, such as sildenafil, tadalafil, and vardenafil, which should not be used with nitrates (within 24 h) because of the risk of cGMP-induced hypotension, obstructive hypertrophic cardiomyopathy, severe aortic stenosis, constrictive pericarditis, mitral stenosis, or closed-angle glaucoma.

Warnings: NGN-induced reflex tachycardia may be countered by combination with a β-blocker, diltiazem, or verapamil. Nitrates and CCBs are effective in vasospastic (Prinzmetal) angina, whereas response to β-blockers is variable or unlikely. Aspirin may worsen ischemic attacks in this variant.

Table 6
Commonly used β-adrenergic blockers in stable ischemic heart disease[a]

Drug (Drugs with Partial Agonist Activity not Included)	Selectivity	Time to Peak Action After Oral Intake (h)	Elimination Half-Life (h)	Dose	Notes
Atenolol	β_1	2–4	6–9	50–200 mg/d	Begin with 50 mg daily and titrate upward; hydrophilic-renal excretion.
Metoprolol	β_1	1–2	3–6	50–200 mg twice daily	An extended-release formulation may be begun at 100 mg daily. Antiarrhythmic class I effect. Lipophilic-hepatic excretion via CYP2D6, which exhibits polymorphisms; fast metabolizers may require 2–3 fold the dose of poor metabolizers.
Bisoprolol	β_1	2–4	9–12	10 mg/d	Inhibits renin secretion ≈ 65%.
Nebivolol	β_1	1.5–4	10	5–10 mg/d	β_1-Blocking action, additional NO-mediated vasodilatory effect. Above 10 mg loses selectivity, or in poor metabolizers, or with CYP2D6 inhibitors.
Esmolol	β_1	2–5 min	9 min	50–300 μg/kg/min IV	IV use
Carvedilol	None	1.0–1.5	7–10	3.125–25 mg Twice daily	Combined α_1-, β_1-, and β_2-blocking activity; antiarrhythmic class I effect; genetic polymorphisms in metabolism.
Labetalol	None	2–4	3–6	200–600 mg Twice daily	Combined α_1-, β_1-, and β_2-blocking activity, maximizing hypotensive action; side effects of postural hypotension and retrograde ejaculation.
Timolol	None	1–2	4–5	10 mg Twice daily	High potency.
Nadolol	None	3–4	14–24	40–80 mg/d	Hydrophilic-renal excretion.
Propranolol	None	1–2	3–5	80–120 mg Twice daily	Antiarrhythmic class I effect; lipophilic; genetic polymorphisms in metabolism.

Absolute contraindications: severe bradycardia, sinus node dysfunction/high-grade AV block, asthma, peripheral arterial disease with rest ischemic, worsening HF.

Relative contraindications: less severe forms of the above, PR interval greater than 0.24 s, systolic BP less than 100 mm Hg, Raynaud syndrome, pregnancy, nightmares, fatigue, mild depression, lack of motivation, impotence, rise in triglyceride level, reduced levels of high-density lipoprotein cholesterol, masking of tachycardia during hypoglycemia in diabetics, hypertension or seizures with cocaine users, worsening of Prinzmetal angina due to unopposed α-adrenergic effect. Use cardioselective agents in asthma, diabetes, and peripheral arterial disease; in these and HF, may need to substitute CCBs. β-Adrenergic receptors may be up-regulated in patients treated with β-blockers, so they should not be stopped abruptly lest rebound vasoconstriction occur.

[a] FDA approval for specific indications of each β-blocker may differ.

effects, with properties summarized in **Table 7**. Although they are effective against angina, they do not modify the natural progression of the disease or mortality. Using verapamil versus atenolol, the number of patients with angina falls from 65% to 25% with no difference in mortality.[27] When dihydropyridines (eg, amlodipine) are used in combination with β-blockers, reflex tachycardia from the CCB is blunted, and exercise duration is optimized. A combination of a second generation CCB (amlodipine or nicardipine) with a β-blocker is frequently underutilized. Nifedipine sustained-release (SR) safely relieves angina and prolongs event-free survival in patients with stable angina, Prinzmetal angina, and hypertension.[28]

Comparing nitrates, β-blockers, and CCBs, β-blockers lowered the frequency of anginal attacks better than CCBs, not including amlodipine and felodipine. The combination of β-blockers with nitrates is beneficial because they both lower myocardial oxygen demand and raise subendocardial blood flow differently, whereas the β-blockers minimize reflex tachycardia from nitrates, and nitrates blunt any potential rise in LV end-diastolic pressure from negative inotropic actions of the β-blockers. Approximately 5% to 15% of patients are refractory to triple therapy.

NEWER, NONTRADITIONAL, UNIQUE, ANTI-ISCHEMIC AGENTS
Nicorandil

Nicorandil is structurally a nicotinamide ester with a nitrate moiety, exhibiting dual mechanisms of action. In addition to activating cGMP for smooth muscle relaxation, it opens ATP-sensitive potassium channels, hyperpolarizing the membrane, preventing activation of the voltage-dependent calcium channel and, hence, free calcium accumulation. Nicorandil also reduces preload through venodilation, lowers afterload, promotes expression of endothelial NO synthase,[29] improves myocardial function during ischemia-reperfusion, and protects against ischemic cell damage.

Nicorandil lowers hospitalization rates for chest pain, MI, and CAD death by 17%.[30] The drug prolongs exercise time to ischemia, reverses ischemia-related impairment in regional wall motion, and is noninferior to isosorbide mononitrate when treating angina.[31] A dose of 10 to 40 mg twice daily controlled 70% to 80% of stable chronic angina patients, with an effect maintained for approximately 12 hours. When used in patients with proven IHD, the drug lowered all-cause and MI mortality by 35%.[32] Nicorandil benefits the coronary microcirculation and Prinzmetal angina. Pretreatment of SIHD patients having stents placed attenuated post-PCI rises in microcirculatory resistance, troponin levels,[33] and progression to MI.[34]

Ivabradine

Ivabradine selectively and specifically inhibits the inward sodium-potassium I_f current carried by hyperpolarization-activated cyclic nucleotide-gated ion channels, a unique pacemaking current in SAN cells, to slow the rate of diastolic depolarization and lower heart rate in tandem with intracellular cyclic adenosine monophosphate levels, themselves cycled by β-receptor or muscarinic discharge.[34] Ivabradine does not affect contractility or AV nodal conduction nor does it alter hemodynamics. The recommended dose is 5 mg twice daily. The drug is metabolized by hepatic cytochrome CYP3A4; its affinity for the enzyme is low, and there is no clinically relevant inhibition or induction, but other CYP3A4 inhibitors or inducers may lower ivabradine levels.

When treating angina, ivabradine compared well with amlodipine or atenolol. In patients with LV dysfunction, heart rates greater than 70, and optimal antianginal treatment, ivabradine still lowered risk of MI and need for revascularization by one-third, but in patients without high heart rates, results are variable. In patients taking 50 mg atenolol daily, ivabradine titrated to 7.5 mg twice a day after 4 months increased total exercise duration and falls in the rate-pressure product at rest and at peak exercise.[35] Ivabradine can be added to nitrates and β-blockers or as add-on therapy when β-blockers are not controlling angina but may be accepted for first-line use.

Ivabradine is a uniquely helpful agent to slow inappropriate sinus tachycardia, because it lowers the intrinsic SAN firing rate and responses to autonomic variation.[36] Other adverse reactions, including conduction abnormalities, occur in ≤10% of cases. Ivabradine is contraindicated in patients with sinus node dysfunction, discouraged with CYP3A4 inhibitors, and rarely needs to be discontinued because of a visual aberrance caused by a retinal current similar to I_f.

Trimetazidine

Trimetazidine, a member of the class of 3-KAT inhibitors, is a metabolic modulator that improves myocardial energetics at several levels, partially inhibiting β-oxidation of fats by lowering activity of mitochondrial enzyme, 3-ketoacyl coenzyme A thiolase.[37] Shifting mitochondrial metabolism from fatty acids to glucose lowers oxygen consumption per unit of ATP produced.[38] Trimetazidine raises myocardial glucose utilization, prevents a fall in ATP and phosphocreatine levels in response to

Table 7
Calcium channel blockers used for stable ischemic heart disease

Drug	Duration of Action	Usual Dose	Common Side Effects	Clinical Notes
Dihydropyridines				
Nifedipine SR	Long	90, 120 mg/d	Hypotension, edema, dizziness, flushing, nausea, constipation	Add β-blocker to counter reflex tachycardia; fewer conduction, contractility effects than diltiazem or verapamil; contraindicated in hypotension, advanced aortic stenosis, and HF. Cimetidine and phenytoin raise levels. Prinzmetal rebound.
Amlodipine	Very long (blood pressure changes delayed 24–48 h, steady state levels at 7–8 d)	5–20 mg qd	Headache, edema.	Leg edema unrelated to HF; begin with 5 mg in the elderly or with liver disease; longest half-life of the CCBs at 35–50 h; preferred in patients with sinus bradycardia, sick sinus syndrome, AV block. Clinical experience substantial.
Felodipine SR	Long	5–10 mg qd	Headache, edema	Not FDA approved for angina. Well-studied.
Isradipine SR	Medium	2.5–10 mg bid	Headache, fatigue	Not FDA approved for angina
Nicardipine	Short	20–40 mg tid	Headache, edema, dizziness, flushing	Hemodynamic and clinical effects similar to nifedipine. Lower frequency of adverse effects with nicardipine versus nifedipine, particularly dizziness.

Nonhydropyridines

Diltiazem immediate-release	Short	30–80 mg qid	Hypotension, dizziness, flushing, bradycardia, edema	Interaction with cimetidine, flecainide, cyclosporine, lithium carbonate, carbamazepine, digoxin, disopyramide. Caution when using verapamil and diltiazem with amiodarone.
Diltiazem slow-release	Long	120–320 qd	Hypotension, dizziness, flushing, bradycardia, edema	Begin with 120 mg bid and titrate upward. Blood pressure effects may be delayed 1–2 wk; relatively safe but caution with β-blockers and isosorbide dinitrate. See above.
Verapamil immediate-release	Short	80–160 mg tid	Hypotension, negative inotropism, HF bradycardia, edema	Not in patients with depressed contractility and SN, AV conduction, HF, digoxin or quinidine toxicity; caution using with β-blockers.
Verapamil slow-release	Long	120–480 mg qd	Hypotension, negative inotropism, HF, bradycardia, edema	See above.

Side effects: headache, dizziness, flushing, and edema are due to vasodilation. Interaction with other negative chronotropic or inotropic agents to produce bradycardia, heart block, or HF has been reported. β-Blockers are avoided with verapamil of diltiazem due to excessive depressions in contractility, bradycardia, AV block, or fatigue. CCBs may also suppress lower esophageal sphincter contraction and worsen symptoms of GERD. CCBs inhibit hepatic CYP3A4 and therefore, may raise blood levels of statins and other drugs. Cimetidine and grapefruit juice may increase the effective level of CCBs. Interactions occur between verapamil, dofetilide, quinidine, digoxin, prazosin, and cyclosporine. Because magnesium is a calcium antagonist, magnesium intake may enhance the actions of CCBs, in particular nifedipine. Delayed gingival hyperplasia has been described after using verapamil, amlodipine, and nifedipine. Both verapamil and diltiazem are contraindicated in patients with acute HF because of their negative inotropic effects; amlodipine and felodipine seem safe when LV dysfunction is compensated.

hypoxia or ischemia, preserves ionic pump function, minimizes free radical production, protects against intracellular calcium overload and acidosis, and improves endothelial function. The drug improves coronary flow reserve, lowers frequency of anginal episodes, enhances exercise performance, and spares the use of nitrates without changes in heart rate, vasodilator, or negative inotropic actions. A Cochrane review found that the drug provided relief through intracellular metabolic changes and was effective alone or with conventional antianginal agents, well tolerated, and cost-effective.[39] Metabolic manipulation that uses the central role of mitochondria in transmitting, amplifying, or processing signals that precondition the heart is being sought. Inhibition of the malate-aspartate shuttle is a similar maneuver that translocates reducing power from the cytosol into the mitochondria, thereby connecting glycolysis with the electron transport chain. In essence, it uses the same principle by shifting fuel preference from fatty acid oxidation to glucose.[38,40]

Fasudil

Hypertension results from either increased contractility of remodeled resistance arterioles with greater myocyte calcium entry via L-type voltage-dependent calcium channels and/or enhanced sensitivity to inward bound calcium driven by the RhoA/Rho kinase pathway.[41] Rho kinase (ROCK) is a major downstream effector of the small GTPase RhoA.[42] Chief roles of ROCK involve the actin cytoskeleton, including contraction, cell proliferation, adhesion, migration, proliferation, and gene expression. ROCK functions as a switch, shuttling between the GDP-bound inactive form and the GTP-bound active form. ROCK phosphorylates myosin II light chains and promotes myosin-actin contraction and vasoconstriction. Fasudil is a Rho kinase inhibitor that prevents vasospasm, promotes NO synthesis,[43] and suppresses angiotensin-converting enzyme (ACE) expression and conversion of angiotensin I to II. Fasudil exerts preconditioning and postconditioning effects on the heart, to overcome negative actions of hyperglycemia.[44] The agent prolongs exercise time to ST-segment depression, significantly reduces the number of anginal attacks, and is effective and safe in angina patients already taking traditional agents.[45]

Ranolazine

Ranolazine is a Food and Drug Administration (FDA)-approved antianginal agent with a mechanism of action independent of changes in blood pressure, heart rate, and inotropic action, which also exhibits antiarrhythmic and hypoglycemic actions.

Normally, there is a high electrochemical gradient driving calcium (Ca^{2+}) into myocytes, and removal by ion pumps is necessary to maintain low intracellular calcium concentrations, one of which is the Na^+/Ca^{2+}-exchanger (NCX). When ischemia impairs energy production, ATPase function falls, limiting removal of intracellular Na^+. Intracellular Na^+ overload, followed by intracellular calcium accumulation via reverse-mode NCX-activity, further inhibits mitochondrial ATP output.[46] Sodium enters the myocyte rapidly during the initial upstroke of the action potential but is followed by a small late inward Na^+ current that enlarges significantly during ischemia and heart failure (HF).[47] Continued exposure of actin and myosin to calcium causes a tonic contracture in isolated fibers but diastolic stiffness in the intact heart. The extra contraction wastes energy, compresses the vascular space during diastole, further compromising myocardial oxygen supply. The rise in intracellular sodium concentration promotes electrical instability and arrhythmias.

Ranozaline is a piperazine derivative that inhibits the late sodium channels, lowering not only total inward sodium flux but also the subsequent intracellular calcium overload.[48] At therapeutic concentrations, reduction of late inward sodium current is confined to ischemic or failing myocytes. The drug interrupts the loop that perpetuates myocardial ischemia, sodium influx, loss of potassium, voltage gradient perturbations, and myocardial dysfunction. Ion channel changes induced by ranozaline resemble those of amiodarone. There is a mild increase in the corrected QT interval (QTc), slightly shortened action potential duration, decreased probabilities of early afterdepolarizations, or raised dispersion of ventricular repolarization, hence no increase in sudden death or polymorphic ventricular tachycardia. Ranolazine suppresses arrhythmias associated with ACS, long QT syndrome, HF, ischemia, and reperfusion.[48]

The starting dose of ranolazine is 500 mg twice daily and can be raised to a maximum of 1000 mg twice daily if needed. Dizziness, nausea, constipation, and weakness have been reported, but the drug is generally well tolerated. Peak plasma levels occur 4 to 6 hours after an oral dose, with 50% to 55% bioavailability, and a steady state is attained in approximately 3 days. Ranolazine is cleared by CYP3A4 (70%–85%) and CYP2D6 (10%–15%) but is also a substrate of P-glycoprotein, a membrane transporter protein. P-glycoprotein inhibitors (eg, cyclosporine) reduce the dose of ranolazine needed to produce a given response (**Table 8**).

Table 8
Some clinical drug interactions of ranolazine

Drug or Challenge	Unwanted Effect	Notes
Ketaconazole	CYP3A4 inhibition and a 4.5-rise in ranolazine levels and side effects, such as dizziness, headache, nausea, constipation, weakness	Also applies to clarithromycin, ritonavir, nefazodone, rifampin, rifabutin, rifapentin, barbiturates, carbamazepine, phenytoin, St. John's wort, grapefruit juice, and other CYP3A4 interactants
Ranolazine	Mild inhibition of both CYP3A4 and CYP2D6, with a 2-fold rise in simvistatin levels	
Ranolazine, 750 mg twice daily	May increase levels of immediate-release metopolol, 100 mg, a CYP2D6 substrate, by 1.8-fold.	Other CYP2D6 substrates may act similarly with ranolazine: propafenone, flecainide, or tricyclic antidepressants and antipsychotics.
Paroxetine	CYP2D6 inhibition may raise ranolazine levels 1.2-fold.	
Diltiazem	Inhibition of CYP3A4 may increase ranolazine levels 1.5-fold.	
Verapamil, ≥360 mg/d	P-glycoprotein inhibition may raise ranolazine levels up to 3-fold.	
Ranolazine	P-glycoprotein interaction may raise digoxin levels 1.4–1.6 fold.	
Ranolazine, 2 g/d	Prolongation of QTc, approximately 6 ms	May affect patients with congenital long QT syndrome, or who take drugs that prolong the QTc, including class Ia (eg, quinidine) or class III antiarrhythmic agents (eg, dofetilide, sotalol, and amiodarone), erythromycin, amitriptyline, some antipsychotic agents (eg, thioridazine and ziprasidone), and others. Even though QTc is a determinant of serious arrhythmias, other electrical properties of ranolazine causes less concern compared with other drugs that prolong QTc.

Caution is advised when using ranolazine in patients with hepatic or renal impairment, patients with low weight, the elderly, or those with NYHA class III–IV HF.

Data from Di Monaco A, Sestito A. The patient with chronic ischemic heart disease. Role of ranolazine in the management of stable angina. Eur Rev Med Pharmacol Sci 2012;16(12):1611–36.

Clinically, ranolazine prolongs exercise duration to angina and to ST depression and relieves effort angina despite use of atenolol, diltiazem, amlodipine, and nitrates, some in maximal doses. There is no evidence of reduced mortality. One study suggested an antiarrhythmic effect, and a small reduction in hemoglobin A_{1c} (HbA$_{1c}$) was observed in diabetics.[49] The drug reduced ventricular wall stress in high-risk ST-segment elevation myocardial infarction patients with elevated levels of B-type natriuretic peptide.[50] In summary, ranolazine is indicated as additional treatment of angina patients inadequately controlled or unable to tolerate first line anti-ischemic drugs. It is considered safe but attention must be given to some drug interactions.[51]

SECONDARY PREVENTION

Because atherosclerosis is largely a lifestyle disease, the importance of an educational program and a systematic, mutually reinforced, monitored approach, together with pharmacologic risk factor reduction to slow progression of disease and

Table 9
Population-attributed risks for MI according to INTERHEART

Risk Factor	Population-Attributable Risk (%)
Smoking	35.7
Raised plasma apolipoprotein B/apolipoprotein A ratio	49.2
Hypertension history	17.9
Diabetes	9.9
Abdominal obesity	20.1
Psychosocial factors	32.5
Physical inactivity	12.2
Inadequate consumption of fruits/vegetables	13.7

From Yusuf S, Hawken S, Ounpuu S, et al. Effect of potentially modifiable risk factors associated with myocardial infarction in 52 countries (the INTERHEART study): case-control study. Lancet 2004;364:937–52; with permission.

prevent future events, is essential. The history, priority, benefits, and other aspects of risk and secondary prevention are summarized elsewhere.[52,53] Lifestyle measures and risk reduction, when sufficient, produce excellent results but are vastly underutilized.

The INTERHEART (A Study of Risk Factors for First Myocardial Infarction in 52 Countries and Over 27,000 Subjects) found that the populated-attributed risks for MI were composed largely of 8 variables (**Table 9**).[54]

The American Heart Association (AHA) emphasized prevention in its 2020 goals statement[55] and classified cardiovascular health into poor, intermediate, or ideal, depending on the satisfaction of 7 targets, outlined in **Table 10**.

Since that time, these behaviors and factors have been validated as a means of measuring cardiovascular health, which accurately permit comparison between time periods and evaluation of progress. Except for psychosocial stress, exceptionally difficult to quantitate and compare clinically, all risk factors identified by the INTERHEART are included in the AHA Simple 7 metrics.

MANAGEMENT OF RISK FACTORS

The latest 2012 ACCF/AHA/multisociety guidelines address the management of major modifiable risk factors for SIHD patients, which are summarized in **Table 11**.[17] Separate statements, however, concerning the management of lifestyle,[56]

Table 10
The 7 metrics defining ideal cardiovascular health—4 behaviors and 3 factors

Metric	Prevalence of Metric at Time of Publication
Smoking, abstinence or remote (abstinence $\geq$1 y)	73
Body mass index <25 kg/m^2	33
Exercising regularly, moderate intensity $\geq$150 min, or 75 min at vigorous intensity weekly	45
Consuming a healthy diet: adhering to 4–5 important dietary components • Sodium intake <1.5 g/d • Sugar-sweetened beverage intake <36 oz weekly • $\geq$4.5 Cups of fruits and vegetables/d • $\geq$Three 1-oz servings of fiber-rich whole grains/d • $\geq$Two 3.5-oz servings of oily fish/wk Optional recommendations: $\geq$4 servings of nuts, legumes and seeds/wk; $\leq$2 servings of processed meats/wk; saturated fat <7% total energy intake	<0.5%
Total cholesterol <200 mg/dL	45
Blood pressure <120/80 mm Hg	42
Fasting blood glucose <100 mg/dL	58

Table 11
Selected recommendations regarding risk reduction in patients with SIHD

Risk Factor	Recommendations (To Be Preceded by a Discussion with the Patient)	Notes
Smoking	Smoking discontinuance is an effective way to prevent IHD. Discontinuance should be mentioned at every visit. Secondhand smoke should be avoided. Pharmacotherapy with nicotine, bupropion, and perhaps varenicline should be used along with referral to special programs. The guiding mnemonic is: Ask, Advise, Assess, Assist, and Arrange.	Cessation may lower risk by 30% in 6 mo, 60% in 3 y.
Hypertension	All patients should be counseled about lifestyle modifications to lower blood pressure: weight control, physical activity, low alcohol, sodium intake, high consumption of fresh fruit and vegetables, and low fat dairy. Either the Dietary Approaches to Stop Hypertension (DASH) or Mediterranean diet is acceptable.	
	Blood pressure should be kept <140/90 mm Hg, or <130/80 in patients with diabetes or kidney disease.	These are JNC 7 numbers. Guidelines differ on these numbers.
	For patients with established IHD, use β-blockers or ACEIs first, then other agents.	
Dyslipidemia	In all patients, begin statins, unless there are contraindications, together with lifestyle modifications.	Use high-potency statins.
	Daily exercise, weight control, lower diet saturated fat <7%, eliminate dietary trans–fatty acids, cholesterol intake <200 mg/d. If triglycerides = 200–499 mg/dL, use statins to achieve a non–high-density lipoprotein (HDL) <130 mg/dL.	
	When triglycerides are 200–499 mg/dL, lowering non-HDL <100 mg/dL with statins is reasonable when risk is high. Niacin or fibrates may be used in selected cases. When triglycerides >500 mg/dL, fibrate and or niacin therapy should be begun to avoid pancreatitis.	Non-HDL incorporates the atherogenicity of other particles.
	Omega-3 fish oil, 1 g/d is reasonable. Greater amounts (≥2.5/d) are needed to lower triglyceride levels.	1 g Fish oil means the sum of eicosapentaenoic acid + docosahexaenoic acid, not total marine oil as labeled on bottles. Most people consume far too little. Omega-3 fats are pleiotropic.
Weight control	A diet diary should be kept. Maintain body mass index between 18.5 and 24.0 kg/m². Aim for a 10% reduction first. Be persistent and measure waist circumference. If it is ≥40″ (102 cm) in men or 35″ (89 cm) in women, look for other components of the metabolic syndrome.	Sustained weight control and exercise treat metabolic syndrome. There is no specific pharmacologic therapy for this syndrome; individual components are treated individually.

(continued on next page)

Table 11
(continued)

Risk Factor	Recommendations (To Be Preceded by a Discussion with the Patient)	Notes
Physical activity	Recommend 30–60 min of moderate-intensity aerobic activity, 7 d/wk, a minimum of 5 d/wk, supplemented by an increase in daily activities, as tolerated or prudent. An activity diary should be kept, and an exercise test performed to guide the exercise prescription. A cardiac rehabilitation programs should be considered in all eligible patients. Resistance training 2 d/wk may be reasonable	3 d Of strength training, 45–60 min each session, is usually the eventual goal if medically appropriate.
Diabetes	Simultaneous reduction of other risk factors (weight, physical activity, dyslipidemia, and blood pressure) should be vigorously pursued as recommended. Keep HbA1c levels ≤7. Metformin is considered first-line therapy unless contraindicated. Looser control may be considered with a history of hypoglycemia, comorbidities, advanced complications.	
Antiplatelet agents	Aspirin should be used, 72–162 mg in all patients, and continued indefinitely unless contraindicated. Clopidogrel, 75 mg, is an alternative for those intolerant or allergic to aspirin. Use with warfarin is not recommended unless a separate indication exists (eg, atrial fibrillation or deep vein thrombosis).	Platelet hyporesponsiveness may be encountered. Genetic variation in responsiveness is of clinical importance.
Renin-angiotensin-aldosterone system blockers	ACEIs should be used in all patients with LV ejection fraction (LVEF) ≤40% in all patients and in those with hypertension, diabetes, or chronic kidney disease. *Angiotensin receptor blockers* should be used for patients who cannot tolerate ACEIs, have HF, or are post-MI with LVEF ≤40%. Aldosterone blockers should be used in post-MI patients without creatinine >2.5 mg/dL in men, >2 mg/dL in women, or potassium levels >5 mEq/L, who are receiving adequate doses of an ACEI and a β-blocker, have LVEF ≤40%, and have either diabetes or HF.	
β-Blockers	β-Blockers should be used in all patients, unless contraindicated, with LVEF ≤40% with HF or prior MI. Carvedilol, metoprolol succinate, and bisoprolol have been shown to increase survival. In patients with normal LVEF who have had ACS or MI, β-blockers may be continued beyond 3 y (reasonable) or indefinitely (considered).	
Vaccination	Influenza vaccination recommended annually	

Data from Fihn SD, Gardin JM, Abrams J, et al. 2012 ACCF/AHA/ACP/AATS/PCNA/SCAI/SCA/STS guideline for the diagnosis and management of patients with stable ischemic heart disease. Circulation 2012;126:e354–471.

weight,[57] assessment of risk,[58] and cholesterol[59] in patients have been issued recently, as well as a science advisory concerning hypertension,[60] with a definitive hypertension guideline to be released later. Other guidelines available include management of diabetes[61] and a choice of several alternative guidelines for hypertension and dyslipidemia. The surprising and paradigm-changing difference has occurred concerning assessment and dyslipidemia, using new pooled risk equations and the elimination of goals for low-density lipoprotein, which primarily apply to primary prevention.[58,59] Controversy and differences in these areas have been substantial and ongoing. Changes have not yet specifically appeared with respect to guidelines for secondary prevention but may affect the frequency of lipid measurement and the use of agents other than statins.

REFERENCES

1. Sheps DS, Creed F, Clouse RE. Chest pain in patients with cardiac and noncardiac disease. Psychosom Med 2004;66:861–7.

2. Eslick GD, Coulshed DS, Talley NJ. Diagnosis and treatment of noncardiac chest pain. Nat Clin Pract Gastroenterol Hepatol 2005;2:463–72.

3. Cayley WE Jr. Diagnosing the cause of chest pain. Am Fam Physician 2005;72:2012–21.

4. Parker JO, Chiong MA, West RO, et al. Sequential alterations in myocardial lactate metabolism, S-T segments, and left ventricular function during angina induced by atrial pacing. Circulation 1969; 40(1):113–31.

5. Scirica BM, Morrow DA, Budaj A, et al. Ischemia detected on continuous electrocardiography after acute coronary syndrome: observations from the MERLIN-TIMI 36 (Metabolic efficiency with ranolazine for less ischemia in non-ST-elevation acute coronary syndrome-thrombolysis in myocardial infarction 36) Trial. J Am Coll Cardiol 2009;53: 1411–21.

6. Yano K, MacLean CJ. The Incidence and prognosis of unrecognized myocardial infarction in the Honolulu, Hawaii, Heart Program. Arch Intern Med 1989;149:1528–32.

7. Deedwania PC, Carbajal EV. Silent ischemia during daily life is an independent predictor of mortality in stable angina. Circulation 1990;81:748–56.

8. Norgaard BL, Andersen K, Dellborg M, et al, The TRIM Study Group. Admission risk assessment by cardiac Troponin T in unstable coronary artery disease: additional prognostic information from continuous ST segment monitoring. J Am Coll Cardiol 1999;33:1519–27.

9. Gotto AM Jr. Statin therapy and the elderly: SAGE Advice? Circulation 2007;115:681–3.

10. Tjia J, Allison J, Saczyynski JS, et al. Encouraging trends in acute myocardial infarction survival in the oldest old. Am J Med 2013;126:798–804.

11. Campeau L. The Canadian Cardiovascular Society grading of angina pectoris revisited 30 years later. Can J Cardiol 2002;18:371–9.

12. Goldman L, Hashimoto B, Cook EF, et al. Comparative reproducibility and validity of systems for assessing cardiovascular functional class: advantages of a new specific activity scale. Circulation 1981;64: 1227–34.

13. Shub C, Click RL, Goon MD. Myocardial ischemia clinical syndromes; B: angina pectoris and coronary heart disease. In: Giuliani ER, Gersh BJ, McGoon MD, et al, editors. Mayo clinic practice of cardiology. 3rd edition. Mosby; 1996. p. 1160–90. Chapter 29.

14. Kones R. Metabolism of the acutely ischemic and hypoxic heart. Crit Care Med 1973;1:321–30.

15. Kones R. Pathogenesis of cardiogenic shock II. N Y State J Med 1973;73:1662–70.

16. Fox K, Garcia MA, Ardissino D, et al, Task Force on the Management of Stable Angina pectoris of the European Society of Cardiology, ESC Committee for Practice Guidelines (CPG). Guidelines on the management of stable angina pectoris: executive summary: the Task Force on the Management of Stable Angina Pectoris of the European Society of Cardiology. Eur Heart J 2006;27:1341–81.

17. Fihn SD, Gardin JM, Abrams J, et al. 2012 ACCF/AHA/ACP/AATS/PCNA/SCAI/SCA/STS guideline for the diagnosis and management of patients with stable ischemic heart disease. Circulation 2012;126:e354–471.

18. Diamond GA, Forrester JS. Analysis of probability as an aid in the clinical diagnosis of coronary-artery disease. N Engl J Med 1979;300:1350–8.

19. Califf RM, Harrell FE, Lee KL, et al. The evolution of medical and surgical therapy for coronary artery disease. JAMA 1989;261:2077–86.

20. O'Connor RE, Brady W, Brooks SC, et al. AHA Guidelines for Cardiopulmonary Resuscitation and Emergency Cardiovascular Care, Part 8: stabilization of the patient with acute coronary syndromes. Circulation 2005;112(Suppl 4):S787–817.

21. Kezerashvilli A, Marzo K, De Leon J. Beta blocker use after acute myocardial infarction in the patient with normal systolic function: when is it "Ok" to discontinue? Curr Cardiol Rev 2012;8:77–84.

22. Münzel T, Gori T. Nitrate therapy and nitrate tolerance in patients with coronary artery disease. Curr Opin Pharmacol 2013;13:251–9.

23. Lacoste LL, Theroux P, Lidon RM, et al. Antithrombotic properties of transdermal nitroglycerin in stable angina pectoris. Am J Cardiol 1994;73:1058–62.

24. Schiffrin EL. Oxidative stress, nitric oxide synthase, and superoxide dismutase: a matter of imbalance

underlies endothelial dysfunction in the human coronary circulation. Hypertension 2008;51:31–2.

25. Huige LI, Förstermann U. Uncoupling of endothelial NO synthase in atherosclerosis and vascular disease. Curr Opin Pharmacol 2013;13:161–7.

26. Pepine CJ, Cohn PF, Deedwania PC, et al. Effects of treatment on outcome in mildly symptomatic patients with ischemia during daily life. The Atenolol Silent Ischemia Study (ASIST). Circulation 1994; 90:762–8.

27. Pepine CJ, Handberg EM, Cooper-DeHoff RM, et al, INVEST Investigators. A calcium antagonist vs a non-calcium antagonist hypertension treatment strategy for patients with coronary artery disease. The International Verapamil-Trandolapril Study (INVEST): a randomized controlled trial. JAMA 2003;290:2805–16.

28. Sierra C, Coca A. The ACTION Study: nifedipine in patients with symptomatic stable angina and hypertension. Expert Rev Cardiovasc Ther 2008;6: 1055–62.

29. Jahangir A, Terzic A, Shen WK. Potassium channel openers: therapeutic potential in cardiology and medicine. Expert Opin Pharmacother 2001;2: 1995–2010.

30. IONA Study Group. Effect of nicorandil on coronary events in patients with stable angina: the Impact of Nicorandil in Angina (IONA) randomised trial. Lancet 2002;359:1269–75.

31. Ciampricotti R, Schotborgh CE, de Kam PJ, et al. A comparison of nicorandil with isosorbide mononitrate in elderly patients with stable coronary heart disease: the SNAPE Study. Am Heart J 2000;139: 939–43.

32. Horinaka S, Yabe A, Yahi H, et al. Effects of nicorandil on cardiovascular events in patients with coronary artery disease in the Japanese Coronary Artery Disease (JCAD) Study. Circ J 2010;74:503–9.

33. Hirohata A, Yamamoto K, Hirose E, et al. Nicorandil prevents microvascular dysfunction resulting from PCI in patients with stable angina pectoris: a randomised study. EuroIntervention 2014;9:1058–66.

34. Ito N, Nanto S, Doi Y, et al. Beneficial effects of intracoronary nicorandil on microvascular dysfunction after primary percutaneous coronary intervention: demonstration of its superiority to nitroglycerin in a cross-over study. Cardiovasc Drugs Ther 2013;27: 279–87.

35. Khan W, Borer JS. Critical evaluation of ivabradine for the management of chronic stable angina. Res Reports Clin Cardiol 2011;2:87–98. Available at: https://www.dovepress.com/critical-evaluation-of-ivabradine-for-the-management-of-chronic-stable-peer-reviewed-article-RRCC-recommendation1.

36. Cappato R, Castelvecchio S, Ricci C. Clinical efficacy of ivabradine in patients with inappropriate sinus tachycardia. A prospective, randomized,

placebo-controlled, double-blind, crossover evaluation. J Am Coll Cardiol 2012;60:1323–9.

37. Marzilli M. Does timetazidine prevent myocardial injury after percutaneous coronary intervention? Nat Clin Pract Cardiovasc Med 2008;5:16–7.

38. Safer B. The metabolic significance of the malate–aspartate shuttle cycle in the heart. Circ Res 1975; 37:527–33.

39. Ciapponi A, Pizarro R, Harrison J. Trimetazidine for stable angina. Cochrane Database Syst Rev 2005;(4):CD003614.

40. Beadle RM, Frenneaux M. Modification of myocardial substrate utilisation: a new therapeutic paradigm in cardiovascular disease. Heart 2010;96:824–30.

41. Zicha J, Behuliak M, Pintérová M, et al. The interaction of calcium entry and calcium sensitization in the control of vascular tone and blood pressure of normotensive and hypertensive rats. Physiol Res 2014;63(Suppl 1):S19–27.

42. Wang Y, Zheng XR, Riddick N, et al. ROCK isoform regulation of myosin phosphatase and contractility in vascular smooth muscle cells. Circ Res 2009; 104:531–40.

43. Surma M, Wei L, Shi J. Rho kinase as a therapeutic target in cardiovascular disease. Future Cardiol 2011;7:657–71.

44. Ichinomiya T, Cho S, Higashijima U, et al. High-dose fasudil preserves postconditioning against myocardial infarction under hyperglycemia in rats: role of mitochondrial KATP channels. Cardiovasc Diabetol 2012;11:28.

45. Dong M, Yan BP, Liao JK, et al. Rho-kinase inhibition: a novel therapeutic target for the treatment of cardiovascular diseases. Drug Discov Today 2010;15:622–9.

46. Barth AS, Tomaselli GF. Cardiac metabolism and arrhythmias. Circ Arrhythm Electrophysiol 2009;2: 327–35.

47. Belardinelli L, Antzelevitch C, Fraser H. Inhibition of late (sustained/persistent) sodium current: a potential drug target to reduce intracellular sodium dependent calcium overload and its detrimental effects on cardiomyocyte function. Eur Heart J 2004; 6:13–7.

48. Antzelevitch C, Burashnikov A, Sicouri S, et al. Electrophysiological basis for the antiarrhythmic actions of ranolazine. Heart Rhythm 2011;8:1281–90.

49. Khan K, Jones M. Ranolazine in the management of chronic stable angina. Br J Cardol 2011;18:1–7.

50. Morrow DA, Scirica BM, Sabatine MS, et al. B-Type Natriuretic peptide and the effect of ranolazine in patients with non-st-segment elevation acute coronary syndromes. Observations from the MERLIN-TIMI 36 Trial. J Am Coll Cardiol 2010;55:1189–96.

51. Truffa AA, Newby LK, Melloni C. Extended-release ranolazine: critical evaluation of its use in stable angina. Vasc Health Risk Manag 2011;7:535–9.

52. Kones R. Is prevention a fantasy, or the future of medicine? A panoramic view of recent data, status, and direction in cardiovascular prevention. Ther Adv Cardiovasc Dis 2011;5:51–61.

53. Kones R. Molecular sources of residual cardiovascular risk, clinical signals, and innovative solutions: relationship with subclinical disease, undertreatment, and poor adherence: implications of new evidence upon optimizing cardiovascular patient outcomes. Vasc Health Risk Manag 2013; 9:617–70.

54. Yusuf S, Hawken S, Ounpuu S, et al. Effect of potentially modifiable risk factors associated with myocardial infarction in 52 countries (the INTER-HEART study): case-control study. Lancet 2004; 364:937–52.

55. Lloyd-Jones DM, Hong Y, Labarthe D, et al, on behalf of the American Heart Association Strategic Planning Task Force and Statistics Committee. Defining and Setting National Goals for Cardiovascular Health Promotion and Disease Reduction: the American Heart Association's Strategic Impact Goal Through 2020 and Beyond. Circulation 2010;121:586–613.

56. Eckel RH, Jakicic JM, Ard JD, et al. 2013 AHA/ACC Guideline on Lifestyle Management to Reduce Cardiovascular Risk: a Report of the American College of Cardiology/American Heart Association Task Force on Practice Guidelines. J Am Coll Cardiol 2014. http://dx.doi.org/10.1016/j.jacc.2013.11.003.

57. Jensen MD, Ryan DH, Apovian CM, et al. 2013 AHA/ACC/TOS Guideline for the Management of Overweight and Obesity in Adults: a Report of the American College of Cardiology/American Heart Association Task Force on Practice Guidelines and The Obesity Society. J Am Coll Cardiol 2014. http://dx.doi.org/10.1016/j.jacc.2013.11.004.

58. Goff DC, Lloyd-Jones DM, Bennett G, et al. 2013 ACC/AHA Guideline on the Assessment of Cardiovascular Risk: a Report of the American College of Cardiology/American Heart Association Task Force on Practice Guidelines. J Am Coll Cardiol 2014. http://dx.doi.org/10.1016/j.jacc.2013.11.005.

59. Stone NJ, Robinson J, Lichtenstein AH, et al. 2013 ACC/AHA Guideline on the Treatment of Blood Cholesterol to Reduce Atherosclerotic Cardiovascular Risk in Adults. A Report of the American College of Cardiology/American Heart Association Task Force on Practice Guidelines. J Am Coll Cardiol 2014. http://dx.doi.org/10.1016/j.jacc.2013.11.002.

60. Go AS, Bauman MA, King SM, et al. AHA/ACC/CDC Science Advisory: an effective approach to high blood pressure control a science advisory from the American Heart Association, the American College of Cardiology, and the Centers for Disease Control and Prevention. J Am Coll Cardiol 2014. http://dx.doi.org/10.1016/j.jacc.2013.11.007.

61. American Diabetes Association. Standards of medical care in diabetes—2014. Diabetes Care 2014; 37(Suppl 1):S14–80.

Acute Coronary Syndromes
Unstable Angina and Non–ST Elevation Myocardial Infarction

Sukhdeep S. Basra, MD, MPH[a], Salim S. Virani, MD, PhD[b],
David Paniagua, MD[b], Biswajit Kar, MD[b], Hani Jneid, MD[b],*

KEYWORDS

- Unstable angina • Non–ST elevation MI • Acute coronary syndromes • Management
- Revascularization • Antiplatelet • Antithrombotic

KEY POINTS

- Improvements in primary prevention and acute management strategies have led to a reduction in in-hospital mortality associated with non–ST elevation acute coronary syndromes (NSTE-ACS); however, the incidence of NSTE-ACS continues to be stable, largely because of an aging population and use of highly sensitive biomarkers for diagnosis of myocardial injury.
- Newer antiplatelet agents, including prasugrel and ticagrelor, have been shown to have superior efficacy compared with clopidogrel and have been approved for the treatment of patients with NSTE-ACS as an alternative to clopidogrel and as part of oral dual antiplatelet therapy.
- Early invasive strategy with diagnostic angiography and intervention within 12 to 24 hours is a reasonable treatment strategy in all NSTE-ACS, especially in the highest-risk patients.
- Early revascularization after NSTE-ACS is beneficial in patients with mild to moderate chronic kidney disease.
- A statin of high to moderate intensity should be administered to all patients with NSTE-ACS by hospital discharge without using the low-density lipoprotein–cholesterol as a target goal.

Unstable angina (UA) and non–ST elevation myocardial infarction (NSTEMI) are collectively known as non–ST elevation acute coronary syndromes (NSTE-ACSs). Improvements in prevention strategies and acute treatments for NSTE-ACSs led to marked improvement in their outcomes. According to data from the National Registry of Myocardial Infarction (1990–2006), in-hospital NSTEMI mortality declined significantly from 7.1% to 5.2%, which was partially attributable to improvements in acute treatments.[1] In the Worcester registry, the 1-year postdischarge case fatality rates for NSTEMI declined from 23.1% in 1997 to 18.7% in 2005.[2] In contrast, the increased sensitivity of new biomarkers for the diagnosis of myocardial infarction (MI) and the increasing prevalence of cardiovascular (CV) risk factors (such as diabetes and obesity) resulted in their increased incidence and prevalence (**Fig. 1**). Data from Kaiser Permanente Northern California showed that the adjusted mortality decreased significantly for NSTEMI between 1999 and 2008, but the age-adjusted and sex-adjusted incidence rate of hospitalizations did not change significantly over time.[3] Therefore, NSTE-ACSs remain common causes of morbidity and mortality in the United States.

[a] Division of Cardiology, Baylor College of Medicine, Houston, TX 77030, USA; [b] Division of Cardiology, Baylor College of Medicine, The Michael E. DeBakey VA Medical Center, 2002 Holcombe Boulevard, Houston, TX 77030, USA
* Corresponding author.
E-mail address: jneid@bcm.edu

Cardiol Clin 32 (2014) 353–370
http://dx.doi.org/10.1016/j.ccl.2014.04.010
0733-8651/14/$ – see front matter Published by Elsevier Inc.

cardiology.theclinics.com

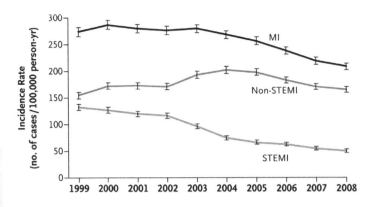

Fig. 1. Age-adjusted and sex-adjusted incidence rates of acute MI, 1999 to 2008. STEMI, ST elevation MI. (*From* Yeh RW, Sidney S, Chandra M, et al. Population trends in the incidence and outcomes of acute myocardial infarction. N Engl J Med 2010;362(23): 2155–65; with permission.)

PATHOPHYSIOLOGY

UA and NSTEMI are characterized by an acute imbalance between myocardial oxygen supply and demand. The most common cause is coronary artery narrowing from a disrupted atherosclerotic plaque with superimposed acute thrombosis that suddenly and significantly compromises coronary blood flow but is usually not 100% occlusive (as in ST elevation MI [STEMI]).[4] Additional causes include coronary artery spasm, severe luminal narrowing from atherosclerosis or restenosis after percutaneous coronary intervention (PCI), and coronary dissection as well as extrinsic factors (such as severe hypotension, tachycardia, anemia, and thyrotoxicosis) in the setting of underlying luminal narrowing of the coronary arteries by atherosclerosis.

DIAGNOSIS AND RISK STRATIFICATION

Medical history, physical examination, electrocardiograms (ECGs), and an initial measurement of cardiac biomarkers should be done rapidly to develop a working diagnosis, establish the acuity of the event and the hazards of death and adverse events, and promptly triage patients to the appropriate treatment strategy. Serial ECGs and measurements of cardiac biomarkers of necrosis are critical to the accurate diagnosis of NSTE-ACS and are complemented by echocardiography, coronary angiography, and other imaging modalities. NSTE-ACS usually presents with ischemic symptoms (angina pectoris or its equivalent) along with new ST segment depression or prominent T-wave inversion on the ECG. The presence of increased biomarkers, usually an increase and/or decrease in cardiac troponin (cTn) value exceeding the 99th percentile upper limits of normal, confirms myonecrosis and differentiates NSTEMI from UA (**Box 1**).[5]

Risk stratification using various scoring systems such as the TIMI (Thrombolysis in Myocardial Infarction),[6] GRACE (Global Registry of Acute Coronary Events),[7] and the PURSUIT (Platelet glycoprotein IIb/IIIa in Unstable agina: Receptor Suppression Using Integrilin)[8] risk scores have been developed to assess patients' prognosis and help guide clinical decision making. All patients with NSTE-ACSs should undergo initial medical stabilization; early administration of antiplatelet, antithrombotic, and anti-ischemic drugs; and should be treated appropriately with either an early invasive or initial conservative strategy depending on their initial risk assessment (**Fig. 2**).

ANTIPLATELET THERAPY
Aspirin

Multiple trials have shown the benefits of aspirin, including improved survival, in patients with ACS.[9–12] Aspirin inhibits cyclooxygenase-1 within the platelet preventing the formation of thromboxane A2 and thus inhibiting platelet aggregation.[13] Aspirin should be administered to all patients with NSTE-ACS as soon as possible after hospital presentation and continued indefinitely thereafter.[14] Doses of aspirin between 75 mg and 1500 mg showed similar reduction in vascular effects but are associated with a dose-dependent increase in bleeding hazards. Thus, following the acute hospitalization period, it is reasonable to use a maintenance dose of 81 mg of aspirin per day in preference to higher maintenance doses in patients with NSTE-ACS. Patients allergic to aspirin should be placed on clopidogrel indefinitely or should undergo aspirin desensitization.

Clopidogrel

Clopidogrel, the most widely used thienopyridine, causes irreversible inhibition of the $P2Y_{12}$ receptor and inhibits platelet aggregation by a different

---

Box 1
Third universal definition of MI

Criteria for acute MI

The term acute MI should be used when there is evidence of myocardial necrosis in a clinical setting consistent with acute myocardial ischemia. Under these conditions any of the following criteria meet the diagnosis for MI:

- Detection of an increase and/or decrease of cardiac biomarker values (preferably cTn) with at least 1 value more than the 99th percentile upper reference limit (URL) and with at least 1 of the following:
  - Symptoms of ischemia
  - New or presumed new significant ST segment–T-wave changes or new left bundle branch block (LBBB)
  - Development of pathologic Q waves in the ECG
  - Imaging evidence of new loss of viable myocardium or new regional wall motion abnormality
  - Identification of an intracoronary thrombus by angiography or autopsy
- Cardiac death with symptoms suggesting myocardial ischemia and presumed new ischemic ECG changes or new LBBB, but death occurred before cardiac biomarkers were obtained or before cardiac biomarker values would be increased.
- PCI-related MI is arbitrarily defined by increase of cTn values (>5 × 99th percentile URL) in patients with normal baseline values (≤99th percentile URL) or an increase of cTn values greater than 20% if the baseline values are increased and are stable or decreasing. In addition, (1) symptoms suggesting myocardial ischemia, (2) new ischemic ECG changes, (3) angiographic findings consistent with a procedural complication, or (4) imaging demonstration of new loss of viable myocardium or new regional wall motion abnormality are required.
- Stent thrombosis associated with MI when detected by coronary angiography or autopsy in the setting of myocardial ischemia and with an increase and/or decrease of cardiac biomarker values with at least 1 value more than the 99th percentile URL.
- CABG-related MI is arbitrarily defined by increase of cardiac biomarker values (>10 × 99th percentile URL) in patients with normal baseline cTn values (≤99th percentile URL). In addition, (1) new pathologic Q waves or new LBBB, (2) angiographic documented new graft or new native coronary artery occlusion, or (3) imaging evidence of new loss of viable myocardium or new regional wall motion abnormality.

Criteria for prior MI

Any of the following criteria meets the diagnosis for prior MI:

- Pathologic Q waves with or without symptoms in the absence of nonischemic causes
- Imaging evidence of a region of loss of viable myocardium that is thinned and fails to contract, in the absence of a nonischemic cause
- Pathologic findings of a prior MI

Adapted from Thygesen K, Alpert JS, Jaffe AS, et al, Joint ESC/ACCF/AHA/WHF Task Force for the Universal Definition of Myocardial Infarction. Third universal definition of myocardial infarction. Circulation 2012;126(16):2022; with permission.

---

mechanism than aspirin. It is widely used with aspirin as part of dual antiplatelet therapy (DAPT) for patients with NSTE-ACS (see **Fig. 2**, **Table 1**).[15,16] Current American College of Cardiology/American Heart Association (ACC/AHA) guidelines recommend that patients with definite NSTE-ACS who are at medium or high-risk should receive 12 months of DAPT with aspirin and clopidogrel on presentation, irrespective of whether they are treated with an invasive or a conservative strategy.[4] A loading dose of clopidogrel of 300 to 600 mg is recommended for all patients; however, patients with NSTE-ACS undergoing invasive therapy should receive a 600-mg loading dose as soon as possible before or at the time of PCI.

Clopidogrel is a prodrug that undergoes conversion to its active metabolite in the liver by the CYP2C19 system. It is therefore prone to significant variability in antiplatelet response and drug-drug interactions. At least 3 major genetic

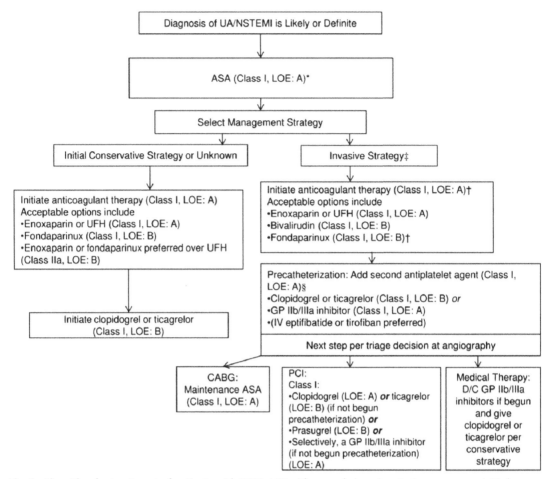

Fig. 2. Algorithm for treatment of patients with NSTE-ACS with an early invasive strategy versus an initial conservative approach. ASA, aspirin; CABG, coronary artery bypass graft; GP IIb/IIIa, glycoprotein IIb/IIIa inhibitor; PCI, percutaneous coronary intervention. (*From* Anderson JL, Adams CD, Antman EM, et al. 2012 ACCF/AHA focused update incorporated into the ACCF/AHA 2007 guidelines for the management of patients with unstable angina/non-ST-elevation myocardial infarction: a report of the American College of Cardiology Foundation/American Heart Association Task Force on Practice Guidelines. Circulation 2013;127(23):e663–828; with permission.)

polymorphisms associated with clopidogrel metabolism and loss of function of the CYP2C19 isoenzyme have been described.[17–19] Current ACC/AHA guidelines do not strongly recommend genotype testing in patients with ACS, but suggest that they may be considered on a case-by-case basis in patients with NSTE-ACS treated with clopidogrel and who have recurrent ischemia.[20] Drug interactions between clopidogrel and proton pump inhibitors (PPIs) have been reported, with a significant reduction in the inhibition of platelet aggregation by clopidogrel caused by inhibition of CYP2C19 by the PPIs. Although multiple retrospective analyses and observational studies suggested that the concomitant use of clopidogrel and PPIs is associated with worse clinical outcomes,[21,22] the COGENT (Clopidogrel

and the Optimization of Gastrointestinal Events Trial) randomized clinical trial failed to show any significant increase in CV events with the combination of clopidogrel and omeprazole.[23] The ACC/AHA expert statement on the use of PPI agents in combination with clopidogrel did not prohibit the use of PPI agents in appropriate clinical settings, but highlighted the potential risks and benefits from their use in combination with clopidogrel.[24]

Prasugrel

Prasugrel is a more potent and faster acting thienopyridine than clopidogrel. It has a 30-minute onset of action (to achieve 50% inhibition of platelet aggregation), compared with 2 to 4 hours for clopidogrel. Prasugrel is a prodrug requiring a 1-step metabolism (unlike the 2-step metabolism of clopidogrel). However, it is not affected by CYP2C19 polymorphisms and is not known to have interactions with PPIs.[25] Since its approval by the US Food and Drug Administration (FDA) in 2009, it is recommended in patients with NSTE-ACS in whom PCI is planned and after the coronary anatomy is delineated as part of DAPT (in addition to aspirin, and as an alternative to clopidogrel). A loading dose of 60 mg is usually followed by a maintenance dose of 10 mg once daily. In patients 75 years of age or older and less than 60 kg in weight, a prasugrel dose of 5 mg/d is usually recommended to minimize the bleeding hazards.

Prasugrel was superior to clopidogrel in the TRITON-TIMI 38 trial[26] (Trial to Assess Improvement in Therapeutic Outcomes by Optimizing Platelet Inhibition with Prasugrel–Thrombolysis in Myocardial Infarction), which was a multicenter trial of 13,608 patients with moderate and high-risk ACS who were randomized to prasugrel or clopidogrel. Compared with clopidogrel, prasugrel reduced the primary composite end point (CV death, nonfatal MI, or nonfatal stroke) over 6 to 15 months (9.9% vs 12.1%; $P<.001$). This finding was driven by a 24% significant reduction in nonfatal MI (7.3% vs 9.5%; $P<.001$), but no differences in CV death or stroke were observed.[26] Prasugrel was associated with reduced urgent target-vessel revascularization (3.7% vs 2.5%; $P<.001$) and stent thrombosis (2.4% vs 1.1%; $P<.001$). Prasugrel was also associated with an increased risk of TIMI major bleeding that was not related to coronary artery bypass graft (CABG), the key safety end point (2.4% vs 1.8%; $P = .03$), as well as increased life-threatening bleeding (1.4% vs 0.9%; $P = .01$). Prasugrel carries a boxed warning against its use in patients with prior transient ischemic accident or stroke, in whom net clinical harm was observed according to the TRITON-TIMI 38 trial.[26] Post hoc analyses from TRITON-TIMI 38 also revealed no net clinical benefit in elderly patients (>75 years) and those with a low body weight (<60 kg). The magnitude of effect on the primary end point was largest (30% risk reduction) in diabetic patients (prasugrel vs clopidogrel: 12.2% vs 17.0%; $P<.001$).[27]

The TRILOGY-ACS (Targeted Platelet Inhibition to Clarify the Optimal Strategy to Medically Manage Acute Coronary Syndromes) trial evaluated the use of prasugrel versus clopidogrel in 9326 patients with unstable angina or NSTEMI undergoing medical management.[28] Prasugrel did not significantly reduce the frequency of the primary end point (vascular death, MI, or stroke), compared with clopidogrel, and similar risks of bleeding were observed.[27]

Ticagrelor

Ticagrelor is a nucleoside-analogue, nonthienopyridine, reversible, direct-acting oral antagonist of the $P2Y_{12}$ receptor that does not require transformation to an active metabolite. Ticagrelor has a faster onset of action (30 minutes to achieve 50% inhibition of platelet aggregation) and provides more potent antiplatelet effects than clopidogrel.[29] A 180-mg loading of ticagrelor followed by 90 mg twice daily is recommended in all patients with NSTE-ACS in addition to aspirin as part of DAPT (as an alternative to clopidogrel) according to the ACC/AHA guidelines.

The Platelet Inhibition and Patient Outcomes (PLATO) trial assessed the safety and efficacy of ticagrelor relative to clopidogrel in more than 18,000 patients admitted with ACS.[30] The primary composite end point occurred less frequently in patients receiving ticagrelor (9.8%) compared with those receiving clopidogrel (11.7%; hazard ratio [HR], 0.84; 95% confidence interval [CI], 0.77–0.92). This finding was driven by significant reductions in both secondary end points of vascular death and MI with ticagrelor. The benefits of ticagrelor were observed irrespective of clopidogrel pretreatment and whether patients initially received invasive or medical management. Most notably, ticagrelor was associated with a 1.4% statistically significant absolute risk reduction in all-cause mortality, which has not been encountered with other antiplatelet agents. Although there was no increase in major bleeding rates according to the PLATO trial or TIMI criteria, ticagrelor was associated with higher incidence of non-CABG bleeding (4.5% vs 3.8%; $P = .03$), including fatal intracranial bleeding. In addition, dyspnea and a higher incidence of ventricular pauses on Holter monitoring were seen more frequently in the ticagrelor arm, although the pauses were rarely associated with symptoms. The benefit of ticagrelor seemed to be attenuated in patients with low body weight, those not taking lipid-lowering drugs at randomization, and those enrolled in North America. Mahaffey and colleagues[31] noted that a significantly higher proportion of patients in the United States received a median aspirin dose greater than 300 mg daily compared with the rest of the world (53.6% vs 1.7%). After multiple analyses factoring all other variables, the geographic variation in outcomes was likely attributable to higher aspirin dosing used in North America,[31] and the current recommended maintenance dose of aspirin while on ticagrelor is 81 mg daily.[14]

Table 1
Landmark clinical trials of oral antiplatelet agents

Clinical Trial	Number of Patients	Study Type	Patient Groups	Outcomes	Results
CURE[15]	12,562	Double blind, randomized	Clopidogrel (300 mg loading dose followed by 75 mg PO QD daily) vs placebo in addition to aspirin	Primary outcome: composite of death from CV causes, nonfatal MI, and stroke Bleeding (life-threatening or hemorrhagic stroke)	Decreased risk of primary outcome with clopidogrel vs placebo (P<.001) Increased risk of major bleeding with clopidogrel (P<.001) but no increase in life-threatening or hemorrhagic strokes
CREDO[76]	2116	Double blind, randomized	Clopidogrel (300-mg loading dose 3–24 h before PCI or placebo. Thereafter, all patients received clopidogrel, 75 mg/d, through day 28. From day 29 through 12 mo, patients in the loading-dose group received clopidogrel, 75 mg/d, and those in the control group received placebo	One-year incidence of the composite of death, MI, or stroke	At 1 y, long-term clopidogrel therapy was associated with a 26.9% relative reduction in the combined risk of death, MI, or stroke (95% confidence interval, 3.9%–44.4%; P = .02; absolute reduction, 3%) Clopidogrel at least 6 h before PCI led to a relative risk reduction of 38.6%
CURRENT-OASIS 7[77]	17,263	Double blind, randomized	Double-dose vs standard-dose clopidogrel and high-dose vs low-dose aspirin in individuals undergoing PCI	Primary outcome was composite of CV death, MI, or stroke from randomization to day 30	Primary outcome of CV death, MI, or stroke at 30 days was reduced in those randomized to higher-dose clopidogrel Major bleeding was more common with higher-dose clopidogrel but not with higher-dose ASA

Trial	N	Design	Intervention	End points	Results
TRITON-TIMI 38[26]	13,608	Double blind, randomized	Prasugrel (60-mg loading dose and 10-mg PO QD maintenance dose) compared with clopidogrel (300-mg loading dose and 75-mg PO QD maintenance dose) among patients undergoing PCI for ACS	Primary end points were death from CV causes, nonfatal MI, or nonfatal stroke; Key safety end point was major bleeding	Prasugrel was associated with a reduction in the composite ischemic event rate, including stent thrombosis, but it was associated with a significantly increased rate of bleeding
TRILOGY-ACS[28]	7243	Double blind, randomized	Prasugrel (10 mg daily) vs clopidogrel (75 mg daily) in patients with ACS not undergoing revascularization	Primary end point of death from CV causes, MI, or stroke; Rates of severe and intracranial bleeding	No significant difference in primary outcome (P = .21). Similar rates of bleeding observed
PLATO[30]	18,624 patients (of whom 11,598 patients had UA/NSTEMI)	Randomized, double blind	Ticagrelor (180 mg LD, 90 mg BID thereafter) and clopidogrel (300–600 mg LD, 75 mg daily thereafter)	Primary efficacy end point: 12-mo composite of death from vascular causes, MI, or stroke; Primary safety end point: any major bleeding event at 12 mo	Ticagrelor reduced primary and secondary end points in patients taking ticagrelor compared with clopidogrel; Ticagrelor was associated with an increase in the rate of non–procedure-related bleeding, but no increase in the rate of overall major bleeding compared with clopidogrel

Abbreviations: ASA, aspirin; BID, twice a day; CREDO, Clopidogrel for the Reduction of Events During Observation Trial; CURE, Clopidogrel in Unstable Angina to Prevent Recurrent Events Trial; CURRENT-OASIS 7, Clopidogrel Optimal Loading Dose Usage to Reduce Recurrent Events/Optimal Antiplatelet Strategy for Interventions 7 Trial; LD, loading dose; PLATO, Study of Platelet Inhibition and Patient Outcomes; PO, by mouth; QD, once daily; TRILOGY-ACS, Targeted Platelet Inhibition to Clarify the Optimal Strategy to Medically Manage Acute Coronary Syndromes; TRILOGY TIMI 38, Trial to Assess Improvement in Therapeutic Outcomes by Optimizing Platelet Inhibition with Prasugrel–Thrombolysis in Myocardial Infarction 38 trial.

Data from Refs.[15,26,28,30,76,77]

Glycoprotein IIb/IIIa Inhibitors

Glycoprotein IIb/IIIa inhibitors have been well established in the treatment of patients with NSTE-ACS, particularly among patients with increased troponins, in diabetics, and in those undergoing early revascularization.[32–34] However, their role as an additive agent to aspirin was established before the contemporary era of oral DAPT and few trials have evaluated their role in the setting of concomitant therapy with P2Y$_{12}$ inhibitors. Two recent trials, EARLY-ACS (Early Glycoprotein IIb/IIIa Inhibition in Non–ST-Segment Elevation Acute Coronary Syndrome) and ACUITY (Acute Catheterization and Urgent Intervention Triage Strategy) trials[35,36] investigated their role as part of triple therapy in addition to aspirin and clopidogrel. In EARLY-ACS, there was no significant difference in the primary CV end point at 30 days in patients randomized to early or deferred therapy with glycoprotein IIb/IIIa inhibitors, but a higher risk of TIMI major bleeding in the early infusion group was observed.[35] There was no interaction noted with clopidogrel administration in the study. The ACUITY trial[36] similarly showed a statistically nonsignificant increase in ischemic events with deferred therapy with glycoprotein IIb/IIIa inhibitors compared with upstream administration, but was associated with a reduction in major bleeding. Current ACC/AHA guidelines support a more selective use rather than the routine use of glycoprotein IIb/IIIa inhibitors as triple therapy in patients with NSTE-ACS.

Cangrelor

Cangrelor is an intravenous agent that selectively and reversibly inhibits the platelet P2Y$_{12}$ receptor. It is a nonthienopyridine with a rapid onset and offset of action. Its plasma half-life is 3 to 6 minutes and the platelet function normalizes within 30 to 60 minutes of infusion discontinuation.[37] As of the time of publication of this article, Cangrelor has not been approved by the FDA.

Cangrelor was studied in 2 large trials with PCI, but did not show superiority compared with clopidogrel or placebo.[38,39] A subsequent pooled-data analysis from these trials, which applied the third universal definition of MI[5] to adjudicate events, showed that cangrelor significantly reduced death, MI, or ischemia-driven revascularization (including stent thrombosis) compared with clopidogrel.[40] The CHAMPION-PHOENIX (Clinical Trial Comparing Cangrelor to Clopidogrel Standard of Care Therapy in Subjects Who Require Percutaneous Coronary Intervention) trial randomized 11,145 patients undergoing urgent or elective PCI to cangrelor versus clopidogrel.[41] Cangrelor was associated

with a 22% statistically significant reduction in the primary efficacy end point (48-hour composite of death, MI, ischemia-driven revascularization, or stent thrombosis), a 38% reduction in stent thrombosis, and a similar primary safety end point to clopidogrel.[41] Substituting the use of oral P2Y$_{12}$ inhibitors with cangrelor in patients with NSTE-ACS who are likely to undergo CABG may be a useful strategy once it becomes FDA approved, but this requires further assessment in clinical trials.

ANTICOAGULANT THERAPY
Unfractionated Heparin

Unfractionated heparin (UFH) potentiates the action of the circulating antithrombin (which inactivates factors IIa, IXa and Xa) and thus prevents thrombus propagation. Meta-analyses investigating the use of UFH in patients with UA/NSTEMI showed a 33% to 56% reduction in early ischemic events with the use of UFH.[42,43] The duration of UFH therapy in most of these trials was 2 to 5 days. Current ACC/AHA guidelines recommend a heparin infusion for at least 48 hours. A weight-adjusted dosing regimen using a standardized nomogram provides more predictable anticoagulation than a fixed-dose regimen.[44]

Enoxaparin

Enoxaparin is a low-molecular-weight heparin (LMWH) with more selective factor Xa inhibition than UFH. Its advantages compared with UFH include its longer half-life, subcutaneous dosing, lack of need for laboratory monitoring, decreased incidence of heparin-associated thrombocytopenia, and decreased binding to plasma protein leading to a more predictable and sustained anticoagulation. Multiple trials comparing LMWH and UFH in patients with NSTE-ACS have shown similar or reduced rates of death or nonfatal MI with the use of LMWH, predominantly driven by a reduction in nonfatal MI.[45–47] The use of enoxaparin is associated with more minor, but not major, bleeding. A post hoc analysis from the SYNERGY (Superior Yield of the New Strategy of Enoxaparin, Revascularization and Glycoprotein IIb/IIIa Inhibitors) trial suggested that this excess bleeding was caused by a crossover to UFH at the time of PCI in patients receiving enoxaparin.[48] Thus the current ACC/AHA guidelines recommend maintaining a consistent anticoagulation agent from the time of presentation to PCI.

Fondaparinux

Fondaparinux is a synthetic pentasaccharide that selectively inhibits factor Xa, and thus inhibits thrombin generation and clot formation and reduces CV risk.[49] It is administered subcutaneously once daily and does not need monitoring. The OASIS-5 (Optimal Antiplatelet Strategy for Interventions) trial evaluated 20,078 patients with ACS randomized to enoxaparin versus fondaparinux, and showed the noninferiority of fondaparinux with respect to the primary composite of death, MI, or recurrent ischemia at 9 days, a trend toward superiority at 30 and 180 days, and lesser bleeding complications.[50] The current ACC/AHA guidelines recommended fondaparinux as the preferred antithrombotic agent in patients with conservatively treated NSTE-ACS who are at a higher bleeding risk. Overall, fondaparinux is recommended in all patients with NSTE-ACS, whether treated invasively or with initial conservative strategy. Fondaparinux should always be complemented in the catheterization laboratory with an anticoagulant with anti–factor IIa activity to avoid catheter-associated thrombosis.

Bivalirudin

Bivalirudin is a short-acting direct thrombin inhibitor that has predictable linear pharmacokinetics with a half-life of 25 minutes.[51] The ACUITY trial was a large-scale (13,819 patients), prospective, multicenter trial in moderate-risk to high-risk patients with ACS that compared bivalirudin to a combination of heparin plus glycoprotein IIb/IIIa inhibitors.[52] It showed the noninferiority of bivalirudin with respect to the ischemic end point as well as significantly reduced major bleeding events with bivalirudin.[52] Because of the comparable efficacy on ischemic outcomes and less bleeding with bivalirudin, it is increasingly being used in patients with NSTE-ACS. Current ACC/AHA guidelines give bivalirudin a class I recommendation for use in patients with NSTE-ACS undergoing initial invasive management with PCI. There is a paucity of data supporting its use in medically managed patients.

Novel Oral Anticoagulants

Long-term anticoagulation with oral factor Xa inhibitors provides an opportunity to further decrease ischemic events after hospital discharge. The challenge is to accomplish this on the background of concomitant DAPT without increasing bleeding hazards. Novel oral anticoagulants provide several practical benefits compared with warfarin, including a more stable pharmacokinetic profile, lack of significant food-drug and drug-drug interactions, and the lack of need for routine monitoring (**Table 2**). Rivaroxaban and apixaban have been evaluated in clinical trials in patients with NSTE-ACS (**Table 3**), but as yet

have not been approved for this indication. Dabigatran, a direct thrombin inhibitor, was also evaluated for reducing ischemic outcomes in patients on DAPT and resulted in a dose-dependent increase in bleeding with no improvement in CV events (the study was not powered for this outcome).[53] Dabigatran is currently not approved by the FDA for the treatment of patients with NSTE-ACS.

ANTI-ISCHEMIC THERAPY
β-Blockers

The routine use of intravenous β-blockers in patients with NSTE-ACS is no longer recommended because of a modest reduction in reinfarction and ventricular fibrillation that was counterbalanced by an increase in cardiogenic shock observed in the large-scale COMMIT (Clopidogrel and Metoprolol in Myocardial Infarction Trial) study.[54] β-Blockers should be initiated orally, within 24-hours, in the absence of contraindications to their use (eg, hypotension, bradycardia, heart failure).

Inhibitors of the Renin-Angiotensin-Aldosterone System

Angiotensin-converting enzyme inhibitors (ACE-Is) have been shown to reduce mortality in patients with acute MI, particularly among those with left ventricular (LV) systolic dysfunction and diabetes mellitus [55–57]. Patients intolerant to ACE-Is may benefit from angiotensin receptor blockers.[58] The use of aldosterone receptor antagonists in patients with MI and LV dysfunction or diabetes has also been associated with improved mortality and morbidity.[59]

Calcium Channel Blockers

Calcium channel blockers may be used to control ischemic symptoms in patients unresponsive to or intolerant of nitrates and β-blockers, and in patients with variant angina. Rapid-release short-acting dihydropyridines should be avoided because of their rapid hypotensive effects.[60] Verapamil or diltiazem should be avoided in patients with heart failure and/or LV systolic dysfunction.[61,62]

Nitrates

Nitrates increase myocardial blood flow through coronary vasodilation, redistribute coronary blood flow to ischemic regions, and reduce myocardial oxygen demand. Intravenous nitroglycerin is particularly useful when the NSTE-ACS event is complicated by heart failure, pulmonary edema,

Table 2
Novel anticoagulants

Drug	Route	Dose	Route of Elimination	Half-life (h)	Indications	Contraindications	Comments
Rivaroxaban	Oral	2.5–5 mg PO BID (based on ATLAS-ACS 2 TIMI 51)	Renal	4–11	Not approved by FDA for NSTEMI/UA; Approved for venous thromboembolism, stroke in nonvalvular AF	Renal impairment (Cr Cl<30), caution with hepatic impairment	No HIT, no laboratory follow-up
Apixaban	Oral	5–10 mg per day (based on APPRAISE-2 trial)	Renal/liver	10–14	Not approved by FDA for NSTEMI/UA; Approved for stroke in nonvalvular AF	Not yet reported	No HIT, no laboratory follow-up
Dabigatran	Oral	50–150 mg BID (based on RE-DEEM trial)	Renal	12–17	Not yet approved by FDA for NSTEMI/UA; Approved for venous thromboembolism, stroke in nonvalvular AF	Severe renal impairment (Cr Cl<30)	No HIT, no laboratory follow-up

Abbreviations: AF, atrial fibrillation; APPRAISE, Apixaban for Prevention of Acute Ischemic Events trial; ATLAS-ACS 2 TIMI, Anti-Xa Therapy to Lower Cardiovascular Events in Addition to Standard Therapy in Subjects with Acute Coronary Syndrome 2–Thrombolysis in Myocardial Infarction 51 (ATLAS-ACS TIMI 51); Cr Cl, creatinine clearance; HIT, heparin-induced thrombocytopenia; RE-DEEM, Dabigatran vs Placebo in Patients with Acute Coronary Syndromes on Dual Antiplatelet Therapy.

Data from Mega JL, Braunwald E, Wiviott SD, et al. Rivaroxaban in patients with a recent acute coronary syndrome. N Engl J Med 2012;366(1):9–19; and Alexander JH, Lopes RD, James S, et al. Apixaban with antiplatelet therapy after acute coronary syndrome. N Engl J Med 2011;365(8):699–708.

Table 3
Clinical trials of the new oral anticoagulants in patients with ACS

Clinical Trial	Number of Patients	Study Type	Patient Groups	Outcomes	Results
ATLAS-ACS TIMI 46[80]	3491	Double blind, randomized, dose escalation	Rivaroxaban (5–20 mg PO QD or BID) vs placebo	Clinically significant bleeding: death MI, stroke, or recurrent ischemia requiring revascularization	Rivaroxaban ↑ bleeding (dose dependent). No effect on death, MI, or recurrent ischemia
ATLAS ACS2 TIMI 51[78]	15,526	Double blind, randomized	Rivaroxaban (2.5–5 mg PO BID) vs placebo	Death from CV causes, MI, or stroke	Rivaroxaban ↓ death from CV causes, MI, or stroke ($P = .008$). Rivaroxaban 2.5 mg ↓ death from CV causes and all-cause mortality. Rivaroxaban ↑ major bleeding and ICH (dose dependent)
APPRAISE[81]	1715	Double blind, randomized, dose escalation	Apixaban (2.5–20 mg PO QD or BID) vs placebo	Major or nonmajor bleeding	Apixaban ↑ major or nonmajor bleeding, $P = .005$). Trend toward ↓ in death, MI, ischemic stroke, and recurrent ischemia
APPRAISE-2[79]	7392	Double blind, randomized	Apixaban (5.0 mg PO BID) vs placebo	CV death, MI, or stroke: major bleeding	Apixaban ↑ major bleeding ($P = .001$); no effect on CV death, MI, or stroke
RE-DEEM[53]	1861	Double blind, randomized, dose escalation	Dabigatran (50–150 mg PO BID) vs placebo	Major or minor bleeding	Dabigatran ↑ major or minor bleeding (dose dependent)

Abbreviations: ATLAS-ACS TIMI 46, Rivaroxaban versus placebo in patients with acute coronary syndromes–Thrombolysis in Myocardial Infarction 46 Trial; ATLAS-ACS 2 TIMI 51, Comparison of the Efficacy and Safety of 2 Rivaroxaban Doses in Acute Coronary Syndrome trial; ICH, intracranial hemorrhage.
Data from Refs.[53,78–81]

and hypertension. Relief of symptoms, but no survival benefit, is achieved with nitrates.

Ranolazine

Ranolazine is a novel antianginal drug that is FDA approved for use in patients with chronic stable angina. Ranolazine affects the late sodium current inhibitor channels and diminishes calcium cellular overload without a clinically significant effect on heart rate or blood pressure. The MERLIN-TIMI 36 (Metabolic Efficiency With Ranolazine for Less Ischemia in Non–ST-Elevation Acute Coronary Syndromes–TIMI 36) trial investigated its use in 6560 patients with NSTE-ACS and showed a trend toward reduction in the primary end point (composite of CV death, MI, or recurrent ischemia).[63] Ranolazine was associated with a significantly lower incidence of recurrent ischemia and clinically significant arrhythmias, but no differences in cardiac death, MI, or sudden cardiac death.[63] Although it may be of benefit, ranolazine is not yet approved by the FDA and is not recommended by the ACC/AHA guidelines for the treatment of patients with NSTE-ACS.

LIPID-LOWERING THERAPY

The 2013 ACC/AHA Guideline on the Treatment of Blood Cholesterol recommended treatment with a high-dose statin (atorvastatin 40–80 mg or rosuvastatin 20–40 mg once daily) in all patients with clinical atherosclerotic CV disease (including NSTE-ACS).[64] Among patients aged 75 years or older and in those who are intolerant to high-dose statins or have drug-drug interactions, a moderate-dose statin should be used.[64] All patients with NSTEMI-ACS should have a statin prescribed at hospital discharge, which is a clinical performance measure for all patients with acute MI.[65]

EARLY INVASIVE STRATEGY VERSUS INITIAL CONSERVATIVE APPROACH

Two treatment strategies are always entertained in initially stabilized patients with NSTE-ACS. An early invasive strategy entails diagnostic coronary angiography and revascularization, preferably within 24 hours of presentation, as the first treatment strategy in initially stabilized patients with NSTE-ACS (see **Fig. 2**). Patients with ongoing ischemia, hemodynamic instability, or arrhythmias should be taken as soon as possible to the cardiac catheterization laboratory for coronary angiography and revascularization. The early invasive approach helps identify patients with left main or triple vessel coronary artery disease who derive survival benefit from revascularization with CABG. In addition, it helps reduce recurrent MI, subsequent hospitalizations, and the need for antianginal medication in patients undergoing revascularization with PCI. As an alternative, an initial conservative approach entails medical optimization with recourse to angiography only in the setting of failure of medical therapy or objective evidence of recurrent or latent ischemia (ie, selectively invasive approach). Patients being treated with an initial conservative approach benefit from an early echocardiogram to evaluate LV function, and should undergo risk stratification with a stress test (preferably pharmacologically induced and with an imaging modality) before or shortly after discharge to identify patients who would benefit from revascularization.

A contemporary meta-analysis comparing early invasive versus initial conservative strategies in a total of 8375 patients showed a 25% significant improvement in 2-year all-cause mortality with early invasive strategy, as well as reduction in nonfatal MI and hospitalization.[66] In contrast, the Invasive versus Conservative Treatment in Unstable coronary Syndromes (ICTUS) trial showed no difference in the composite ischemic end point at 3 years in 1200 patients with NSTE-ACS and suggested that an initially conservative strategy may be considered as a reasonable treatment.[67] The current ACC/AHA guideline delineated general principles for favoring an early invasive strategy or initial conservative strategy in different patient groups (**Box 2**).[20]

TIMING OF INVASIVE THERAPY

The timing of coronary angiography in patients being treated with an early invasive strategy was evaluated by the ISAR-COOL (Intracoronary Stenting with Antithrombotic Regimen Cooling Off),[68] TIMACS (Timing of Interventions in Patients with Acute Coronary Syndromes),[69] and the ABOARD (Angioplasty to Blunt the Rise of Troponin in Acute Coronary Syndromes Randomized for an Immediate or Delayed Intervention)[70] clinical trials. The pivotal TIMACS trial, randomized moderate-risk to high-risk patients with NSTE-ACS presenting within 24 hours of ischemic symptoms to routine early angiography/intervention within 24 hours (median time, 14 hours) versus delayed angiography/intervention after at least 36 hours of randomization (median time, 50 hours). Early intervention did not differ greatly from delayed intervention in preventing the primary composite outcome of death, MI, or stroke at 6 months.[69] However, early intervention reduced the rate of the composite secondary outcome of death, MI, or refractory ischemia (9.5% vs 12.9%; HR, 0.72;

Box 2
Selection of initial treatment strategy: invasive versus conservative strategy

Early invasive strategy

    Recurrent angina or ischemia at rest or with low-level activities despite intensive medical therapy

    Increased cardiac biomarkers (TnT or TnI)

    New or presumably new ST segment depression

    Signs or symptoms of HF or new or worsening mitral regurgitation

    High-risk findings from noninvasive testing

    Hemodynamic instability

    Sustained ventricular tachycardia

    PCI within 6 months

    Prior CABG

    High-risk score (eg, TIMI, GRACE)

    Mild to moderate renal dysfunction

    Diabetes mellitus

    Reduced LV function (LVEF $\leq$ 40%)

Initial Conservative Strategy

    Low-risk score (eg, TIMI, GRACE)

    Patient or physician preference in the absence of high-risk features

Abbreviations: HF, heart failure; LVEF, LV ejection fraction; TnI, troponin I; TnT, troponin T.

Adapted from Jneid H, Anderson JL, Wright RS, et al. 2012 ACCF/AHA focused update of the guideline for the management of patients with unstable angina/non-ST-elevation myocardial infarction (updating the 2007 guideline and replacing the 2011 focused update): a report of the American College of Cardiology Foundation/American Heart Association Task Force on Practice Guidelines. J Am Coll Cardiol 2012;60(7):645–81; with permission.

95% CI, 0.58 to 0.89; $P = .003$), and was particularly superior to delayed intervention in the high-risk patients with GRACE score greater than or equal to 140.[69] There was no benefit from immediate therapy with angiography and revascularization in patients with NSTE-ACS,[70] akin to their STEMI counterparts. The aforementioned trials formed the basis for the current ACC/AHA guideline recommendation of early invasive therapy (angiography and intervention within 12–24 hours of presentation) as a reasonable and preferred strategy rather than a more delayed invasive approach in initially stabilized patients with NSTE-ACS.

ADDITIONAL CONSIDERATIONS AND PATIENT SUBGROUPS
Diabetes Mellitus

The 2012 ACC/AHA guideline for NSTE-ACS recommended that the treatment and decisions on whether to perform stress testing, angiography, and revascularization should be similar in patients with and without diabetes mellitus.[20] Based on the results of the NICE-SUGAR (Normoglycemia in Intensive Care Evaluation and Surviving Using Glucose Algorithm Regulation) trial, it is currently recommended to keep the blood glucose less than 180 mg/dL while avoiding hypoglycemia in patients with UA/NSTEMI.[71] In addition, in patients with multivessel disease, CABG with use of the internal mammary arteries is currently preferred rather than PCI in patients with diabetes mellitus.[72]

Chronic Kidney Disease

The SWEDEHEART (Swedish Web-System for Enhancement and Development of Evidence-Based Care in Heart Disease Evaluated According to Recommended Therapies) study, a large national registry of 23,262 patients hospitalized with NSTEMI, evaluated whether early revascularization within 14 days of admission for NSTEMI improved outcomes at all stages of kidney function.[73] SWEDEHEART showed a survival benefit from early revascularization at 1-year in patients with NSTEMI with mild to moderate (stages 1 and 2) chronic kidney disease (CKD), but no clear benefit in patients with stages 4 and 5 (small numbers and underpowered analyses). In a subsequent meta-analysis in patients with NSTE-ACS, including SWEDEHEART, Huang and colleagues[74] showed reduced mortality with early revascularization in appropriately selected patients with CKD. In the aforementioned meta-analysis, the mortality reduction with early revascularization occurred in advance, was evident across all CKD stages (including patients with severe CKD and dialysis), and was independent of the influence of any single study (including SWEDEHEART).[74]

Creatinine clearance should be estimated in patients with NSTE-ACS, and the doses of renally cleared medications should be adjusted according to the pharmacokinetic data for specific medications.[75] Patients undergoing coronary angiography should receive intravenous hydration and minimal doses of contrast media should be used.[14]

SUMMARY

UA and NSTEMI represent around 70% of all ACS events. Despite advances in primary prevention, the incidence of NSTE-ACS has remained stable over the past decade, driven particularly by the aging population, the increase in certain CV risk factors, and the widespread adoption of the highly sensitive and specific biomarkers of necrosis, cardiac troponins. Newer antiplatelet therapies have evolved, including the more potent and faster acting $P2Y_{12}$ receptor inhibitors, prasugrel and ticagrelor, which showed superior efficacy compared with clopidogrel. The direct thrombin inhibitor bivalirudin is associated with less bleeding and better safety profile compared with older anticoagulants. Early invasive strategy within 12 to 24 hours is a reasonable treatment strategy in all NSTE-ACS, especially in the highest-risk patients. Early revascularization after NSTE-ACS is beneficial in patients with diabetes mellitus, in those with moderate CKD, and possibly in selected patients with even more advanced CKD. A statin of high to moderate intensity should be administered to all patients with NSTE-ACS by hospital discharge without using the low-density lipoprotein–cholesterol as a target goal.

REFERENCES

1. Peterson ED, Shah BR, Parsons L, et al. Trends in quality of care for patients with acute myocardial infarction in the National Registry of Myocardial Infarction from 1990 to 2006. Am Heart J 2008; 156(6):1045–55.

2. McManus DD, Gore J, Yarzebski J, et al. Recent trends in the incidence, treatment, and outcomes of patients with STEMI and NSTEMI. Am J Med 2011;124(1):40–7.

3. Yeh RW, Sidney S, Chandra M, et al. Population trends in the incidence and outcomes of acute myocardial infarction. N Engl J Med 2010; 362(23):2155–65.

4. Anderson JL, Adams CD, Antman EM, et al. 2012 ACCF/AHA focused update incorporated into the ACCF/AHA 2007 guidelines for the management of patients with unstable angina/non-ST-elevation myocardial infarction: a report of the American College of Cardiology Foundation/American Heart Association Task Force on Practice Guidelines. Circulation 2013;127(23):e663–828.

5. Thygesen K, Alpert JS, Jaffe AS, et al. Third universal definition of myocardial infarction. Circulation 2012;126(16):2020–35.

6. Pollack CV Jr, Sites FD, Shofer FS, et al. Application of the TIMI risk score for unstable angina and non-ST elevation acute coronary syndrome to an unselected emergency department chest pain population. Acad Emerg Med 2006;13(1):13–8.

7. Granger CB, Goldberg RJ, Dabbous O, et al. Predictors of hospital mortality in the global registry of acute coronary events. Arch Intern Med 2003; 163(19):2345–53.

8. Boersma E, Pieper KS, Steyerberg EW, et al. Predictors of outcome in patients with acute coronary syndromes without persistent ST-segment elevation. Results from an international trial of 9461 patients. The PURSUIT Investigators. Circulation 2000;101(22):2557–67.

9. Lewis HD Jr, Davis JW, Archibald DG, et al. Protective effects of aspirin against acute myocardial infarction and death in men with unstable angina. Results of a Veterans Administration Cooperative Study. N Engl J Med 1983;309(7):396–403.

10. Risk of myocardial infarction and death during treatment with low dose aspirin and intravenous heparin in men with unstable coronary artery disease. The RISC Group. Lancet 1990;336(8719): 827–30.

11. Theroux P, Ouimet H, McCans J, et al. Aspirin, heparin, or both to treat acute unstable angina. N Engl J Med 1988;319(17):1105–11.

12. Antithrombotic Trialists Collaboration. Collaborative meta-analysis of randomised trials of antiplatelet therapy for prevention of death, myocardial infarction, and stroke in high risk patients. BMJ 2002; 324(7329):71–86.

13. Jneid H, Bhatt DL. Advances in antiplatelet therapy. Expert Opin Emerg Drugs 2003;8(2):349–63.

14. Writing Committee M, Jneid H, Anderson JL, et al. 2012 ACCF/AHA focused update of the guideline for the management of patients with unstable angina/non-ST-elevation myocardial infarction (updating the 2007 guideline and replacing the 2011 focused update): a report of the American College of Cardiology Foundation/American Heart

Association Task Force on Practice Guidelines. Circulation 2012;126(7):875–910.

15. Yusuf S, Zhao F, Mehta SR, et al. Effects of clopidogrel in addition to aspirin in patients with acute coronary syndromes without ST-segment elevation. N Engl J Med 2001;345(7):494–502.

16. Jneid H, Bhatt DL, Corti R, et al. Aspirin and clopidogrel in acute coronary syndromes: therapeutic insights from the CURE study. Arch Intern Med 2003;163(10):1145–53.

17. Holmes DR Jr, Dehmer GJ, Kaul S, et al. ACCF/AHA clopidogrel clinical alert: approaches to the FDA "boxed warning": a report of the American College of Cardiology Foundation Task Force on Clinical Expert Consensus Documents and the American Heart Association endorsed by the Society for Cardiovascular Angiography and Interventions and the Society of Thoracic Surgeons. J Am Coll Cardiol 2010;56(4):321–41.

18. Guidotti TL. Preventive medicine, public health, and the environmental movement. Am J Prev Med 1991;7(2):124–5.

19. Giusti B, Gori AM, Marcucci R, et al. Relation of cytochrome P450 2C19 loss-of-function polymorphism to occurrence of drug-eluting coronary stent thrombosis. Am J Cardiol 2009;103(6):806–11.

20. Jneid H, Anderson JL, Wright RS, et al. 2012 ACCF/AHA focused update of the guideline for the management of patients with unstable angina/non-ST-elevation myocardial infarction (updating the 2007 guideline and replacing the 2011 focused update): a report of the American College of Cardiology Foundation/American Heart Association Task Force on Practice Guidelines. J Am Coll Cardiol 2012;60(7):645–81.

21. Ho PM, Maddox TM, Wang L, et al. Risk of adverse outcomes associated with concomitant use of clopidogrel and proton pump inhibitors following acute coronary syndrome. JAMA 2009;301(9):937–44.

22. O'Donoghue ML, Braunwald E, Antman EM, et al. Pharmacodynamic effect and clinical efficacy of clopidogrel and prasugrel with or without a proton-pump inhibitor: an analysis of two randomised trials. Lancet 2009;374(9694):989–97.

23. Bhatt DL, Cryer BL, Contant CF, et al. Clopidogrel with or without omeprazole in coronary artery disease. N Engl J Med 2010;363(20):1909–17.

24. Abraham NS, Hlatky MA, Antman EM, et al. ACCF/ACG/AHA 2010 expert consensus document on the concomitant use of proton pump inhibitors and thienopyridines: a focused update of the ACCF/ACG/AHA 2008 expert consensus document on reducing the gastrointestinal risks of antiplatelet therapy and NSAID use: a report of the American College of Cardiology Foundation Task Force on Expert Consensus Documents. Circulation 2010;122(24):2619–33.

25. Mega JL, Close SL, Wiviott SD, et al. Cytochrome P450 genetic polymorphisms and the response to prasugrel: relationship to pharmacokinetic, pharmacodynamic, and clinical outcomes. Circulation 2009;119(19):2553–60.

26. Wiviott SD, Braunwald E, McCabe CH, et al. Prasugrel versus clopidogrel in patients with acute coronary syndromes. N Engl J Med 2007;357(20):2001–15.

27. Wiviott SD, Braunwald E, Angiolillo DJ, et al. Greater clinical benefit of more intensive oral antiplatelet therapy with prasugrel in patients with diabetes mellitus in the trial to assess improvement in therapeutic outcomes by optimizing platelet inhibition with prasugrel-Thrombolysis in Myocardial Infarction 38. Circulation 2008;118(16):1626–36.

28. Roe MT, Armstrong PW, Fox KA, et al. Prasugrel versus clopidogrel for acute coronary syndromes without revascularization. N Engl J Med 2012;367(14):1297–309.

29. Husted S, Emanuelsson H, Heptinstall S, et al. Pharmacodynamics, pharmacokinetics, and safety of the oral reversible P2Y12 antagonist AZD6140 with aspirin in patients with atherosclerosis: a double-blind comparison to clopidogrel with aspirin. Eur Heart J 2006;27(9):1038–47.

30. Wallentin L, Becker RC, Budaj A, et al. Ticagrelor versus clopidogrel in patients with acute coronary syndromes. N Engl J Med 2009;361(11):1045–57.

31. Mahaffey KW, Wojdyla DM, Carroll K, et al. Ticagrelor compared with clopidogrel by geographic region in the Platelet Inhibition and Patient Outcomes (PLATO) trial. Circulation 2011;124(5):544–54.

32. Boersma E, Harrington RA, Moliterno DJ, et al. Platelet glycoprotein IIb/IIIa inhibitors in acute coronary syndromes: a meta-analysis of all major randomised clinical trials. Lancet 2002;359(9302):189–98.

33. Hamm CW, Heeschen C, Goldmann B, et al. Benefit of abciximab in patients with refractory unstable angina in relation to serum troponin T levels. c7E3 Fab Antiplatelet Therapy in Unstable Refractory Angina (CAPTURE) Study Investigators. N Engl J Med 1999;340(21):1623–9.

34. Roffi M, Chew DP, Mukherjee D, et al. Platelet glycoprotein IIb/IIIa inhibitors reduce mortality in diabetic patients with non-ST-segment-elevation acute coronary syndromes. Circulation 2001;104(23):2767–71.

35. Giugliano RP, White JA, Bode C, et al. Early versus delayed, provisional eptifibatide in acute coronary syndromes. N Engl J Med 2009;360(21):2176–90.

36. Stone GW, Bertrand ME, Moses JW, et al. Routine upstream initiation vs deferred selective use of glycoprotein IIb/IIIa inhibitors in acute coronary

syndromes: the ACUITY Timing trial. JAMA 2007; 297(6):591–602.

37. Storey RF, Wilcox RG, Heptinstall S. Comparison of the pharmacodynamic effects of the platelet ADP receptor antagonists clopidogrel and AR-C69931MX in patients with ischaemic heart disease. Platelets 2002;13(7):407–13.

38. Bhatt DL, Lincoff AM, Gibson CM, et al. Intravenous platelet blockade with cangrelor during PCI. N Engl J Med 2009;361(24):2330–41.

39. Harrington RA, Stone GW, McNulty S, et al. Platelet inhibition with cangrelor in patients undergoing PCI. N Engl J Med 2009;361(24):2318–29.

40. White HD, Chew DP, Dauerman HL, et al. Reduced immediate ischemic events with cangrelor in PCI: a pooled analysis of the CHAMPION trials using the universal definition of myocardial infarction. Am Heart J 2012;163(2):182–90.e4.

41. Bhatt DL, Stone GW, Mahaffey KW, et al. Effect of platelet inhibition with cangrelor during PCI on ischemic events. N Engl J Med 2013;368(14):1303–13.

42. Cohen M, Adams PC, Parry G, et al. Combination antithrombotic therapy in unstable rest angina and non-Q-wave infarction in nonprior aspirin users. Primary end points analysis from the ATACS trial. Antithrombotic Therapy in Acute Coronary Syndromes Research Group. Circulation 1994; 89(1):81–8.

43. Oler A, Whooley MA, Oler J, et al. Adding heparin to aspirin reduces the incidence of myocardial infarction and death in patients with unstable angina. A meta-analysis. JAMA 1996;276(10):811–5.

44. Becker RC, Ball SP, Eisenberg P, et al. A randomized, multicenter trial of weight-adjusted intravenous heparin dose titration and point-of-care coagulation monitoring in hospitalized patients with active thromboembolic disease. Antithrombotic Therapy Consortium Investigators. Am Heart J 1999;137(1):59–71.

45. Low-molecular-weight heparin during instability in coronary artery disease, Fragmin during Instability in Coronary Artery Disease (FRISC) study group. Lancet 1996;347(9001):561–8.

46. Cohen M, Theroux P, Borzak S, et al. Randomized double-blind safety study of enoxaparin versus unfractionated heparin in patients with non-ST-segment elevation acute coronary syndromes treated with tirofiban and aspirin: the ACUTE II study. The Antithrombotic Combination Using Tirofiban and Enoxaparin. Am Heart J 2002;144(3):470–7.

47. Blazing MA, de Lemos JA, White HD, et al. Safety and efficacy of enoxaparin vs unfractionated heparin in patients with non-ST-segment elevation acute coronary syndromes who receive tirofiban and aspirin: a randomized controlled trial. JAMA 2004; 292(1):55–64.

48. Ferguson JJ, Califf RM, Antman EM, et al. Enoxaparin vs unfractionated heparin in high-risk patients with non-ST-segment elevation acute coronary syndromes managed with an intended early invasive strategy: primary results of the SYNERGY randomized trial. JAMA 2004;292(1):45–54.

49. Alban S. From heparins to factor Xa inhibitors and beyond. Eur J Clin Invest 2005;35(Suppl 1): 12–20.

50. Fifth Organization to Assess Strategies in Acute Ischemic Syndromes Investigators, Yusuf S, Mehta SR, Chrolavicius S, et al. Comparison of fondaparinux and enoxaparin in acute coronary syndromes. N Engl J Med 2006;354(14):1464–76.

51. Eikelboom J, White H, Yusuf S. The evolving role of direct thrombin inhibitors in acute coronary syndromes. J Am Coll Cardiol 2003;41(4 Suppl S): 70S–8S.

52. Stone GW, McLaurin BT, Cox DA, et al. Bivalirudin for patients with acute coronary syndromes. N Engl J Med 2006;355(21):2203–16.

53. Oldgren J, Budaj A, Granger CB, et al. Dabigatran vs. placebo in patients with acute coronary syndromes on dual antiplatelet therapy: a randomized, double-blind, phase II trial. Eur Heart J 2011; 32(22):2781–9.

54. Chen ZM, Pan HC, Chen YP, et al. Early intravenous then oral metoprolol in 45,852 patients with acute myocardial infarction: randomised placebo-controlled trial. Lancet 2005;366(9497):1622–32.

55. Indications for ACE inhibitors in the early treatment of acute myocardial infarction: systematic overview of individual data from 100,000 patients in randomized trials. ACE Inhibitor Myocardial Infarction Collaborative Group. Circulation 1998;97(22): 2202–12.

56. Gustafsson I, Torp-Pedersen C, Kober L, et al. Effect of the angiotensin-converting enzyme inhibitor trandolapril on mortality and morbidity in diabetic patients with left ventricular dysfunction after acute myocardial infarction. Trace Study Group. J Am Coll Cardiol 1999;34(1):83–9.

57. Jneid H, Moukarbel GV, Dawson B, et al. Combining neuroendocrine inhibitors in heart failure: reflections on safety and efficacy. Am J Med 2007;120(12):1090.e1–8.

58. Pfeffer MA, McMurray JJ, Velazquez EJ, et al. Valsartan, captopril, or both in myocardial infarction complicated by heart failure, left ventricular dysfunction, or both. N Engl J Med 2003;349(20): 1893–906.

59. Pitt B, Remme W, Zannad F, et al. Eplerenone, a selective aldosterone blocker, in patients with left ventricular dysfunction after myocardial infarction. N Engl J Med 2003;348(14):1309–21.

60. Furberg CD, Psaty BM, Meyer JV. Nifedipine. Dose-related increase in mortality in patients with

coronary heart disease. Circulation 1995;92(5): 1326–31.

61. Gibson RS, Boden WE, Theroux P, et al. Diltiazem and reinfarction in patients with non-Q-wave myocardial infarction. Results of a double-blind, randomized, multicenter trial. N Engl J Med 1986; 315(7):423–9.

62. Hansen JF, Hagerup L, Sigurd B, et al. Treatment with verapamil and trandolapril in patients with congestive heart failure and angina pectoris or myocardial infarction. The DAVIT Study Group. Danish Verapamil Infarction Trial. Am Heart J 1997;134(2 Pt 2):S48–52.

63. Morrow DA, Scirica BM, Karwatowska-Prokopczuk E, et al. Effects of ranolazine on recurrent cardiovascular events in patients with non-ST-elevation acute coronary syndromes: the MERLIN-TIMI 36 randomized trial. JAMA 2007; 297(16):1775–83.

64. Stone NJ, Robinson J, Lichtenstein AH, et al. 2013 ACC/AHA guideline on the treatment of blood cholesterol to reduce atherosclerotic cardiovascular risk in adults: a report of the American College of Cardiology/American Heart Association Task Force on Practice Guidelines. Circulation 2013. [Epub ahead of print].

65. Krumholz HM, Anderson JL, Bachelder BL, et al. ACC/AHA 2008 performance measures for adults with ST-elevation and non-ST-elevation myocardial infarction: a report of the American College of Cardiology/American Heart Association Task Force on Performance Measures (writing committee to develop performance measures for ST-elevation and non-ST-elevation myocardial infarction): developed in collaboration with the American Academy of Family Physicians and the American College of Emergency Physicians: endorsed by the American Association of Cardiovascular and Pulmonary Rehabilitation, Society for Cardiovascular Angiography and Interventions, and Society of Hospital Medicine. Circulation 2008;118(24):2596–648.

66. Bavry AA, Kumbhani DJ, Rassi AN, et al. Benefit of early invasive therapy in acute coronary syndromes: a meta-analysis of contemporary randomized clinical trials. J Am Coll Cardiol 2006;48(7): 1319–25.

67. Hirsch A, Windhausen F, Tijssen JG, et al. Long-term outcome after an early invasive versus selective invasive treatment strategy in patients with non-ST-elevation acute coronary syndrome and elevated cardiac troponin T (the ICTUS trial): a follow-up study. Lancet 2007;369(9564): 827–35.

68. Neumann FJ, Kastrati A, Pogatsa-Murray G, et al. Evaluation of prolonged antithrombotic pretreatment ("cooling-off" strategy) before intervention in patients with unstable coronary syndromes: a randomized controlled trial. JAMA 2003;290(12): 1593–9.

69. Mehta SR, Granger CB, Boden WE, et al. Early versus delayed invasive intervention in acute coronary syndromes. N Engl J Med 2009;360(21): 2165–75.

70. Montalescot G, Cayla G, Collet JP, et al. Immediate vs delayed intervention for acute coronary syndromes: a randomized clinical trial. JAMA 2009; 302(9):947–54.

71. NICE-SUGAR Study Investigators, Finfer S, Chittock DR, Su SY, et al. Intensive versus conventional glucose control in critically ill patients. N Engl J Med 2009;360(13):1283–97.

72. Hlatky MA, Boothroyd DB, Bravata DM, et al. Coronary artery bypass surgery compared with percutaneous coronary interventions for multivessel disease: a collaborative analysis of individual patient data from ten randomised trials. Lancet 2009;373(9670):1190–7.

73. Szummer K, Lundman P, Jacobson SH, et al. Influence of renal function on the effects of early revascularization in non-ST-elevation myocardial infarction: data from the Swedish Web-System for Enhancement and Development of Evidence-Based Care in Heart Disease Evaluated According to Recommended Therapies (SWEDEHEART). Circulation 2009;120(10):851–8.

74. Huang HD, Alam M, Hamzeh I, et al. Patients with severe chronic kidney disease benefit from early revascularization after acute coronary syndrome. Int J Cardiol 2013;168(4):3741–6.

75. Basra SS, Tsai P, Lakkis NM. Safety and efficacy of antiplatelet and antithrombotic therapy in acute coronary syndrome patients with chronic kidney disease. J Am Coll Cardiol 2011;58(22):2263–9.

76. Steinhubl SR, Berger PB, Mann JT 3rd, et al. Early and sustained dual oral antiplatelet therapy following percutaneous coronary intervention: a randomized controlled trial. JAMA 2002;288(19): 2411–20.

77. Mehta SR, Tanguay JF, Eikelboom JW, et al. Double-dose versus standard-dose clopidogrel and high-dose versus low-dose aspirin in individuals undergoing percutaneous coronary intervention for acute coronary syndromes (CURRENT-OASIS 7): a randomised factorial trial. Lancet 2010; 376(9748):1233–43.

78. Mega JL, Braunwald E, Wiviott SD, et al. Rivaroxaban in patients with a recent acute coronary syndrome. N Engl J Med 2012;366(1):9–19.

79. Alexander JH, Lopes RD, James S, et al. Apixaban with antiplatelet therapy after acute coronary syndrome. N Engl J Med 2011;365(8):699–708.

80. Mega JL, Braunwald E, Mohanavelu S, et al. Rivaroxaban versus placebo in patients with acute coronary syndromes (ATLAS ACS-TIMI 46): a

randomised, double-blind, phase II trial. Lancet 2009;374(9683):29–38.

81. APPRAISE Steering Committee and Investigators, Alexander JH, Becker RC, Bhatt DL, et al. Apixaban, an oral, direct, selective factor Xa inhibitor, in combination with antiplatelet therapy after acute coronary syndrome: results of the Apixaban for Prevention of Acute Ischemic and Safety Events (APPRAISE) trial. Circulation 2009;119(22): 2877–85.

Current State of ST-Segment Myocardial Infarction

Evidence-based Therapies and Optimal Patient Outcomes in Advanced Systems of Care

Joseph L. Thomas, MD[a,b], William J. French, MD[a,b],*

KEYWORDS

- ST-segment myocardial infarction • Fibrinolysis • Primary percutaneous coronary intervention
- Coronary thrombectomy • Antithrombotic therapies • Antiplatelet therapies
- STEMI receiving center

KEY POINTS

- Current management of ST-segment elevation myocardial infarction (STEMI) reflects 3 decades of clinical evidence development.
- Timely reperfusion therapy with fibrinolysis or the preferred treatment of percutaneous coronary intervention is at the core of optimal STEMI care.
- Contemporary treatments and low overall mortality in STEMI represent a significant achievement in modern medicine.
- Providing STEMI care within advanced regional systems is critical to delivering optimal treatment across the population.

INTRODUCTION

Current management of ST-segment elevation myocardial infarction (STEMI) is the product of intensive research and ongoing therapeutic refinement. The cornerstone of contemporary treatment is primary reperfusion therapy, and optimal patient outcomes are based on more than 3 decades of evidence development and widespread implementation of dedicated systems of care. STEMI is a striking example of the achievements possible in collaborative health care delivery involving frontline emergency services, cardiovascular specialists, and tertiary care systems.

This article focuses on 2 critical components in STEMI: the robust clinical evidence that guides current treatment and the care delivery systems in which patients are rapidly triaged and treated. Both reflect a commitment to the individual patient and to broader population health. STEMI care is now a key deliverable for both acute care facilities and cardiologists. STEMI care brings value to interventional cardiology, and in turn, interventional cardiology brings professional value to STEMI care systems.

STEMI represents approximately one-third of all acute myocardial infarction (MI) cases in the

[a] David Geffen School of Medicine, University of California Los Angeles, Los Angeles, CA 90095, USA;
[b] Division of Cardiology, Harbor UCLA Medical Center, 1000 West Carson Street, Torrance, CA 90509, USA
* Corresponding author. Division of Cardiology, Harbor UCLA Medical Center, 1000 West Carson Street, Box 405, Torrance, CA 90509.
E-mail address: wjfrench@labiomed.org

Cardiol Clin 32 (2014) 371–385
http://dx.doi.org/10.1016/j.ccl.2014.04.002
0733-8651/14/$ – see front matter © 2014 Elsevier Inc. All rights reserved.

United States. Data from the Nationwide Inpatient Sample demonstrated a decline in STEMI discharges from 299,000 in 2002 to 168,000 in 2010.[1] During this 9-year period, treatment with percutaneous coronary intervention (PCI) increased markedly (**Fig. 1**). On a more regional basis, STEMI care has become a high-profile issue, despite documentation of similar declines in STEMI incidence within local health systems.[2]

Reperfusion strategies have evolved rapidly and primary PCI is the guideline-recommended choice over fibrinolysis.[3] There has been a greater than 3-fold increase in the use of PCI for STEMI since 2000.[1] Despite regional and interhospital variations in adoption, the use of PCI for STEMI continues to increase, and risk-adjusted in-hospital mortality for STEMI has settled at approximately 5.5%.[4,5]

Early Evidence in STEMI Reperfusion

Current reperfusion strategies are all based on iterative advances over early fibrinolytic and aspirin data. The *Second International Study of Infarct Survival* (ISIS-2) demonstrated a remarkable 25% reduction in vascular death with the use of aspirin and streptokinase. Together, the use of both agents in synergy produced a 42% reduction in vascular death.[6] The first GISSI (Gruppo Italiano per lo Studio della Streptochinasi nell'Infarto Miocardico) study demonstrated a similar 18% mortality benefit with fibrinolysis.[7] These and other landmark studies have served

as the basis for STEMI reperfusion over the ensuing 3 decades.[8] Of added importance to cardiovascular care, these investigations established both the feasibility and the value of rigorously designed mega-trials.

The move toward fibrin-specific thrombolytics was propelled by accumulating evidence that supported novel agents and modified dosing strategies. Recombinant tissue plasminogen activator (t-PA) was shown to provide a 24.5% reduction in short-term mortality versus placebo in patients with an abnormal electrocardiogram (ECG).[9] The first Global Utilization of Streptokinase and Tissue Plasminogen Activator for Occluded Coronary Arteries (GUSTO) study demonstrated the superiority of an accelerated t-PA regimen (more than 1.5 hours) plus intravenous heparin over streptokinase. Accelerated t-PA was associated with a 6.3% 30-day mortality and a 14% relative risk reduction as compared with the streptokinase regimen.[10] Subsequent studies including the Assessment of the Safety and Efficacy of a New Thrombolytic Regimen (ASSENT) series evaluated tenecteplase in MI with ST-segment elevation.[11,12] In a further evolution of fibrinolytic treatment, the utility of low-molecular-weight heparins was initially evaluated in the third ASSENT trial. Later, EXTRACT TIMI-25 definitively proved that enoxaparin in fibrinolytic-treated patients significantly reduced nonfatal MI and major bleeding in comparison to unfractionated heparin.[13,14]

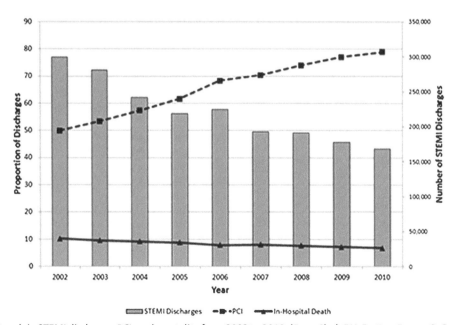

Fig. 1. Trends in STEMI discharge, PCI, and mortality from 2002 to 2010. (*From* Shah RU, Rutten-Ramos S, Garberich R, et al. STEMI trends in the United States 2002–2010: increasing use of PCI and declining mortality. Circ Cardiovasc Qual Outcomes 2013;6:A22; with permission.)

Although fibrinolysis was the first true STEMI intervention, the introduction of coronary angioplasty by Andreas Gruentzig enabled the next (and most currently relevant) evolution in STEMI treatment. In the 1980s, pioneers such as Geoff Hartzler overcame great skepticism and proved that the acutely occluded coronary artery was amenable to angioplasty.[15] The techniques and devices of the 1980s and 1990s may bear little resemblance to contemporary PCI, but the leading role of angioplasty in STEMI was clearly defined in the 1990s.

Angioplasty was directly compared with an accelerated t-PA regimen in the GUSTO IIb trial. This study was the largest early comparison of the 2 approaches. Time to treatment did not approach contemporary standards, although this reflected the era of study enrollment between 1994 and 1996. Primary angioplasty occurred nearly 2 hours after randomization, and the door-to-balloon (DTB) time was likely substantially longer. Despite long treatment intervals, angioplasty was associated with a 33% reduction in the composite endpoint of death, nonfatal MI, and disabling stroke.[16] A seminal meta-analysis by Keeley and coworkers[17] reinforced the superiority of primary angioplasty over pharmacologic reperfusion with either streptokinase or fibrin-specific agents (**Fig. 2**).

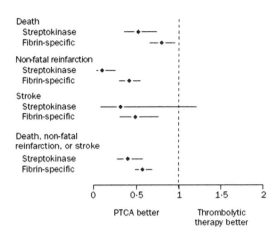

Fig. 2. Meta-analysis of fibrinolytic agents versus primary angioplasty. PTCA, percutaneous coronary transluminal angioplasty. (*From* Keeley EC, Boura JA, Grines C. Primary angioplasty versus intravenous thrombolytic therapy for acute myocardial infarction: a quantitative review of 23 randomised trials. Lancet 2003;361:17; with permission.)

23 Study Meta-Analysis	Primary Angioplasty vs Fibrinolysis (%)
Death, MI, stroke	8 vs 14
Short-term death	7 vs 9
Nonfatal MI	3 vs 7
Stroke	1 vs 2

A preference for PCI reperfusion is now supported by US guidelines when angioplasty can be performed within 90 minutes at PCI-capable hospitals or within 120 minutes of first medical contact (FMC) for patients needing transfer for PCI (**Fig. 3**).[3] An increasing preference for primary PCI is present in reports from across the world, although substantial variation exists in delivery within certain regions, hospital types, and populations.[18–20] In the National Cardiovascular Data Registry (NCDR) analysis by Fazel and colleagues,[5] variation also persists in primary PCI utilization by gender, race, time of presentation, and patient clinical characteristics (**Fig. 4**).

Coronary Stents and Contemporary Primary PCI

Following nearly 2 decades of experience with balloon angioplasty, the introduction of metallic coronary stents rapidly expanded the scope and safety of interventional procedures. Stents have almost completely obviated risks of dissection, recoil, and acute closure that were present with balloon angioplasty alone. In addition, restenosis rates after angioplasty are significantly reduced with coronary stents.

A randomized trial comparing bare-metal stents (BMS) and angioplasty did not show a significant reduction in the individual endpoints of MI or death. Reduction in major adverse events with stent implantation was entirely due to a 55% reduction in target vessel revascularization (TVR) with a number needed to treat of only 11 patients to prevent one revascularization at 6 months. Furthermore, recurrent angina was significantly reduced with stenting.[21] The benefit of stenting in primary angioplasty was reinforced in the CADILLAC (Controlled Abciximab and Device Investigation to Lower Late Angioplasty Complications) trial that evaluated the potential synergy of the glycoprotein IIb/IIIa inhibitor (GPI) abciximab with stents versus angioplasty. A similar 10% absolute reduction in TVR was demonstrated in the stent arm of this study, although the benefit of abciximab was strongest in the balloon angioplasty only arm.[22]

The introduction of drug-eluting stents (DES) 1 decade ago has resulted in widespread acceptance of DES as the stent of choice over BMS for most indications. Currently, 85% of PCI in the United States use DES. Nonetheless, significant concerns existed regarding the safety and appropriateness of DES in STEMI. First-generation DES

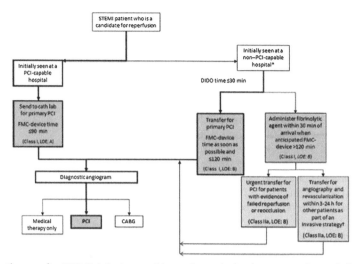

Fig. 3. Reperfusion therapy for STEMI. * Patients with cardiogenic shock or severe heart failure seen initially at a non-PCI capable hospital should be transferred as soon as possible for cardiac catheterization and revascularization. † Angiography and revascularization should not be performed within the first 2 to 3 hours after administration of thrombolytic agents. (*From* O'Gara PT, Kushner FG, Ascheim DD, et al. 2013 ACCF/AHA guideline for the management of ST-elevation myocardial infarction. A report of the American College of Cardiology Foundation/American Heart Association task force on practice guidelines. Circulation 2013;127:e362–425; with permission.)

were evaluated in a series of studies that were primarily powered to evaluate restenosis and not necessarily individual clinical endpoints. Randomized study of sirolimus and paclitaxel stents supported the anti-restenotic effect of DES but did not fully clarify the role of DES in STEMI.[23–25]

Coincident with concerns about DES safety and stent thrombosis (ST), registry data suggested harm with DES in STEMI.[26] These concerns have now been largely dismissed. The HORIZONS-AMI (The Harmonizing Outcomes with Revascularization and Stents in Acute Myocardial Infarction Trial) stent arm compared paclitaxel-eluting DES versus BMS. In this trial, there was no signal of harm at 1 year or during extended follow-up. Consistent with the known benefits of DES, TVR was reduced significantly. It is important to note that while ST occurred in more than 3% of patients at 1 year, there was no difference between DES

and BMS.[27] Palmerini and colleagues[28] have since published a meta-analysis of 22 trials with more than 12,000 patients randomized to DES or BMS. Everolimus-eluting, sirolimus-eluting, and paclitaxel-eluting stents were shown to have lower 1-year TVR with no excess risk of ST. Everolimus-eluting stents were specifically shown to be superior to BMS with respect to cardiac death, MI, and ST. Based on this data, DES are considered a safe and efficacious first-line choice in primary PCI.

With 2 decades of broad, worldwide experience with coronary stent implantation, the benefits of stenting over angioplasty are obvious whether for STEMI or other indications. Although the risk of ST is higher after primary PCI than for elective PCI, it is necessary to recognize that ST as the cause of STEMI is an increasing problem. Primary PCI for STEMI due to ST is associated with lower rates of successful reperfusion, higher rates of

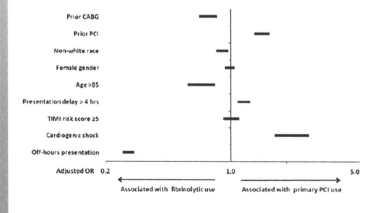

Fig. 4. Predictors of reperfusion strategy in NCDR 2000 to 2006. (*From* Fazel R, Krumholz HM, Bates ER, et al. Choice of reperfusion strategy at hospitals with primary percutaneous coronary intervention: a national registry of myocardial infarction analysis. Circulation 2009;120:2460; with permission.)

distal embolization, and more in-hospital major adverse cardiac events (MACE) than primary PCI for de novo STEMI culprit lesions.[29] An analysis of more than 3000 consecutive STEMI patients treated between 2003 and 2010 revealed 3 important findings: 8.5% of STEMI are due to ST; ST patients have higher long-term risks of recurrent ST and MI; and the frequency of ST causing STEMI is increasing (**Fig. 5**).[30] In short, ST causing STEMI is frequent enough and divergent enough to be considered a unique clinical problem.

Protection of the microvascular circulation during primary PCI is an issue requiring further clarification. Analysis of the original STENT PAMI (Primary Angioplasty for Acute Myocardial Infarction) study demonstrated a trend toward lower rates of Thrombolysis in Myocardial Infarction (TIMI) 3 flow after stent implantation.[21] Although that concern was not borne out in future studies, 2 new concepts in primary PCI address this phenomenon. A micro-mesh-covered metallic stent (MGuard; InspireMD, Tel Aviv, Israel) (**Fig. 6**) designed to trap thrombus and friable atherosclerotic debris is currently under investigation in the United States. This device has been compared with standard metallic stents and produced superior rates of ST-segment resolution (STR) and TIMI 3 flow.[31] Furthermore, a proof-of-concept evaluation of deferred stenting after restoration of coronary flow with thrombectomy or balloon angioplasty yielded significantly less slow-flow/no-reflow and greater myocardial salvage by magnetic resonance imaging (MRI). In that study, deferred stenting was performed at a median of 9 hours after the initial procedure.[32] It is likely that future improvements in stents used for primary PCI will address the relationship between stent implantation and microvascular obstruction.

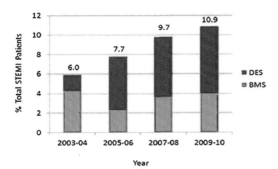

Fig. 5. Frequency of STEMI due to stent thrombosis as a percentage of total STEMI between 2003 and 2010. (*From* Brodie BR, Hansen C, Garberich RF, et al. ST-segment elevation myocardial infarction resulting from stent thrombosis. J Am Coll Cardiol 2012;60:1989; with permission.)

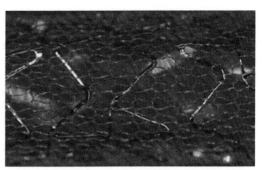

Fig. 6. MGuard stent with micromesh covering. (*From* Stone GW, Abizaid A, Silber S, et al. Prospective, randomized, multicenter evaluation of a polyethylene terephthalate micronet mesh-covered stent in st-segment elevation myocardial infarction: the MASTER trial. J Am Coll Cardiol 2012;60:1977; with permission.)

Surrogate Markers of Reperfusion in STEMI

Infarct size can be assessed by nuclear perfusion or quantitative MRI and is directly related to clinical outcome. Surrogates such as cardiac biomarker levels, angiographic indices including TIMI blush grade, and ECG STR can assist in prognostication following STEMI. In the interest of testing new therapies and adjunctive treatments, surrogate endpoints have been quite useful in allowing the practical conduct of smaller clinical investigations.

Thrombectomy and Embolic Protection Devices

Distal embolization and microvascular obstruction are known complications of primary PCI. Large thrombus burden predisposes to increased risk of distal embolization. Microvascular obstruction is postulated to result from platelet plugging, cellular debris, endothelial damage, and cytokine generation. Both distal embolization and microvascular obstruction are associated with the slow-flow and no-reflow phenomena.

In the early 1990s, embolic protection devices (EPD) were developed. Initial study in saphenous vein graft PCI demonstrated a substantial reduction in death and MI with EPD.[33] EPD technology has enhanced the safety of interventions on bypass grafts and has been extended into endovascular lower extremity and carotid interventions. Intuitively, EPD could offer similar benefits in STEMI.

The pivotal EMERALD (Enhanced Myocardial Efficacy and Recovery by Aspiration of Liberated Debris) study of the Guardwire Plus (Medtronic Corporation, Santa Rosa, CA, USA) in 501 patients with STEMI was well-conducted with short-term coprimary endpoints of STR and infarct size by nuclear imaging.[34] The use of EPD during primary PCI did not have any effect on any surrogate or clinical endpoint. Since that time, no EPD have been shown to be efficacious in improving outcomes in native coronary artery PCI.

Unlike EPD, thrombectomy has taken a leading role in primary PCI. Thrombectomy addresses the same problems as EPD, such as embolization, no-reflow, and adverse clinical events. Both mechanical and aspiration thrombectomy techniques aim to remove thrombotic and atheromatous debris. Aspiration thrombectomy uses simple suction with a noncomplex device. Mechanical thrombectomy devices like the Angiojet (Possis/Medrad, Warrendale, PA, USA) are more complex but retain ease-of-use and setup.

The Thrombus Aspiration during Percutaneous Coronary Intervention in Acute Myocardial Infarction (TAPAS) trial demonstrated improved STR, myocardial blush grade, and, uniquely, improved mortality at 30 days and 1 year.[35,36] No other study has demonstrated a mortality benefit with thrombus aspiration, and the results of thrombectomy on microvascular function and infarct size have been mixed. A prominent meta-analysis of thrombectomy trials did not demonstrate improvements in most individual clinical endpoints (**Table 1**), although a mortality advantage was present and entirely driven by TAPAS results.[37] Thrombectomy had no effect on short-term 30-day mortality in a recent randomized study nested within the Swedish national registry and including 7244 patients.[38]

Mechanical or rheolytic thrombectomy (RT) has had a long but even more limited role in primary PCI. The JETSTENT (The Angiojet Rheolytic Thrombectomy Before Direct Infarct Artery Stenting in Patients Undergoing Primary PCI for Acute Myocardial Infarction Trial) randomized study showed superior STR with RT but no difference in other surrogate endpoints.[39] In a meta-analysis including JETSTENT and 6 other RT trials, there was no reduction in any component of MACE or total MACE.[37]

Novel Adjunctive Therapies

Various adjunctive therapies to limit infarct size have been evaluated, although none have, as yet, become part of contemporary primary PCI. The search for a way to reduce myonecrosis and infarct size is a complex challenge that is exceptionally detailed in a review by Gerczuk and Kloner.[40] Novel adjunctive therapies that have been studied include

- Medications: cyclosporine, nicorandil, adenosine, natriuretic peptides
- Intermittent balloon occlusion, post-ischemic conditioning
- Supersaturated aqueous oxygen
- Mild therapeutic hypothermia

These studies have relied primarily on surrogate endpoints and the results have been mixed. Thus, primary PCI continues to rely on standard balloon dilation, thrombectomy, and stent implantation.

The most recent evaluation of induced hypothermia via cold saline infusion and endovascular cooling was the CHILL-MI study. Cooling commenced before PCI and was continued for 1 hour after reperfusion. The mean temperature during treatment was 34.7°C. Mild hypothermia was safe but did not reduce the primary endpoint of infarct size, although the subgroup of early anterior MI seemed to enjoy a greater benefit. A signal toward reduced subsequent heart failure events with hypothermia was also present.[41] Ongoing studies of mild hypothermia are being conducted using surface, intravascular, and alternative methods, such as intraperitoneal cooling. At this time, the role of adjunctive therapies remains in question.

Antiplatelet and Antithrombotic Therapies in STEMI

There has been extensive research into oral and intravenous antiplatelet agents used in STEMI, in primary PCI, and for long-term management after stent implantation. Aspirin has been the cornerstone of therapy since the earliest MI studies.[6,8] The focus on intravenous agents during PCI has decreased in recent years because of greater understanding of existing oral agents, more potent novel oral agents, and a reliance on the direct thrombin inhibitor bivalirudin. Care guidelines

Table 1
Effect of aspiration thrombectomy at 6 months: results of a meta-analysis of 18 trials

	Relative Risk	P Value
All-cause mortality	0.71	.049
Reinfarction	0.68	NS
Stroke	1.31	NS
TVR	0.79	.06
MACE	0.76	.006

Adapted from Kumbhani DJ, Bavry AA, Desai MY, et al. Role of aspiration and mechanical thrombectomy in patients with acute myocardial infarction undergoing primary angioplasty: an updated meta-analysis of randomized trials. J Am Coll Cardiol 2013;62:1409–18; with permission.

currently support long-term maintenance with low-dose aspirin after an initial loading dose. For PCI in STEMI, clopidogrel and the newer agents, ticagrelor and prasugrel, share equivalent recommendations despite their differential antiplatelet potency and clinical efficacy.

Clopidogrel has been part of PCI and acute coronary syndrome treatment for well over a decade. In the CLARITY (clopidogrel to aspirin and fibrinolytic therapy for myocardial infarction) TIMI-28 study, the addition of clopidogrel to fibrinolysis reduced the likelihood of the combined angiographic/clinical composite endpoint of occluded artery and death or MI before angiography. The benefit of clopidogrel with fibrinolysis was driven by an increased frequency of normal TIMI 3 flow at initial angiography.[42] Another mega-trial looked at clinical outcomes with short-term clopidogrel in more than 45,000 patients who primarily presented with STEMI. It is important to recognize that nearly half of the patients in this study received no reperfusion therapy, but a significant reduction in MACE, including individual endpoints of death and nonfatal MI, was observed with the addition of clopidogrel.[43]

Prasugrel is a thienopyridine agent similar to clopidogrel but with more rapid onset and greater antiplatelet effect. Prasugrel loading and maintenance at standard doses were compared with clopidogrel at commonly accepted doses in acute patients undergoing PCI. The STEMI subgroup in the TRITON (Trial to Assess Improvement in Therapeutic Outcomes by Optimizing Platelet Inhibition with Prasugrel) TIMI 38 Trial analysis demonstrated a 6.5% MACE rate with prasugrel versus 9.5% (hazard ratio 0.68, $P = .0017$) with clopidogrel. Major bleeding was similar and prasugrel was also associated with a 50% reduction in ST.[44] The current data support prasugrel as the most effective oral antiplatelet agent for primary PCI patients.

Ticagrelor is a nonthienopyridine antiplatelet agent that has demonstrated superiority over clopidogrel in both medically and invasively managed acute coronary syndrome patients. Subgroup analysis of the STEMI population in the PLATO (Study of Platelet Inhibition and Patient Outcomes) trial reinforced a trend toward enhanced efficacy with ticagrelor.[45,46]

The use of the direct thrombin inhibitor, bivalirudin, is endorsed by guidelines and has replaced unfractionated heparin with or without GPI in many centers. Recent NCDR data suggest that it is used in more than 20% of primary PCI, although its utilization is likely greater.[47] In comparison with heparin plus GPI, bivalirudin reduced net adverse clinical events (NACE = MACE plus bleeding). The benefit was driven by a reduction in bleeding, although it is important to also note that bivalirudin was associated with improved survival at 1 year (**Fig. 7**). One caveat is that early ST is significantly more frequent with bivalirudin, although total ST at 30 days and 1 year is equivalent.[48]

The negative consequences of bleeding complications on both short-term and long-term outcomes are an area of intense recent focus. Bleeding concerns dictate not only antiplatelet and antithrombotic choices but also the selection of vascular access. The negative consequences of a major bleeding event are potentially greater

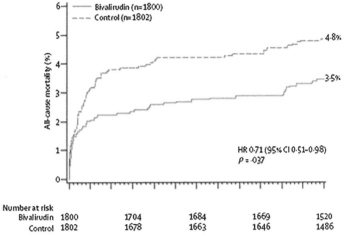

Fig. 7. Effect of bivalirudin in STEMI on mortality at 1 year. (*From* Mehran R, Lansky AJ, Witzenbichler B, et al, for the HORIZONS-AMI Trial Investigators. Bivalirudin in patients undergoing primary angioplasty for acute myocardial infarction (HORIZONS-AMI): 1-year results of a randomised controlled trial. Lancet 2009;374:1154; with permission.)

than traditionally accepted adverse events, such as nonfatal MI. HORIZONS patients with in-hospital major bleeding had an absolute 20% greater risk of death at 3 years as compared with those without an in-hospital major bleeding event. The reduction in bleeding with bivalirudin still provides only a partial explanation for its associated mortality benefit.[49,50]

When considering trends in vascular access for STEMI, an important concept is that access site bleeding accounts for only 50% of major bleeding events. Non-access site bleeding is thought to be prognostically more important. Nonetheless, the choice between radial access and femoral access with or without a vascular closure device (VCD) is important. Three main trials have evaluated the effect of radial access in STEMI. Bleeding is consistently reduced in all studies with radial access. In the RIVAL (The RadIal Vs femorAL access for coronary intervention Trial) trial, radial access was also associated with reduced MACE and all-cause mortality in the STEMI subgroup. In RIFLE-STEACS (Radial Versus Femoral Randomized Investigation in ST-Elevation Acute Coronary Syndrome Trial), cardiac mortality was reduced with radial access. In the STEMI-RADIAL (ST-segment elevation myocardial infarction treated by radial or femoral approach in a multicenter randomized clinical trial) study, radial access was associated with dramatic reductions in bleeding events but there was no effect on mortality.[51–53] With respect to femoral access, there is likely a synergistic effect of both bivalirudin use and VCD use in reducing access site bleeding.[54] The use of radial access in STEMI is increasing, although this remains an area of debate.

New Challenges in STEMI

Although multivessel disease is more common in patients with MI without ST-segment elevation, multivessel disease beyond the obvious culprit lesion is a common finding during primary PCI. Guidelines have for many years been quite clear about PCI of nonculprit lesions during primary PCI. PCI of a nonculprit lesion continues to receive a class III (contraindicated) recommendation in the guidelines.[3] The recent publication of a trial looking at "preventive" angioplasty of nonculprit vessels during primary PCI has brought into question this recommendation. "Preventive" PCI was associated with significant long-term reduction in MACE and the individual components of MACE, including cardiac death and MI.[55] Many questions remain regarding multivessel disease in STEMI. The PRAMI (Preventive Angioplasty in Myocardial Infarction) study excluded patients with chronic total occlusions (CTO) and this is a critical point because the presence of a nonculprit CTO in STEMI has profound prognostic implications well beyond the presence of multivessel disease (**Fig. 8**).[56]

The initial management of out-of-hospital cardiac arrest (OOHCA) patients has been dramatically altered by therapeutic hypothermia and increased awareness and interest within cardiology. STEMI complicated by OOHCA represents an ongoing challenge to emergency medical services (EMS), cardiology, and health care systems. The prognosis of the unresponsive or minimally responsive postarrest STEMI patient is significantly worse than the general STEMI population.[57] With evidence-based therapies, including hypothermia and PCI, survival and neurologic function can be improved, although the potential impacts on STEMI systems and publicly reported outcomes for PCI are significant.

Cardiogenic Shock and Ventricular Assistive Devices in STEMI

The intra-aortic balloon pump (IABP) has a long track record and is relatively inexpensive, safe,

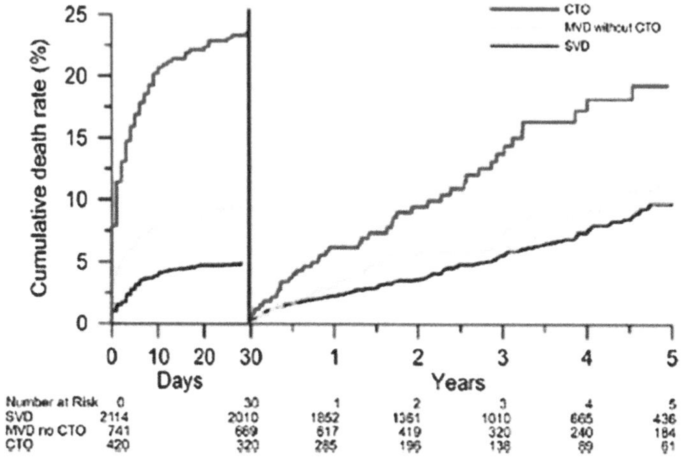

Fig. 8. Mortality differences in STEMI patients with single-vessel disease, multivessel disease, or CTO of nonculprit vessel. MVD, multi-vessel disease; SVD, single vessel disease. (From Claessen BE, van der Schaaf RJ, Verouden NJ, et al. Evaluation of the effect of concurrent chronic total occlusion on long-term mortality and left ventricular function after primary percutaneous coronary intervention. JACC Cardiovasc Interv 2009;2:1131; with permission.)

and easy to use. Although the hemodynamic effects of IABP are modest, it remains the most widely used ventricular assistive device. The utility of IABP was recently evaluated in patients with anterior STEMI but without cardiogenic shock. There was no improvement in final infarct size or any clinical endpoint.[58]

Similar to the OOHCA patient, the patient with cardiogenic shock remains a tremendous challenge and an outlier to the reported low mortality in large STEMI cohorts. The findings of the original SHOCK (Should We Emergently Revascularize Occluded Coronaries for Cardiogenic Shock Trial) trial have guided treatment decisions for nearly 2 decades. SHOCK was a landmark study in an extreme risk population (nearly 50% mortality at 30 days) that showed a modest survival benefit with revascularization at 6 months. Most patients in both the revascularization and the control arms did have an IABP placed. However, this trial was relatively small and the revascularization strategies bear little resemblance to the current state.[59] SHOCK was an extremely insightful study, although it did betray a negative effect of revascularization in subgroup analysis of the small number of patients aged 75 years and over. This finding remained in the care guidelines until recently.

The IABP-SHOCK II study was designed to assess the effect of routine IABP placement in patients with MI complicated by cardiogenic shock. Patients were undergoing angiography with revascularization at the discretion of the operator, although only two-thirds of the study population had STEMI. The trial was successful in selecting truly high-risk patients as reflected by the short-term mortality rate of 40%. However, there was no benefit to routine IABP placement in cardiogenic shock. One overlooked finding of this study was that there was no excess of bleeding or vascular complications with routine balloon pump use.[60]

Newer and more powerful assistive devices, such as Tandem Heart (CardiacAssist, Inc, Pittsburgh, PA, USA) and Impella (Abiomed, Inc, Danvers, MA, USA), have not been rigorously studied in STEMI complicated by cardiogenic shock, although they can provide substantially more hemodynamic support than the IABP. Although the role of revascularization in cardiogenic shock is clear, the role and choice of ventricular assist devices remain unanswered.

Timely Reperfusion and Patient Outcomes

Longer ischemic times are directly linked to larger infarcts and worse outcomes. Treatment delays can be variably attributed to the patients themselves, providers, hospital facilities, and even the organization of local EMS and health systems. These sources of delay have been formidable obstacles preventing efficient and timely delivery of reperfusion across large populations (**Box 1**). The improvements of the past 2 decades are significant, especially from the vantage point of the 1990s.

In 1990, only half of all eligible patients received any form of reperfusion therapy. Less than 3% of patients were treated with primary PCI. Median door-to-needle time for thrombolytic administration was 59 minutes. DTB time for PCI was first collected in the National Registry of Myocardial Infarction (NRMI) in 1994, and the median DTB time was 111 minutes. The status of STEMI care presented a great opportunity for improvement, and over the next decade, treatment intervals declined steadily.[61] Despite that progress, between 1999 and 2002, less than half of the PCI patients had DTB times within the recommended 90 minutes, and only higher volume PCI facilities were achieving significant improvement in DTB intervals.[62]

By 2004, PCI and thrombolytic treatment were used in equal numbers of patients.[61] The NRMI-2 analysis demonstrated a 41% to 62% relative increase in short-term mortality with DTB greater than 120 minutes.[63] NRMI-3 and NRMI-4 analyses more clearly conveyed a direct relationship between treatment delay and mortality (**Fig. 9**) with a low in-hospital mortality of only 3% for those with DTB less than 90 minutes.[64] The mortality benefit of timely primary PCI was broadly appreciated and the need to improve treatment was obvious for individual patients and system-wide as a mark of quality care.

With evidence of a direct correlation between treatment delay and death, the imperative to

---

Box 1
Modifiable sources of delay in reperfusion therapy

Patient, public
  Delay in recognizing cardiac symptoms
  Delay in seeking FMC
Emergency services
  Delay in transport, triage, and transfer
  Delay in ECG transmission
  Delay in identification and diagnosis of STEMI
Medical and cardiovascular providers
  Delay in response and availability
  Delay in diagnosis and activation
  Delay in treatment

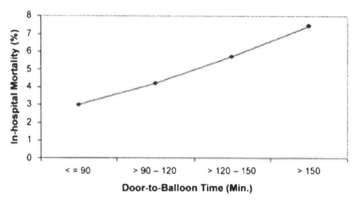

Fig. 9. Relationship between DTB and mortality in NRMI 3-4. (*From* McNamara RL, Wang Y, Herrin J, et al. Effect of door-to-balloon time on mortality in patients with st-segment elevation myocardial infarction. J Am Coll Cardiol 2006;47:2184; with permission.)

improve care delivery was evident. This call to action has been partly answered. The percentage of patients treated inside a DTB time less than 90 minutes in the latest NCDR report increased from 60% in 2005 to 83% in 2009.[47] Since 2010, the percentage of patients with a DTB less than 90 minutes has exceeded 90%.[65] Despite the fact that median DTB times are well below 90 minutes, short-term mortality has been flat at approximately 5% (**Fig. 10**). A reasonable assumption is that total ischemic time and symptom duration trump relatively smaller improvements in reperfusion speed once the DTB decreases to less than 90 minutes. Alternatively, greater inclusion of lower risk STEMI patients in recent years and other statistical limitations could cloud the direct link between treatment time and mortality.[66]

Treating STEMI in Regional Systems of Care

The rapid improvements in STEMI care are attributable to several critical occurrences in the past decade: national initiatives to improve patient outcomes via the surrogate marker of treatment intervals, ambitious goals for PCI performance, integrated regional systems of care, and the prioritization of STEMI care in the cardiovascular community. Successful deployment of an advanced system of care requires community infrastructure, planning, system support, evidence-based therapies, and continuous quality assessment.[67]

The American College of Cardiology–sponsored D2B Alliance was initiated as a collaborative effort promoting these evidence-based treatments,

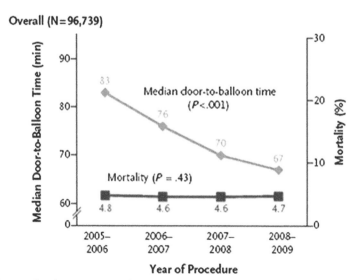

Fig. 10. In-hospital mortality from STEMI and DTB Time, NCDR 2005 to 2009. (*From* Menees DS, Peterson ED, Wang Y, et al. Door-to-balloon time and mortality among patients undergoing primary PCI. N Engl J Med 2013;369:905; with permission.)

guideline adherence, and dynamic improvement in STEMI care.[68] The D2B Alliance proposed some important practical strategies for improving care delivery:

- Activation of cardiac catheterization laboratory by emergency physicians
- Activation of cardiac catheterization laboratory based on prehospital ECG
- Single-call systems for cardiac catheterization laboratory activation
- Requirement of a 20-minute to 30-minute response time by cardiac catheterization laboratory team
- Administrative and management support for STEMI care and DTB goals
- Closed-loop feedback between emergency and cardiovascular providers
- Team-based approach from EMS FMC to PCI

The use of prehospital ECG has fulfilled several predicated requirements in the formation and execution of regional systems of care. ECGs of high diagnostic quality performed in the field enable early diagnosis and triage to specialized STEMI receiving centers (SRC) (**Fig. 11**). Based on field ECG diagnosis, early activation of the SRC catheterization laboratory advances the FMC to treatment time by at least 15 minutes. Electronic transmission of prehospital ECGs also provides the opportunity for emergency and specialist physicians to participate in early decision-making, including bypassing the emergency department for direct admission to the catheterization laboratory. Issues related to false-positive prehospital ECGs are important but are far less significant than the benefits of field diagnosis and triage.

Using prehospital ECG with field triage to an SRC for primary PCI has shown dramatic results. This strategy was compared with standard transport and diagnosis in the North Sydney Area Health Service (Australia) and was associated with substantial reductions in both total symptom duration and DTB.[69] Another prospective evaluation of prehospital ECG and field triage demonstrated a median DTB time of 56 minutes compared with 98 minutes ($P<.001$) in the standard evaluation arm.[70] The system-wide improvements in diagnosis and DTB using prehospital ECG and field triage are remarkable and can be sustained over the long term.[71]

An NCDR study of EMS-transported patients has confirmed the generalizability of the effect of prehospital ECG acquisition in the United States. Regardless of whether reperfusion was performed with fibrinolysis or PCI, treatment intervals are shorter when a field ECG is obtained. There was a 10-minute reduction in door-to-needle time ($P = .003$) and a significant 14-minute reduction in DTB ($P<.001$) associated with prehospital ECG performance. Importantly, in the total EMS-transported STEMI population, there was a trend toward reduced mortality with this strategy.[72]

There is a substantial impact in integrating prehospital ECG and field diagnosis with triage to specialized centers while following rigorous guideline-directed goals for FMC to balloon and DTB times. Nearly a dozen regional SRC systems successfully pioneered the concept in the United States. The number of regional SRC systems has increased substantially in recent years, reflecting a commitment toward patients and an ability to harness the assets of EMS, providers, and hospital systems in a cooperative and productive manner. In Los Angeles County, the effect of a regional SRC system has been dramatic with a sustained improvement in DTB (**Fig. 12**).[73] Furthermore, the STEMI infrastructure has provided a model for postcardiac arrest care.

Rapid transfer is a prerequisite for rapid treatment. Interfacility transfer has been a tremendous challenge and historical transfer times are disappointingly long. An additional benefit of regionalized STEMI care is the ability to organize EMS transport between non-PCI and PCI-capable facilities.[74] Clearly defined guideline recommendations have also enhanced the adoption of timely interfacility transfer practices. In addition, bypassing

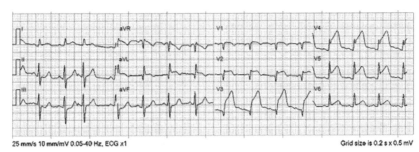

25 mm/s 10 mm/mV 0.05-40 Hz, ECG x1   Grid size is 0.2 s x 0.5 mV

Fig. 11. Prehospital 12-lead ECG, electronically transmitted quality.

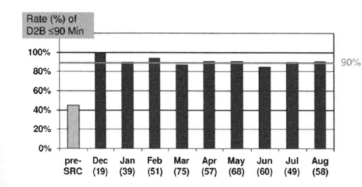

Fig. 12. Effect on DTB of SRC participation with prehospital ECG use in Los Angeles County. (*From* Rokos IC, French WJ, Koenig WJ, et al. Integration of pre-hospital electrocardiograms and ST-elevation myocardial infarction receiving center (SRC) networks. JACC Cardiovasc Interv 2009;2:339–46; with permission.)

emergency departments for direct admission to the catheterization laboratory from the field or in transfer is a safe and effective option.[75]

It is indisputable that advanced systems of care improve the use of reperfusion therapy and reduce treatment delay. Unfortunately, for a patient to enjoy the benefits of an SRC, they must enter into the system (and ideally at the earliest possible point of EMS FMC with a prehospital ECG). Reductions in total ischemic time may be less affected by modern SRCs without intensive public education efforts. Public education is a guideline-recommended component of STEMI care, but it is a challenging task without clarity about how to best achieve it.[3]

Patients who do not use EMS do not derive the same benefit from the evolution of the SRC. An NCDR analysis of STEMI patients between 2007 and 2009 reported that only 60% of STEMI patients availed of EMS transport. As expected, self-transport was associated not only with treatment delay but also longer symptom duration.[76] Reducing the number of self-transported patients will need to be prioritized nationally and within each regional SRC.

SUMMARY

The past 3 decades have witnessed the development of robust clinical data on best practices with fibrinolysis, PCI, and medical therapy with the intent of improving outcomes in STEMI. Successfully applying optimal STEMI care across populations is only made possible by delivering that care within dedicated regional systems, which has required goal-directed and collaborative effort within national and regional organizations. The clinical evidence base of STEMI management will continue to evolve. In coming years, the critical task will be to continue extending the benefits of modern medicine and advanced systems of care to all patients.

REFERENCES

1. Shah RU, Rutten-Ramos S, Garberich R, et al. STEMI trends in the United States 2002-2010: increasing use of PCI and declining mortality. Circ Cardiovasc Qual Outcomes 2013;6:A22.

2. Yeh RW, Sidney S, Chandra M, et al. Population trends in the incidence and outcomes of acute myocardial infarction. N Engl J Med 2010;362: 2155–65.

3. O'Gara PT, Kushner FG, Ascheim DD, et al. 2013 ACCF/AHA guideline for the management of ST-elevation myocardial infarction. A report of the American College of Cardiology Foundation/American Heart Association task force on practice guidelines. Circulation 2013;127:e362–425.

4. Roe MT, Messenger JC, Weintraub WS, et al. Treatments, trends and outcomes of acute myocardial infarction and percutaneous coronary intervention. J Am Coll Cardiol 2010;56:254–63.

5. Fazel R, Krumholz HM, Bates ER, et al. Choice of reperfusion strategy at hospitals with primary percutaneous coronary intervention: a national registry of myocardial infarction analysis. Circulation 2009;120:2455–61.

6. Randomized trial of intravenous streptokinase, oral aspirin, both, or neither among 17187 cases of suspected acute myocardial infarction: ISIS-2.ISIS-2 (Second International Study of Infarct Survival) Collaborative Group. J Am Coll Cardiol 1988;12: 3A–13A.

7. Effectiveness of intravenous thrombolytic therapy in acute myocardial infarction. Gruppo Italiano per lo Studio della Streptochinasi nell'Infarto Miocardico (GISSI). Lancet 1988;2:349–60.

8. Collins R, Peto R, Baigent C, et al. Aspirin, heparin, and thrombolytic therapy in suspected acute myocardial infarction. N Engl J Med 1997;336: 847–60.

9. Wilcox RG, von der Lippe G, Olsson CG, et al. Trial of tissue plasminogen activator for mortality reduction in acute myocardial infarction. Anglo-

scandinavian study of early thrombolysis (ASSET). Lancet 1988;2:525–30.

10. The GUSTO Investigators. An international randomized trial comparing four thrombolytic strategies for acute myocardial infarction. N Engl J Med 1993;329:673–82.

11. Van de Werf F, Cannon CP, Luyten A, et al. Safety assessment of single-bolus administration of TNK tissue-plasminogen activator in acute myocardial infarction: the ASSENT-1 trial. Am Heart J 1999; 137:786–91.

12. Sinnaeve P, Alexander J, Belmans A, et al, ASSENT-2 Investigators. One-year follow-up of the ASSENT-2 trial: a double-blind, randomized comparison of single-bolus tenecteplase and front-loaded alteplase in 16,949 patients ST-elevation acute myocardial infarction. Am Heart J 2003;146:27–32.

13. Assessment of the Safety and Efficacy of a New Thrombolytic Regimen (ASSENT)-3 Investigators. Efficacy and safety of tenecteplase in combination with enxoparin, abciximab, or unfractionated heparin: the ASSENT-3 randomized trial in acute myocardial infarction. Lancet 2001;358:605–13.

14. Antmann EM, Morrow DA, McCabe CH, et al, for the EXTRACT-TIMI 25 Investigators. Enoxaparin versus unfractionated heparin with fibrinolysis st-segment elevation myocardial infarction. N Engl J Med 2006;354:1477–88.

15. O'Keefe JH, Bailey WL, Rutherford BD, et al. Primary angioplasty for acute myocardial infarction in 1,000 consecutive patients. Results in an unselected population and high-risk subgroups. Am J Cardiol 1993;72:107G–15G.

16. A clinical trial comparing coronary angioplasty with tissue plasminogen activator for acute myocardial infarction. The global use of strategies to open occluded coronary arteries in acute coronary syndromes (GUSTO IIb) Angioplasty Substudy Investigators. N Engl J Med 1997;336:1621–8.

17. Keeley EC, Boura JA, Grines C. Primary angioplasty versus intravenous thrombolytic therapy for acute myocardial infarction: a quantitative review of 23 randomised trials. Lancet 2003;361: 13–20.

18. Lawesson SS, Alfredsson J, Fredrikson M, et al. Time trends in STEMI—improved treatment and outcome but still a gender gap: a prospective observational cohort study from the SWEDEHEART register. BMJ Open 2012;2:e000726.

19. Wu KL, Tsui KL, Lee KT, et al. Reperfusion strategy for ST-elevation myocardial infarction: trend over a 10-year period. Hong Kong Med J 2012; 18:276–83.

20. Eagle KA, Nallamothu BK, Mehta RH, et al. Trends in acute reperfusion therapy for ST-segment elevation myocardial infarction from 1999 to 2006: we

are getting better but we have got a long way to go. Eur Heart J 2008;29:609–17.

21. Grines CL, Cox DA, Stone GW, et al, for The Stent Primary Angioplasty in Myocardial Infarction Study Group. Coronary angioplasty with or without stent implantation for acute myocardial infarction. N Engl J Med 1999;341:1949–56.

22. Stone GW, Grines CL, Cox DA, et al, for the Controlled Abciximab and Device Investigation to Lower Late Angioplasty Complications (CADIL-LAC) Investigators. Comparison of angioplasty with stenting, with or without abciximab, in acute myocardial infarction. N Engl J Med 2002;346: 957–66.

23. Spaulding C, Henry P, Teiger E, et al, for the TYPHOON Investigators. Sirolimus-eluting versus uncoated stents in acute myocardial infarction. N Engl J Med 2006;355:1093–104.

24. Laarman GJ, Suttorp MJ, Dirksen MT, et al. Paclitaxel-eluting versus uncoated stents in primary percutaneous coronary intervention. N Engl J Med 2006;355:1105–13.

25. Menichelli M, Parma A, Pucci E, et al. Randomized trial of sirolimus-eluting stent versus bare metal stent in acute myocardial infarction (SESAMI). J Am Coll Cardiol 2007;49:1924–30.

26. Steg PG, Fox KA, Eagle KA, et al, for the Global Registry of Acute Coronary Events (GRACE) Investigators. Mortality following placement of drug-eluting and bare-metal stents for st-segment elevation acute myocardial infarction in the global registry of acute coronary events. Eur Heart J 2009;30:321–9.

27. Stone GW, Lansky AL, Pocock SJ, et al, for the HORIZONS-AMI Trial Investigators. Paclitaxel-eluting stents versus bare-metal stents in acute myocardial infarction. N Engl J Med 2009;360: 1946–59.

28. Palmerini T, Biondi-Zoccai G, Della Riva D, et al. Clinical outcomes with drug-eluting and bare-metal stents in patients with st-segment elevation myocardial infarction: evidence from a comprehensive network meta-analysis. J Am Coll Cardiol 2013;62:496–504.

29. Chechi T, Vecchio S, Vittori G, et al. ST-segment elevation myocardial infarction due to early and late stent thrombosis: a new group of high risk patients. J Am Coll Cardiol 2008;51:2396–402.

30. Brodie BR, Hansen C, Garberich RF, et al. ST-segment elevation myocardial infarction resulting from stent thrombosis. J Am Coll Cardiol 2012;60: 1989–91.

31. Stone GW, Abizaid A, Silber S, et al. Prospective, randomized, multicenter evaluation of a polyethylene terephthalate micronet mesh-covered stent in st-segment elevation myocardial infarction: the master trial. J Am Coll Cardiol 2012. [Epub ahead of print].

32. Carrick D, Oldroyd KG, McEntegart M, et al. A randomized trial of deferred stenting versus immediate stenting to prevent no-or slow reflow in acute st-elevation myocardial infarction (DEFER-STEMI). J Am Coll Cardiol 2014. [Epub ahead of print].

33. Baim DS, Wahr D, George B, et al. Randomized trial of a distal embolic protection device during percutaneous intervention of saphenous vein aorto-coronary bypass grafts. Circulation 2002; 105:1285–90.

34. Stone GW, Webb J, Cox DA, et al, for the Enhanced Myocardial Efficacy and Recovery by Aspiration of Liberated Debris (EMERALD) Investigators. Distal microcirculatory protection during percutaneous coronary intervention in acute st-segment elevation myocardial infarction. JAMA 2005;293:1036–72.

35. Svilaas T, Vlaar PJ, van der Horst IC, et al. Thrombus aspiration during primary percutaneous coronary intervention. N Engl J Med 2008;358: 557–67.

36. Svilaas T, Vlaar PJ, van der Horst IC, et al. Cardiac death and reinfarction after 1 year in the thrombus aspiration during percutaneous coronary intervention in acute myocardial infarction study (TAPAS): a 1-year follow-up study. Lancet 2008;371:1915–20.

37. Kumbhani DJ, Bavry AA, Desai MY, et al. Role of aspiration and mechanical thrombectomy in patients with acute myocardial infarction undergoing primary angioplasty: an updated meta-analysis of randomized trials. J Am Coll Cardiol 2013;62: 1409–18.

38. Frobert O, Lagerqvist B, Olivecrona GK, et al. Thrombus aspiration during ST-segment elevation myocardial infarction. N Engl J Med 2013;369: 1587–97.

39. Migliorini A, Stabile A, Rodriguez AE, et al. Comparison of angiojet rheolytic thrombectomy before direct infarct artery stenting with direct stenting alone in patients with acute myocardial infarction. The JETSTENT trial. J Am Coll Cardiol 2010;56: 1298–306.

40. Gerczuk PZ, Kloner RA. An update on cardioprotection. A review of the latest adjunctive therapies to limit myocardial infarct size in clinical trials. J Am Coll Cardiol 2012;59:969–78.

41. Erlinge D, Gotberg M, Lang I, et al. Rapid endovascular core cooling combined with cold saline as an adjunct to percutaneous coronary intervention for the treatment of acute myocardial infarction (The CHILL-MI Trial). J Am Coll Cardiol 2014. [Epub ahead of print].

42. Sabatine MS, Cannon CP, Gibson CM, et al, for the CLARITY-TIMI 28 Investigators. Addition of clopidogrel to aspirin and fibrinolytic therapy for myocardial infarction with st-segment elevation. N Engl J Med 2005;352:1179–89.

43. COMMIT (Clopidogrel and Metoprolol in Myocardial Infarction Trial) Collaborative Group. Addition of clopidogrel to aspirin in 45,852 patients with acute myocardial infarction: a randomized placebo-controlled trial. Lancet 2005;366:1607–21.

44. Montalescot G, Wiviott SD, Braunwald E, et al, for the TRITON-TIMI 38 Investigators. Prasugrel compared with clopidogrel in patients undergoing percutaneous coronary intervention for ST-segment elevation myocardial infarction (TRITON-TIMI 38): double-blind, randomised controlled trial. Lancet 2009;373:723–31.

45. Cannon CP, Harrington RA, James S, et al, for the PLATlet inhibition and patient Outcomes (PLATO) Investigators. Comparison of ticagrelor with clopidogrel in patients with a planned invasive strategy for acute coronary syndromes (PLATO): a randomised double-blind study. Lancet 2010;375:283–93.

46. Steg PG, James S, Harrington RA, et al. Ticagrelor versus clopidogrel in patients with st-elevation acute coronary syndromes intended for reperfusion with primary percutaneous coronary intervention: a platelet inhibition and patient outcomes (PLATO) trial subgroup analysis. Circulation 2010; 122:2131–41.

47. Menees DS, Peterson ED, Wang Y, et al. Door-to-balloon time and mortality among patients undergoing primary PCI. N Engl J Med 2013;369:901–9.

48. Mehran R, Lansky AJ, Witzenbichler B, et al, for the HORIZONS-AMI Trial Investigators. Bivalirudin in patients undergoing primary angioplasty for acute myocardial infarction (HORIZONS-AMI): 1-year results of a randomised controlled trial. Lancet 2009;374:1149–59.

49. Suh J-W, Mehran R, Claessen BE, et al. Impact of in-hospital major bleeding on late clinical outcomes primary percutaneous coronary interventions in acute myocardial infarction. J Am Coll Cardiol 2011;58:1750–6.

50. Stone GW, Clayton T, Deliagyris EN, et al. Reduction in cardiac mortality in patients with and without major bleeding. J Am Coll Cardiol 2014;63:15–20.

51. Mehta SR, Jolly SS, Cairns J, et al. Effects of radial versus femoral artery access in patients with acute coronary syndromes with or without st-segment elevation. J Am Coll Cardiol 2012;60:2490–9.

52. Romagnoli E, Biondi-Zoccai G, Sciahbasi A, et al. Radial versus femoral randomized investigation in ST-segment elevation acute coronary syndrome. J Am Coll Cardiol 2012;60:2481–9.

53. Bernat I, Horak D, Stasek J, et al. ST elevation myocardial infarction treated by radial or femoral approach in a multicenter randomized clinical trial: the STEMI-radial trial. J Am Coll Cardiol 2014;63: 964–72.

54. Marso SP, Amin AP, House JA, et al. Association between use of bleeding avoidance strategies and risk of periprocedural bleeding among patients undergoing percutaneous coronary intervention. JAMA 2010;303:2156–64.

55. Wald DS, Morris JK, Wald NJ, et al, for the PRAMI Investigators. Randomized trial of preventive angioplasty in myocardial infarction. N Engl J Med 2013;369:1115–23.

56. Claessen BE, van der Schaaf RJ, Verouden NJ, et al. Evaluation of the effect of concurrent chronic total occlusion on long-term mortality and left ventricular function after primary percutaneous coronary intervention. JACC Cardiovasc Interv 2009;2:1128–34.

57. Hosmane VR, Mustafa NG, Reddy VK, et al. Survival and neurologic recovery in patients with ST-segment elevation myocardial infarction resuscitated from cardiac arrest. J Am Coll Cardiol 2009;53:409–15.

58. Patel MR, Smalling RW, Thiele H, et al. Intra-aortic balloon counterpulsation and infarct size in patients with acute anterior myocardial infarction without shock. JAMA 2011;306:1329–37.

59. Hochman JS, Sleeper LA, Webb JG, et al, for the SHOCK Investigators. Early revascularization in acute myocardial infarction complicated by cardiogenic shock. N Engl J Med 1999;341:625–34.

60. Thiele H, Zeymer U, Neumann FJ, et al, for the IABP-SHOCK II Trial Investigators. Intraaortic balloon support for myocardial infarction with cardiogenic shock. N Engl J Med 2012;367:1287–96.

61. Gibson CM, Pride YB, Frederick PD, et al. Trends in reperfusion strategies, door-to-needle and door-to-balloon times, and in-hospital mortality among patients with ST-segment elevation myocardial infarction enrolled in the National Registry of Myocardial Infarction from 1990 to 2006. Am Heart J 2008;156:1035–44.

62. McNamara RL, Herrin J, Bradley EH, et al. Hospital improvement in time to reperfusion in patients with acute myocardial infarction, 1999 to 2002. J Am Coll Cardiol 2006;47:45–51.

63. Cannon CP, Gibson CM, Lambrew CT, et al. Relationship of symptom-onset-to-balloon and door-to-balloon time with mortality in patients undergoing angioplasty for acute myocardial infarction. JAMA 2000;283:2941–7.

64. McNamara RL, Wang Y, Herrin J, et al. Effect of door-to-balloon time on mortality in patients with ST-segment elevation myocardial infarction. J Am Coll Cardiol 2006;47:2180–6.

65. Krumholz HM, Herrin J, Miller LE, et al. Improvements in door-to-balloon time in the United States, 2005 to 2010. Circulation 2011;124:1038–45.

66. Bates ED, Jacobs AK. Time to treatment in patients with STEMI. N Engl J Med 2013;369:889–92.

67. Antman EM. Time is muscle: translation into practice. J Am Coll Cardiol 2008;52:1216–21.

68. Krumholz HM, Bradley EH, Nallamothu BK, et al. A campaign to improve the timeliness of primary percutaneous coronary intervention, door-to-balloon: an alliance for quality. JACC Cardiovasc Interv 2008;1:97–104.

69. Carstensen S, Nelson GC, Hansen PS, et al. Field triage to primary angioplasty combined with emergency department bypass reduces treatment delays and is associated with improved outcome. Eur Heart J 2007;28:2313–9.

70. Hutchison AW, Malaipan Y, Jarvie I, et al. Pre-hospital 12-lead ECG to triage st-segment myocardial infarction and emergency department activation of the infarct team significantly improves door-to-balloon times: ambulance Victoria and monash-HEART Acute Myocardial Infarction (MonAMI) 12-lead ECG project. Circ Cardiovasc Interv 2009;2:528–34.

71. Hutchison AW, Malaipan Y, Cameron JD, et al. Pre-hospital 12-lead ECG to triage ST elevation myocardial infarction and long term improvements in door to balloon times: the first 1000 patients from the MonAMI project. Heart Lung Circ 2013;22:910–6.

72. Diercks DB, Kontos MC, Chen AY, et al. Utilization and impact of pre-hospital electrocardiograms for patients with acute ST-segment elevation myocardial infarction. J Am Coll Cardiol 2009;53:161–6.

73. Rokos IC, French WJ, Koenig WJ, et al. Integration of pre-hospital electrocardiograms and ST-elevation myocardial infarction Receiving Center (SRC) networks. JACC Cardiovasc Interv 2009;2:339–46.

74. Baruch T, Rock A, Koenig WJ, et al. "Call 911" STEMI protocol reduces delays in transfer of patients from non primary percutaneous coronary intervention referral centers. Crit Pathw Cardiol 2010;9:113–5.

75. Bagai A, Jollis JG, Dauerman HL, et al. Emergency department bypass for ST-segment elevation myocardial infarction patients identified with prehospital electrocardiogram: a report from the American Heart Association Mission: lifeline program. Circulation 2013;128:352–9.

76. Mathews R, Peterson ED, Li S, et al. Use of emergency medical service transport among patients with st-segment elevation myocardial infarction. Circulation 2011;124:154–63.

Noninvasive Stress Testing for Coronary Artery Disease

Todd D. Miller, MD*, J. Wells Askew, MD,
Nandan S. Anavekar, MBBCh

KEYWORDS

- Stress testing • Exercise treadmill testing (ETT)
- Single-photon emission computed tomography (SPECT) • Positron emission tomography (PET)
- Myocardial perfusion imaging (MPI) • Exercise echocardiography • Dobutamine echocardiography

KEY POINTS

- The most important use of stress testing is risk stratification.
- Most patients can be accurately classified as low or high risk from treadmill test scores.
- Standard exercise treadmill testing is the preferred initial testing strategy in patients without prior revascularization who can adequately exercise and have a normal or near-normal resting electrocardiogram.
- Selection between imaging modalities depends primarily on patient characteristics and local expertise.
- The usefulness of the ischemic burden identified by stress imaging for categorizing risk and serving as a guide for selection of optimal treatment of coronary artery disease remains uncertain.

INTRODUCTION

Stress testing remains the traditional noninvasive approach for assessing patients with possible or established coronary artery disease (CAD). The most commonly used modalities include standard exercise treadmill testing (ETT); nuclear myocardial perfusion imaging with single-photon emission computed tomography (SPECT) and, less commonly, positron emission tomography (PET); and stress echocardiography. The stress imaging procedures can be performed with exercise stress or pharmacologic stress. Exercise is the preferred approach whenever possible because it provides an opportunity to evaluate the reproducibility of a patient's symptoms and to measure important prognostic variables (especially exercise capacity)

that are not available with pharmacologic stress. Although several exercise modalities including cycle ergometry and arm crank ergometry are available, in the United States the predominant type of exercise is graded treadmill walking. Pharmacologic stress testing can be performed in patients who cannot adequately exercise, generally defined as a workload less than 5 to 7 metabolic equivalents (METs), or in the presence of specific abnormalities on the resting electrocardiogram (ECG), such as left bundle branch block or paced ventricular rhythm. The most commonly used pharmacologic agents with nuclear imaging include the vasodilating agents regadenoson, adenosine, or dipyridamole, and with echocardiography the sympathomimetic agent dobutamine. Individuals who perform stress testing should be familiar with

Division of Cardiovascular Diseases, Mayo Clinic, Gonda 6, 200 First Street, Southwest, Rochester, MN 55905, USA
* Corresponding author.
E-mail address: miller.todd@mayo.edu

Cardiol Clin 32 (2014) 387–404
http://dx.doi.org/10.1016/j.ccl.2014.04.008
0733-8651/14/$ – see front matter © 2014 Elsevier Inc. All rights reserved.

contraindications to exercise and to the use of these pharmacologic agents, which are described elsewhere.[1–4]

Stress Testing for Diagnostic Purposes

Stress testing has traditionally been performed as a diagnostic test. The variable for each modality that has been most commonly used to define an abnormal test includes standard ETT, greater than or equal to 1 mm horizontal or downsloping ST segment depression measured 0.06 to 0.08 seconds after the J point; SPECT or PET, a perfusion abnormality; and echocardiography, a regional wall motion abnormality (**Fig. 1**). Diagnostic test accuracy is expressed in terms of sensitivity (true-positives/true-positives + false-negatives) and specificity (true-negatives/true-negatives + false-positives). Average values for sensitivity are higher for the imaging procedures (SPECT, 87%; echocardiography, 86%) than ETT (68%); values for specificity are similar (SPECT, 73%; echocardiography 81%; ETT, 77%).[1,5,6]

Impact of Verification Bias on Diagnostic Accuracy

The gold standard for diagnosing CAD is the presence of a significant stenosis (defined as ≥50% or ≥70% diameter narrowing) in a major epicardial vessel by invasive coronary angiography. A stress test is not a definitive diagnostic study because the results of the test provide only the posttest probability that CAD is present or absent. The results of the stress test must be verified against the findings at coronary angiography. Nearly all studies that have been performed to address the diagnostic accuracy of stress testing have examined the minority subset of patients who are referred for coronary angiography following stress testing. Because coronary angiography is more likely to be performed in patients with positive versus negative stress test results, the angiographic subset is dominated by patients with positive test results. This concept, known as verification or posttest referral bias, drives sensitivity to 100% (many more true-positives than false-negatives) and specificity to 0% (many more false-positives than true-negatives).[7,8] The only pure approach to avoid the impact of verification bias on sensitivity and specificity is to design a study in which all patients who present for evaluation of CAD are referred for coronary angiography irrespective of the results of stress testing. The single study that applied this design using standard ETT reported test sensitivity of 45%, compared with mean sensitivity of 68% reported by meta-analysis.[9] Another approach to adjust

for verification bias applies a mathematical correction based on statistical modeling to the derived values for sensitivity and specificity.[10–12] Studies performed at the Mayo Clinic using this approach reported substantially lower values for sensitivity after adjustment for referral bias (for men, SPECT 98% to 67% and echocardiography 78% to 39%) and for specificity higher values after adjustment (SPECT 9% to 64%, echocardiography 44% to 81%).[11,12] These findings show that the diagnostic accuracy of all stress testing modalities is only modest. In particular, true test sensitivity is lower than is commonly appreciated.

Stress Testing for Risk Stratification

The major role of stress testing has evolved from use as a diagnostic test to application as a prognostic tool. American College of Cardiology (ACC)/American Heart Association (AHA) guidelines define clinical risk from annual mortality: low (<1%), intermediate (1%–3%), or high (>3%).[13] The results of stress testing can be applied to categorize patients into these risk categories. General recommendations for patient management include referring most high-risk patients to coronary angiography versus proceeding with observation and, when indicated, medical therapy alone for most low-risk patients. Management of patients categorized as intermediate risk is less certain and commonly involves additional testing in an attempt to clarify risk with greater certainty as low or high. For diagnostic purposes the stress testing modalities focus on a single variable (ST segment depression, perfusion abnormality, regional wall motion abnormality) analyzed in a dichotomous manner (positive or negative). For risk stratification purposes the stress testing modalities analyze multiple variables in a continuous fashion. The more severely abnormal the test result, the greater likelihood that the patient has severe anatomic (left main and/or 3-vessel) CAD and worse clinical outcome. In contrast with diagnostic studies that include only the minority subset of patients who are referred for angiography, prognostic studies involve measuring clinical outcome in all patients, except those who undergo early revascularization. Early revascularization is defined as percutaneous coronary intervention (PCI) or coronary artery bypass grafting (CABG) performed within the first 2 to 3 months following the stress test. The results of the stress test are major factors influencing the decision to proceed with early revascularization. By convention, these patients are excluded from analysis because they have received a treatment not administered to the rest of the population that potentially could affect the clinical outcome.

Risk Stratification by Standard ETT

Several variables that can be measured during standard ETT have prognostic value.[14,15] The most important prognostic variable is exercise duration.[1,14–19] Increasing exercise duration is associated with a decreasing risk of left main/ 3-vessel CAD and lower risk of death.[17,18,20] In one study only 0.4% of patients with exercise capacity greater than or equal to 10 METs (completion of the third stage or more of the Bruce protocol) had ischemia measuring greater than or equal to 10% of the left ventricle by SPECT.[21] Other important prognostic variables include abnormal responses of blood pressure or heart rate during or after exercise.[14,15] The most reliable definition of a hypotensive blood pressure response is systolic blood pressure during exercise that is lower than the preexercise measurement.[22] It can indicate inadequate cardiac output during exercise caused by severe CAD and/or poor left ventricular function.[23,24] Chronotropic incompetence is defined as peak exercise heart rate less than 80% of the predicted value,[14] or less than 62% or patients on β-blockers.[25] Impaired heart rate recovery is defined as failure of the heart rate to decrease during the first minute after exercise by 12 beats/min if upright or 15 beats/min if supine.[14] Both chronotropic incompetence and impaired heart rate recovery are adverse prognostic indicators.[25–28] In general, angina and ST segment depression, although useful for diagnosing CAD, are weak prognostic variables. The prognostic significance of frequent ventricular ectopy during or after exercise is controversial.[15]

Risk Stratification by Treadmill Scores

Several years ago McNeer and colleagues[20] showed an association between the combination of treadmill duration and exercise ECG results with severe CAD at angiography (Table 1). Patients who could complete only the first or second stage of the Bruce protocol and who also had an ischemic ECG had an approximate 25% prevalence of left main CAD and a 50% to 75% prevalence of 3-vessel CAD. Since that time several stress test scores that incorporate multiple stress test variables based on statistical multivariable models have been published.[29–31] These scores are designed to determine a single composite variable that can be used to categorize risk. The most extensively validated and widely applied score is the Duke treadmill score.[32,33] This score consists of only 3 variables and can easily be calculated:

Duke treadmill score =
exercise duration (minutes Bruce protocol) -
(5 × ST segment deviation) (mm) -
(4 × angina index) (0 = no angina;
1 = nonlimiting angina; 2 = limiting angina)

The risk categories that are derived using this score include low (score $\geq +5$), intermediate (score -10 to $+4$), and high (score ≤ -11). **Fig. 2** shows that accurate risk stratification can be achieved by applying this score. Annual cardiovascular mortality for low-risk patients is only 0.25%. Studies of primarily outpatients undergoing evaluation of stable CAD have shown that most (60%–80%) patients can be categorized as low risk from the Duke treadmill score.[33,34] The accuracy of the Duke treadmill score can be enhanced by incorporating additional clinical and exercise test variables into the model (**Fig. 3**).[35] The expanded model more accurately risk stratifies a population primarily by correctly identifying more low-risk patients. The disadvantage of the expanded model is its greater complexity, limiting its ease of clinical applicability.

Risk Stratification with SPECT

One of the major strengths of nuclear perfusion imaging is the abundant prognostic literature that has been generated using stress SPECT. A meta-analysis of nearly 70,000 patients showed an approximate 7-fold to 8-fold difference in annual rates of cardiac death or myocardial infarction when test results were analyzed simply as normal/ low risk versus abnormal/high risk (**Fig. 4**).[36] Patients who undergo pharmacologic testing in general are sicker than those who undergo exercise stress. Event rates in pharmacologic patients are modestly higher than in exercise patients. Risk stratification can be further refined when abnormal perfusion images are interpreted from the extent and severity of the perfusion defect. The left ventricle is divided into 17 segments, and a perfusion grade based on the intensity of isotope uptake is assigned to each segment using a 5-point scoring system.[37] This grading scheme can be applied to the stress images (summed stress score [SSS]) and to the rest images (summed rest score [SRS]). The difference between SSS and SRS is the summed difference score (SDS). SSS is a reflection of the extent and severity of combined infarction and ischemia. It is the strongest prognostic perfusion variable and can refine risk stratification of patients within categories of the Duke treadmill score (**Fig. 5**).[38] SDS is a reflection of the extent and severity of ischemia. SDS can be converted into the percent of the left ventricle that is ischemic by dividing SDS by 68 if using the 17-segment model (68 is the theoretic maximal

A
Electrocardiogram - Exercise

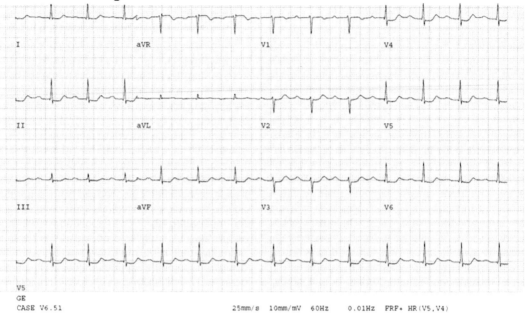

B
Electrocardiogram - Rest

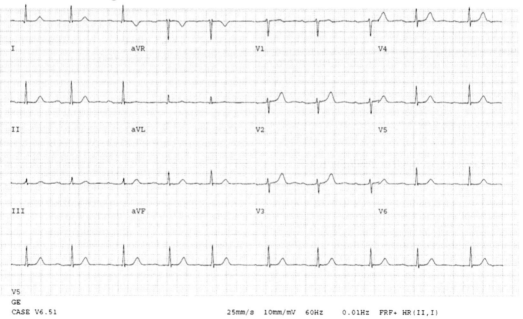

Fig. 1. Examples of abnormal stress test results. (*A, B*) Standard ETT showing 1-mm horizontal ST segment depression. (*C*) SPECT images showing a medium-sized partially reversible inferolateral wall perfusion defect. Top, stress; Bottom, rest. (*D*) Stress echocardiography showing a large reversible anterior, septal, and apical wall motion abnormality. Left-sided images, rest; Right-sided images, stress.

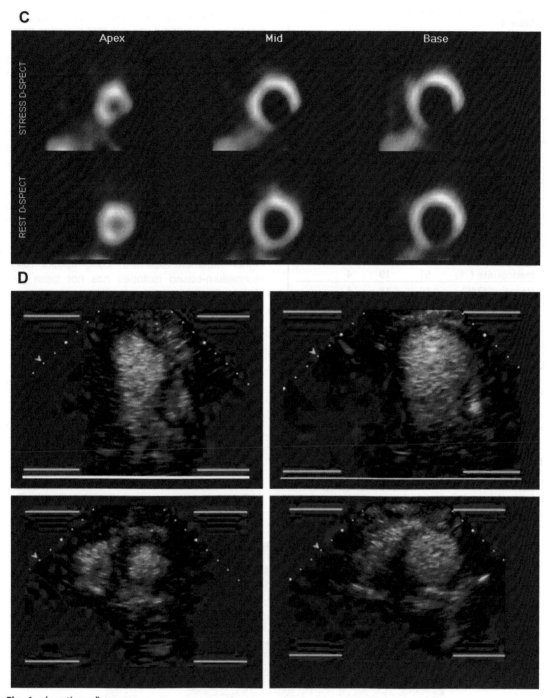

Fig. 1. (*continued*)

value for SDS if the entire left ventricle was severely ischemic). Hachamovitch and colleagues[39] reported in an observational study that an ischemic burden of 10% of the left ventricle was the threshold that separated a survival advantage between treatment with medical therapy (small ischemic burden) versus revascularization (large ischemic burden). This threshold is being applied as the SPECT entry criterion for the International Study of Comparative Health Effectiveness with Medical and Invasive Approaches (ISCHEMIA) trial, which will test the hypothesis that patients with large ischemic burden have improved outcome when treated by optimal medical therapy plus revascularization versus medical therapy alone in a prospective, randomized manner.[40]

Table 1
Relationship of stage entered and ST segment interpretation, in combination, to presence and extent of significant CAD

	CAD	3VD	>50% LMC
Stage I			
Positive (51)	98	73	27
Inadequate (34)	71	40	12
Negative (79)	52	21	10
Stage II			
Positive (159)	97	51	24
Inadequate (104)	65	27	8
Negative (186)	48	21	3
Stage III			
Positive (115)	86	41	10
Inadequate (75)	51	19	4
Negative (248)	46	11	4
≥Stage IV			
Positive (104)	77	29	5
Inadequate (37)	46	14	0
Negative (280)	36	9	1

Abbreviation: 3VD, 3-vessel coronary artery disease; LMC, left main coronary artery disease.

Adapted from McNeer J, Margolis J, Lee K, et al. The role of the exercise test in the evaluation of patients for ischemic heart disease. Circulation 1978;57(1):66.

Other SPECT Prognostic Variables

SPECT can be performed with gating to provide information on left ventricular volumes at rest and after stress, and left ventricular ejection fraction, regional thickening, and wall motion.[41] Ejection fraction is a powerful variable that provides prognostic information independent from the perfusion variables.[42] Significant enlargement of the left ventricle after stress compared with rest is termed transient ischemic dilatation. Transient ischemic dilatation is another important prognostic variable.[43] It can be a marker of left main CAD and can be especially useful to identify the infrequent patient whose SPECT images reveal little or no ischemia,[44] in whom balanced ischemia may be present. In the past, increased lung uptake assessed primarily by planar thallium imaging was also an important prognostic variable but is no longer commonly assessed. Compared with technetium-based isotopes, thallium usage is decreasing because of poor count statistics and higher radiation exposure. Lung uptake using technetium-based isotopes has not been well standardized.

Stress PET for Risk Stratification

Myocardial perfusion imaging can also be performed with PET. The prognostic value of stress PET has been shown but the literature is not as extensive as the SPECT literature.[45,46] Most stress PET is performed using pharmacologic stress. Exercise stress is feasible but challenging because of the short half-lives of PET perfusion agents (rubidium-82, 75 seconds; ammonia-13, 10 minutes). Stress PET is otherwise analogous to stress SPECT with provision of summed rest and stress scores, volumes, and ejection fraction.

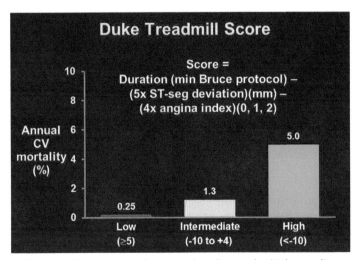

Fig. 2. Clinical outcome for outpatients expressed as annual cardiovascular (CV) mortality according to categories of the Duke treadmill score. (*Data from* Mark DB, Shaw L, Harrell FE Jr, et al. Prognostic value of a treadmill exercise score in outpatients with suspected coronary artery disease [see comments]. N Engl J Med 1991;325(12):852.)

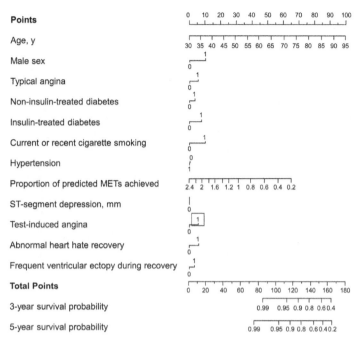

Fig. 3. A more complex nomogram based on clinical and exercise test variables for predicting mortality. (*From* Lauer MS, Pothier CE, Magid DJ, et al. An externally validated model for predicting long-term survival after exercise treadmill testing in patients with suspected coronary artery disease and a normal electrocardiogram. Ann Intern Med 2007;147(12):826; with permission.)

Stress Echocardiography for Risk Stratification

Stress echocardiography for assessment of CAD predominantly uses wall motion abnormalities to detect infarction, ischemia, or their combination.[4,47] The presence or absence of stress-induced ischemia (the development of new wall motion abnormalities or worsening wall motion abnormalities) has been the most commonly used diagnostic criteria and prognostic tool for stress echocardiography. Stress echocardiography responses follow 4 basic patterns centered on wall motion assessment: normal (normal at rest and normal or hyperkinetic during stress); ischemic

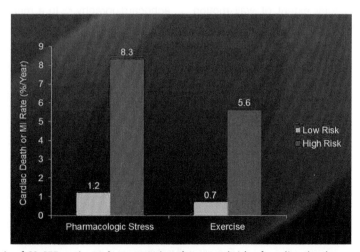

Fig. 4. Meta-analysis of 69,655 patients demonstrating the annual risk of cardiac death or myocardial infarction (MI) for patients with a normal or low-risk SPECT image versus those with a moderately to severely abnormal SPECT image. (*Data from* Shaw LJ, Iskandrian AE. Prognostic value of gated myocardial perfusion SPECT. J Nucl Cardiol 2004;11(2):180.)

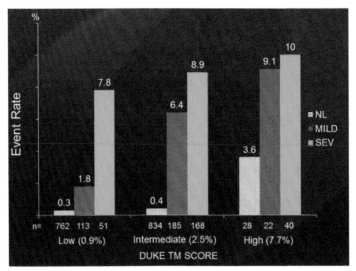

Fig. 5. An observational study from Cedars Sinai Medical Center showing the incremental prognostic value of SPECT imaging across categories of the Duke treadmill (TM) score. NL, normal; SEV, severe. (*Data from* Hachamovitch R, Berman DS, Kiat H, et al. Exercise myocardial perfusion SPECT in patients without known coronary artery disease: incremental prognostic value and use in risk stratification. Circulation 1996;93(5):910.)

(normal at rest to hypokinetic, akinetic, or dyskinetic during stress); infarcted, fixed, or necrotic (resting wall motion abnormality that remains fixed during stress); and viable (resting wall motion abnormalities with sustained improvement or biphasic response during stress).

The left ventricle can be divided into 16 segments with each segment scored on its contractility using a 5-point scale (score 1–5). A wall motion score index (WMSI) can be calculated by summing the scores for each segment and dividing by the total number of segments with a normal WMSI equaling 1. A worsening stress WMSI reflecting the total extent of wall motion abnormalities is associated with an increasing

cardiac event rate (**Fig. 6**).[48–51] Similar to SPECT, stress echocardiography has shown the ability to provide prognostic information that is incremental to clinical characteristics and exercise data as well as the ability to subclassify patients with low-risk, intermediate-risk, and high-risk Duke treadmill scores.[48] Additional prognostic variables of stress echocardiography include the left ventricular end-systolic volume response to stress. An abnormal response (no change or increase) in left ventricular end-systolic volume is an important prognostic variable in predicting cardiac outcome in patients undergoing exercise stress echocardiography.[52] In a meta-analysis involving more than 3000 patients, the annual risk of

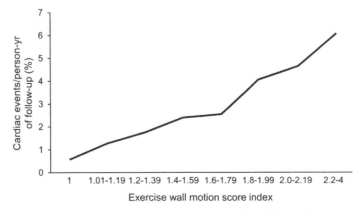

Fig. 6. The association between cardiac event rate and exercise WMSI in 5798 patients who underwent exercise echocardiography. (*From* Arruda-Olson AM, Juracan EM, Mahoney DW, et al. Prognostic value of exercise echocardiography in 5798 patients: is there a gender difference? J Am Coll Cardiol 2002;39(4):630; with permission.)

cardiac death or myocardial infarction with normal exercise echocardiography was 0.54%.[53]

Comparison Between Standard ETT and Stress Imaging

The major advantage of standard ETT is its lower cost. The 2013 Medicare relative value unit (RVU) for ETT is 2.48 (current procedural terminology [CPT] code 93015) versus an RVU for stress echo of 6.78 (CPT code 93351-6) and for stress SPECT 14.38 (CPT code 78452-6).[54] The standard ETT is also more widely available and less technically demanding. The important prognostic variables of exercise duration, symptoms, heart rate and blood pressure readings, ischemic ECG changes, and ventricular ectopy can be accurately measured in all patients. Advantages of the imaging modalities compared with standard ETT include higher diagnostic sensitivity, provision of incremental prognostic information, ability to localize and quantify ischemia, and direct measurement of volumes and ejection fraction.

Standard ETT Versus Stress Imaging in the Presence of a Normal Resting ECG

Although stress imaging is superior to standard ETT for diagnostic and prognostic assessment, a key question is whether these expensive imaging modalities are more accurate and cost-effective for risk stratification in clinical settings in which the standard ETT performs well. To address this issue, Christian and colleagues[55] performed a key study that compared the accuracy of ETT versus SPECT, both for correctly identifying patients with left main/3-vessel CAD at angiography and predicting clinical outcome. The study population consisted of 411 patients, all of whom had a normal resting ECG. The rationale for including only patients with a normal resting ECG was 2-fold: (1) approximately 95% of patients with a normal resting ECG have a normal ejection fraction when directly measured by a variety of imaging techniques,[56–59] and (2) the specificity of the exercise ECG is much higher when the resting ECG is normal.[1,60] The statistical methodology applied a reclassification approach to determine what percentage of the population was correctly classified according to a statistical model consisting of only clinical plus standard ETT variables versus a model that also included the SPECT variables. The results of the study are shown in **Fig. 7**. Only 3% of the population was correctly reclassified by the SPECT model. Most of the correct reclassifications resulted by shifting patients from the intermediate-risk category to the low-risk category. The SPECT model did not detect more

patients with left main/3-vessel CAD. A cost analysis concluded that adding SPECT to standard ETT was not cost-effective for identification of severe CAD in this population. Also, there was no difference in prediction of clinical outcome by either model.

Choosing Between Standard ETT Versus Stress Imaging

The optimal approach for accurate risk stratification involves initially selecting a low-cost test that provides definitive results for most of the population and categorizes a small number of patients as intermediate risk. In general, studies of cost-effectiveness show that applying a low-cost test to an entire population with selective use of more expensive testing at a second stage for patients with intermediate risk or indeterminate results is more cost-effective than applying the more expensive test as the initial step in the entire population. **Table 2** summarizes the ACC/AHA guidelines approach for selecting between standard ETT and stress imaging.[13] Ability to adequately exercise conveys an estimated exercise capacity of at least 5 minutes on the Bruce protocol. Five minutes is the minimal duration necessary to reach a Duke treadmill score of 5 and categorization as low risk in the absence of angina and ischemic ECG changes. Functional capacity can be estimated from a simple clinical questionnaire.[61] An abnormal resting ECG is defined as left bundle branch block, paced ventricular rhythm, ventricular preexcitation, or greater than or equal to 1 mm ST segment depression. Patients with milder abnormalities on the resting ECG including less than 1 mm ST segment deflection and/or T wave inversion are candidates for the standard ETT. The rationale for recommending imaging in patients with prior PCI or CABG relates to the higher prevalence of resting ECG abnormalities in these patients and the importance of localizing ischemia if another revascularization procedure is contemplated.

Choosing Between SPECT and Echocardiography

Although a few studies have compared the diagnostic or prognostic accuracy of SPECT and stress echocardiography,[62,63] there is no large, carefully designed study applying current imaging technologies performed in the setting of well-established imaging laboratories to conclusively prove the superiority of one imaging technique to another. A meta-analysis reported that normal images by both techniques accurately identify low-risk patients: annualized risk of cardiac death or

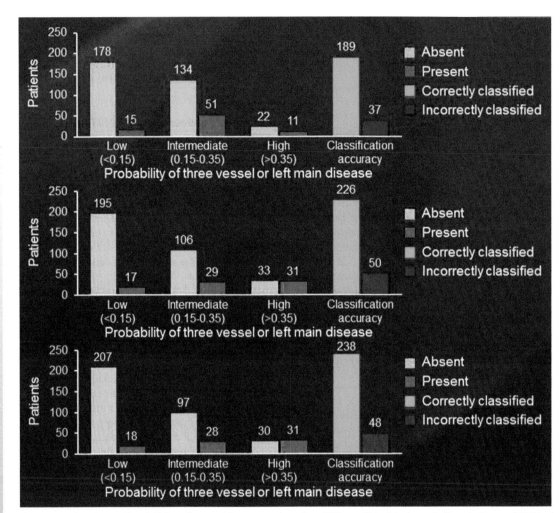

Fig. 7. Results of a study of 411 patients with a normal resting ECG predicted to have left main/3-vessel CAD at angiography by standard ETT and the percentage of the population correctly reclassified by SPECT. Top, clinical variables alone; Middle, clinical plus ETT variables; Bottom, clinical, ETT, plus SPECT variables. Patients were considered to be correctly classified if predicted to have left main/3-vessel CAD and angiography showed left main/3-vessel CAD or if predicted not to have left main/3-vessel CAD and angiography showed that left main/3-vessel CAD was not present. Patients categorized as unclassified were those with intermediate probability of left main/3-vessel CAD. (*Data from* Christian TF, Miller TD, Bailey KR, et al. Exercise tomographic thallium-201 imaging in patients with severe coronary artery disease and normal electrocardiograms [see comments]. Ann Intern Med 1994;121(11):829.)

myocardial infarction by SPECT, 0.45%; and by echocardiography, 0.54%.[53] The Multimodality Appropriate Use Criteria for Stable Ischemic Heart Disease assigned identical appropriateness ratings to both modalities for 79 of 80 test indications.[64] Recommendations for selecting between these modalities are based on local expertise in performing each technique and the characteristics of the patient. Local expertise depends on many factors including the training of the individuals interpreting the studies; the volume of studies performed; and, perhaps most importantly, a center's experience with the reported test results. Selected

patient characteristics can lead to relative advantages for each technique. Relative advantages of SPECT and PET include greater likelihood of technically adequate images in patients with obesity and chronic obstructive pulmonary disease; higher confidence with image interpretation in patients with regional wall motion abnormalities at rest; and more extensive validation of the methodology, including the development of scoring systems that have been prospectively validated in multiple nuclear cardiology imaging laboratories. Relative advantages of echocardiography include modestly lower cost, no exposure to ionizing radiation,

Table 2
Selection of ETT or stress imaging as the initial testing strategy in patients with stable CAD

	ETT	Imaging
Ability to exercise	Able	Unable
Prior PCI/CABG	No	Yes
Resting ECG	Normal/near normal	Abnormal[a]

[a] Left bundle branch block, paced; Wolff-Parkinson-White syndrome, greater than or equal to 1 mm ST decrease.

Adapted from Gibbons RJ, Chatterjee K, Daley J, et al. ACC/AHA/ACP-ASIM guidelines for the management of patients with chronic stable angina: a report of the American College of Cardiology/American Heart Association Task Force on Practice guidelines (Committee on the Management of Patients with Chronic Stable Angina). J Am Coll Cardiol 1999;33:2092–97; with permission.

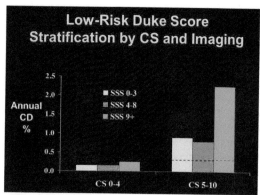

Fig. 8. Annual cardiac death (CD) rates for 1461 patients, all of whom had a low-risk Duke treadmill score, categorized by clinical risk and SPECT image results. For patients with low clinical risk (clinical score [CS] 0–4), cardiac death rates were extremely low even if SPECT images were severely abnormal (SSS 9+). (Adapted from Poornima IG, Miller TD, Christian TF, et al. Utility of myocardial perfusion imaging in patients with low risk treadmill scores. J Am Coll Cardiol 2004;43:196; with permission.)

and more comprehensive evaluation that includes assessment of cardiac valves and diastolic function.

Correct Interpretation of a Stress Imaging Study

A mistake that occasionally happens in clinical practice is overreliance on the image results and minimizing of other important prognostic data. Accurate risk stratification of a patient necessitates interpreting the image results in the context of all available clinical and stress test information. Studies have shown that the same perfusion abnormality on stress SPECT has different prognostic implications based on clinical characteristics of the patient. Poornima and colleagues[65] showed in a study of 1461 patients with a low-risk Duke treadmill score that those with low-risk clinical characteristics had an excellent outcome regardless of the results of SPECT imaging. Seven-year cardiac survival was 99% even for those with severely abnormal SSS (**Fig. 8**). Fine and colleagues[66] similarly reported low annual all-cause mortality (0.84%) and cardiovascular mortality (0.25%) in patients with severe ischemia on echocardiography but with excellent ($\geq$10 METs) exercise capacity. In contrast, normal or equivocally normal SPECT perfusion images may not be associated with a benign outcome in patients with other selected high-risk indicators, including a high-risk Duke treadmill score, an ischemic ECG during pharmacologic stress testing using a vasodilating agent, or transient ischemic dilatation. Hachamovitch and colleagues[38] reported a 19-month event rate of cardiac death or nonfatal myocardial

infarction of 3.6% for patients with normal SPECT images and a high-risk Duke treadmill score, which was substantially higher than the event rate for patients with normal images and either a low-risk (0.3%) or intermediate-risk (0.4%) Duke score. Annual cardiac event rates for patients with normal SPECT images but ischemic ECG changes during adenosine SPECT have been reported to be as high as 4% to 5%, which is considerably more than the rate of less than or equal to 1% that is usually found in patients with normal images.[67,68] Berman and colleagues[44] reported that 13% of 101 patients with left main CAD had a small ($\leq$5% of the left ventricle) perfusion defect. Most of these patients could be identified by transient ischemic dilatation.

Recent Randomized Trials of Stress Testing

Most of the literature evaluating the accuracy and clinical value of stress testing derives from observational data. In the ACC/AHA guidelines addressing standard ETT, SPECT, and echocardiography, less than 1% of studies received the top level of evidence (A) rating.[69] Two recent studies examined the risk stratification value of stress testing in a prospective randomized manner. In the Detection of Ischemia in Asymptomatic Diabetics (DIAD) study, 1123 asymptomatic patients with type II diabetes were randomized to a strategy of screening using adenosine low-level exercise SPECT versus no screening.[70] Although SPECT could effectively risk stratify the population, the annual cardiac event rate for the study population during follow-up was very low at 0.6%, and there were no differences in outcome between the groups (**Fig. 9**).[71] In the What is the Optimal Method for Ischemia Evaluation in Women (WOMEN) trial, 824 symptomatic women with intermediate likelihood of CAD were randomized to a testing strategy of standard ETT versus exercise SPECT.[72] There were only 17 events during an average follow-up of 2 years. There were no differences in outcome between testing arms (survival free of major adverse events 98% for ETT and 97.7% for SPECT; $P = .59$), and cumulative costs were lower with the standard ETT (mean total costs for ETT $337.80 and $643.24 for SPECT; $P<.001$).

Stress Imaging Substudies in Recent Randomized Trials

Three large prospective, randomized trials compared treatment strategies of medical therapy alone with medical therapy plus revascularization in various populations of patients with CAD: Clinical Outcomes Using Revascularization and Aggressive Drug Evaluation (COURAGE),[73] Bypass Angioplasty Revascularization Investigation 2 Diabetes (BARI 2D),[74] and Surgical Treatment for Ischemic Heart Failure (STICH).[75] All 3 trials

contained stress imaging substudies. SPECT was performed in all of the trials, and stress echocardiography was also performed in STICH. COURAGE, BARI 2D, and STICH were designed and performed as randomized controlled trials, but the imaging substudies were not randomized. In COURAGE, 2 imaging substudies applying different methodologies were performed. In the first COURAGE substudy, paired SPECT imaging was performed at baseline and at 1 year of follow-up to measure ischemia reduction (defined as a reduction in the amount of ischemia by at least 5% of the left ventricle on the second study). There was a favorable trend toward 5-year survival free of death or myocardial infarction in patients with versus without ischemia reduction: 13.4% versus 24.7% (unadjusted $P = .037$, risk-adjusted $P = .26$) (**Fig. 10**).[76] Ischemia reduction was more effectively achieved with PCI versus medical therapy alone (33% vs 19% of the population; $P = .004$). However, in the second COURAGE imaging substudy, which examined clinical outcome from the amount of ischemia on the baseline SPECT study according to treatment assignment, 7-year event rates were similar between 18% and 22% for all patient subsets, regardless of the amount of ischemia (small or large) or treatment assignment (medical therapy

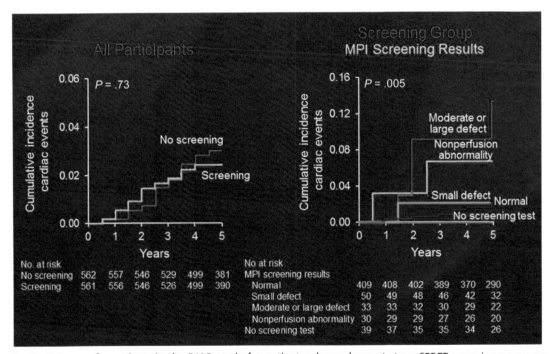

Fig. 9. Outcomes for patients in the DIAD study for patients who underwent stress SPECT screening versus no screening. MPI, myocardial perfusion imaging. (*Data from* Young LH, Wackers FJ, Chyun DA, et al. Cardiac outcomes after screening for asymptomatic coronary artery disease in patients with type 2 diabetes: the DIAD study: a randomized controlled trial. J Am Med Assoc 2009;301:1550.)

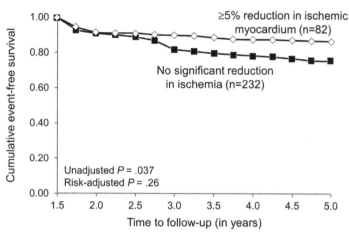

Fig. 10. Results from the first COURAGE imaging substudy showing a trend for better outcome in patients who achieved greater than or equal to 5% reduction in ischemic myocardium over a 1-year period. (*From* Shaw LJ, Berman DS, Maron DJ, et al. Optimal medical therapy with or without percutaneous coronary intervention to reduce ischemic burden: results from the Clinical Outcomes Utilizing Revascularization and Aggressive Drug Evaluation (COURAGE) trial nuclear substudy. Circulation 2008;117(10):1288; with permission.)

alone or PCI) (**Fig. 11**).[77] In the BARI 2D SPECT substudy, SSS and SRS, expressed as percentages of abnormal myocardium, were significantly associated with outcome (SSS, $P = .005$; SRS, $P = .002$). However, the percent ischemic myocardium was not associated with outcome ($P = .271$), and there was no interaction between any of the SPECT variables and treatment assignment.[78] In the STICH imaging substudy, the presence of ischemia by SPECT or echocardiography did not predict outcome ($P = .157$), and there was no

interaction between ischemia and treatment assignment (medical therapy alone or CABG) for the end point of mortality ($P = .643$) or any of the other study end points.[79] The results from these recent imaging studies question the importance of ischemia as a prognostic variable. These results stand in marked contrast with the extensive literature generated earlier from observational studies showing the value of stress SPECT and echocardiography for risk stratification. These results also fail to support the hypothesis that the ischemic

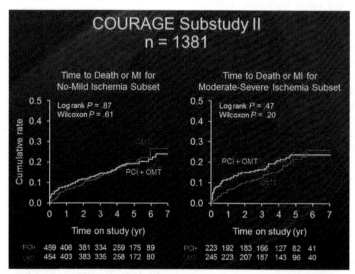

Fig. 11. Results from the second COURAGE imaging substudy showing similar outcomes for all patient subsets regardless of the amount of ischemia by SPECT at baseline or treatment assignment. OMT, optimal medical therapy. (*From* Shaw LJ, Weintraub WS, Maron DJ, et al. Baseline stress myocardial perfusion imaging results and outcomes in patients with stable ischemic heart disease randomized to optimal medical therapy with or without percutaneous coronary intervention. Am Heart J 2012;164(2):247; with permission.)

burden can be used to select optimal treatment of CAD. This hypothesis will be more rigorously tested in the ISCHEMIA trial.

Future Directions

Most studies that have evaluated standard ETT and stress imaging were based on old methodologies. Several newer technologies offer the potential to improve noninvasive assessment of CAD. The use of expanded, more complex algorithms incorporating multiple clinical and exercise variables to maximize the risk stratifying potential of standard ETT is being simplified by the use of hand-held electronic devices that facilitate application of these algorithms in the clinical practice setting. Several advances to enhance the accuracy of stress echocardiography have been developed, including administration of contrast agents, three-dimensional imaging, assessment of stress diastolic function, and strain imaging.[80–85] Advances in SPECT imaging include the introduction of ultrafast camera systems that replace sodium-iodide crystal technology with cadmium-zinc-telluride solid-state detectors, resulting in better image resolution, shorter imaging times, and less radiation exposure.[86,87] PET advances include the introduction of computer software programs for quantification of myocardial blood flow and investigation of a new perfusion agent (flurpiridaz), which has a longer half-life than currently available agents, to facilitate performing exercise PET and as well as potentially improving accuracy.[88] Stress cardiac magnetic resonance imaging represents a newer but increasingly used technique that can assess both perfusion and function, perhaps more comprehensively than any other technique.[89] Computed tomography (CT) angiography represents another noninvasive modality for assessing CAD that is based on coronary artery anatomy rather than physiology. The Prospective Multicenter Imaging Study for Evaluation of Chest Pain (PROMISE) is a prospective, randomized trial comparing CT angiography with stress testing, including ETT, SPECT, or echocardiography.[90] The results of this trial should be available in the near future to help determine which modality most efficiently categorizes specific patient subsets.

REFERENCES

1. Gibbons RJ, Balady GJ, Bricker JT, et al. ACC/AHA 2002 guidelines update for exercise testing: a report of the American College of Cardiology/American Heart Association Task Force on Practice Guidelines (Committee on Exercise Testing). American College of Cardiology website. Available at: http://wwwaccorg/clinical/guidelines/exercise/exercise_cleanpdf. Accessed March 14, 2014.

2. Fletcher GF, Ades PA, Kligfield P, et al. Exercise standards for testing and training: a scientific statement from the American Heart Association. Circulation 2013;128(8):873–934.

3. DePuey EG, Mahmarian JJ, Miller TD, et al. Patient-centered imaging. J Nucl Cardiol 2012;19:185–215.

4. Pellikka PA, Nagueh SF, Elhendy AA, et al. American Society of Echocardiography recommendations for performance, interpretation, and application of stress echocardiography. J Am Soc Echocardiogr 2007;20(9):1021–41.

5. Klocke FJ, Baird MG, Bateman TM, et al. ACC/AHA/ASNC guidelines for the clinical use of cardiac radionuclide imaging: a report of the American College of Cardiology/American Heart Association Task Force on Practice Guidelines (ACC/AHA/ASNC Committee to Revise the 1995 Guidelines for the Clinical Use of Cardiac Radionuclide Imaging). American College of Cardiology website. Available at: http://wwwaccorg/clinical/guidelines/radio/rni_fulltextpdf. Accessed March 14, 2014.

6. Cheitlin MD, Armstrong WF, Aurigemma GP, et al. ACC/AHA/ASE 2003 guideline update for the clinical application of echocardiography. A Report of the American College of Cardiology/American Heart Association Task Force on Practice Guidelines (ACC/AHA/ASE Committee to Update the 1997 Guidelines for the Clinical Application of Echocardiography). J Am Coll Cardiol 2003;42:954–70.

7. Begg CB, Greenes RA. Assessment of diagnostic tests when disease verification is subject to selection bias. Biometrics 1983;39:207–15.

8. Diamond GA. Reverend Bayes' silent majority: an alternative factor affecting sensitivity and specificity of exercise electrocardiography. Am J Cardiol 1986;57(13):1175–80.

9. Froelicher VF, Lehmann KG, Thomas R, et al. The electrocardiographic exercise test in a population with reduced workup bias: diagnostic performance, computerized interpretation, and multivariable prediction. Ann Intern Med 1998;128(1):965–74.

10. Morise AP, Diamond GA. Comparison of the sensitivity and specificity of exercise electrocardiography in biased and unbiased populations of men and women. Am Heart J 1995;130(4):741–7.

11. Roger VL, Pellikka PA, Bell MR, et al. Sex and test verification bias: impact on the diagnostic value of exercise echocardiography. Circulation 1997;95(2):405–10.

12. Miller TD, Hodge DO, Christian TF, et al. Effects of adjustment for referral bias on the sensitivity and specificity of single photon emission computed tomography for the diagnosis of coronary artery disease. Am J Med 2002;112:290–7.

13. Gibbons RJ, Chatterjee K, Daley J, et al. ACC/AHA/ACP-ASIM guidelines for the management of patients with chronic stable angina: a report of the American College of Cardiology/American Heart Association Task Force on Practice guidelines (Committee on the Management of Patients with Chronic Stable Angina). J Am Coll Cardiol 1999;33:2092–97.

14. Kligfield P, Lauer MS. Exercise electrocardiogram testing: beyond the ST segment. Circulation 2006; 114:2070–82.

15. Miller TD. The exercise treadmill test: estimating cardiovascular prognosis. Cleve Clin J Med 2008; 75(6):424–30.

16. Blair SN, Kohl HW 3rd, Paffenbarger RS Jr, et al. Physical fitness and all-cause mortality. A prospective study of healthy men and women. J Am Med Assoc 1989;262(17):2395–401.

17. Gulati M, Black HR, Shaw LJ, et al. The prognostic value of a nomogram for exercise capacity in women. N Engl J Med 2005;353:468–75.

18. Myers J, Prakash M, Froelicher VF, et al. Exercise capacity and mortality among men referred for exercise testing. N Engl J Med 2002;346(11):793–801.

19. Mark DB, Lauer MS. Exercise capacity: the prognostic variable that doesn't get enough respect. Circulation 2003;108(13):1534–6.

20. McNeer J, Margolis J, Lee K, et al. The role of the exercise test in the evaluation of patients for ischemic heart disease. Circulation 1978;57(1):64–70.

21. Bourque JM, Holland BH, Watson DD, et al. Achieving an exercise workload of > or =10 metabolic equivalents predicts a very low risk of inducible ischemia: does myocardial perfusion imaging have a role? J Am Coll Cardiol 2009;54(6):538–45.

22. Dubach P, Froelicher VF, Klein J, et al. Exercise-induced hypotension in a male population. Criteria, causes, and prognosis. Circulation 1988;78(6): 1380–7.

23. Hakki AH, Munley BM, Hadjimiltiades S, et al. Determinants of abnormal blood pressure response to exercise in coronary artery disease. Am J Cardiol 1986;57:71–5.

24. Hammermeister KE, DeRouen TA, Dodge HT, et al. Prognostic and predictive value of exertional hypotension in suspected coronary artery disease. Am J Cardiol 1983;51:1261–5.

25. Khan MN, Pothier CE, Lauer MS. Chronotropic incompetence as a predictor of death among patients with normal electrograms taking beta blockers (metoprolol or atenolol). Am J Cardiol 2005;96:1328–33.

26. Lauer MS, Francis GS, Okin PM, et al. Impaired chronotropic response to exercise stress testing as a predictor of mortality. J Am Med Assoc 1999;281:524–9.

27. Lauer MS, Okin PM, Larson MG, et al. Impaired heart rate response to graded exercise: prognostic implications of chronotropic incompetence in the Framingham Heart Study. Circulation 1996;93: 1520–6.

28. Cole CR, Foody JM, Blackstone EH, et al. Heart rate recovery after submaximal exercise testing as a predictor of mortality in a cardiovascular healthy cohort. Ann Intern Med 2000; 132:552–5.

29. Froelicher VF, Morrow K, Brown M, et al. Prediction of atherosclerotic cardiovascular death in men using a prognostic score. Am J Cardiol 1994;73(2): 133–8.

30. Prakash M, Myers J, Froelicher VF, et al. Clinical and exercise test predictors of all-cause mortality: results from >6,000 consecutive referred male patients. Chest 2001;120(3):1003–13.

31. Morise AP, Jalisi F. Evaluation of pretest and exercise test scores to assess all-cause mortality in unselected patients presenting for exercise testing with symptoms of suspected coronary artery disease. J Am Coll Cardiol 2003;42:842–50.

32. Mark DB, Hlatky MA, Harrell FE Jr, et al. Exercise treadmill score for predicting prognosis in coronary artery disease. Ann Intern Med 1987;106(6): 793–800.

33. Mark DB, Shaw L, Harrell FE Jr, et al. Prognostic value of a treadmill exercise score in outpatients with suspected coronary artery disease [see comments]. N Engl J Med 1991;325(12):849–53.

34. Kwok JM, Miller TD, Christian TF, et al. Prognostic value of a treadmill exercise score in symptomatic patients with nonspecific ST-T abnormalities on resting ECG. J Am Med Assoc 1999;282(11): 1047–53.

35. Lauer MS, Pothier CE, Magid DJ, et al. An externally validated model for predicting long-term survival after exercise treadmill testing in patients with suspected coronary artery disease and a normal electrocardiogram. Ann Intern Med 2007; 147(12):821–8.

36. Shaw LJ, Iskandrian AE. Prognostic value of gated myocardial perfusion SPECT. J Nucl Cardiol 2004; 11(2):171–85.

37. Cerqueira MD, Weissman NJ, Dilsizian V, et al. Standardized myocardial segmentation and nomenclature for tomographic imaging of the heart. A statement for healthcare professionals from the Cardiac Imaging Committee of the Council on Clinical Cardiology of the American Heart Association. Circulation 2002;105:539–42.

38. Hachamovitch R, Berman DS, Kiat H, et al. Exercise myocardial perfusion SPECT in patients without known coronary artery disease: incremental prognostic value and use in risk stratification. Circulation 1996;93(5):905–14.

39. Hachamovitch R, Hayes SW, Friedman JD, et al. Comparison of the short-term survival benefit

associated with revascularization compared with medical therapy in patients with no prior coronary artery disease undergoing stress myocardial perfusion single photon emission computed tomography. Circulation 2003;107:2900–7.

40. Available at: https://ischemiatrial.org. Accessed March 14, 2014.

41. Abidov A, Germano G, Hachamovitch R, et al. Gated SPECT in assessment of regional and global left ventricular function: major tool of modern nuclear imaging. J Nucl Cardiol 2006;13(2):261–79.

42. Sharir T, Germano G, Kavanagh PB, et al. Incremental prognostic value of post-stress left ventricular ejection fraction and volume by gated myocardial perfusion single photon emission computed tomography. Circulation 1999;100(10):1035–42.

43. Abidov A, Germano G, Berman D. Transient ischemic dilation ratio: a universal high-risk diagnostic marker in myocardial perfusion imaging. J Nucl Cardiol 2007;14(4):497–500.

44. Berman D, Kang X, Slomka P, et al. Underestimation of extent of ischemia by gated SPECT myocardial perfusion imaging in patients with left main coronary artery disease. J Nucl Cardiol 2007; 14(4):521–8.

45. Dorbala S, Di Carli MF, Beanlands RS, et al. Prognostic value of stress myocardial perfusion positron emission tomography results from a multicenter observational registry. J Am Coll Cardiol 2013; 61(2):176–84.

46. Bourque JM, Beller GA. Stress myocardial perfusion imaging for assessing prognosis: an update. JACC Cardiovasc Imaging 2011;4(12):1305–19.

47. Sicari R, Nihoyannopoulos P, Evangelista A, et al. Stress echocardiography expert consensus statement—executive summary: European Association of Echocardiography (EAE) (a registered branch of the ESC). Eur Heart J 2009;30(3):278–89.

48. Marwick TH, Case C, Vasey C, et al. Prediction of mortality by exercise echocardiography: a strategy for combination with the Duke treadmill score. Circulation 2001;103(21):2566–71.

49. Arruda-Olson AM, Juracan EM, Mahoney DW, et al. Prognostic value of exercise echocardiography in 5,798 patients: is there a gender difference? J Am Coll Cardiol 2002;39(4):625–31.

50. Sicari R, Pasanisi E, Venneri L, et al. Stress echo results predict mortality: a large-scale multicenter prospective international study. J Am Coll Cardiol 2003;41(4):589–95.

51. Shaw LJ, Vasey C, Sawada S, et al. Impact of gender on risk stratification by exercise and dobutamine stress echocardiography: long-term mortality in 4234 women and 6898 men. Eur Heart J 2005;26(5):447–56.

52. McCully RB, Roger VL, Mahoney DW, et al. Outcome after abnormal exercise echocardiography for patients with good exercise capacity: prognostic importance of the extent and severity of exercise-related left ventricular dysfunction. J Am Coll Cardiol 2002;39(8):1345–52.

53. Metz LD, Beattie M, Hom R, et al. The prognostic value of normal exercise myocardial perfusion imaging and exercise echocardiography: a meta-analysis. J Am Coll Cardiol 2007;49(2):227–37.

54. Available at: http://www.cms.gov/Medicare/Medicare-Fee-for-Service-Payment/PhysicianFeeSched/PFS-Federal-Regulation-Notices.html. Accessed March 14, 2014.

55. Christian TF, Miller TD, Bailey KR, et al. Exercise tomographic thallium-201 imaging in patients with severe coronary artery disease and normal electrocardiograms [see comments]. Ann Intern Med 1994;121(11):825–32.

56. O'Keefe JH Jr, Zinsmeister AR, Gibbons RJ. Value of normal electrocardiographic findings in predicting resting left ventricular function in patients with chest pain and suspected coronary artery disease. Am J Med 1989;86(6 Pt 1):658–62.

57. Rihal CS, Davis KB, Ward Kennedy J, et al. The utility of clinical, electrocardiographic, and roentgenographic variables in the prediction of left ventricular function. Am J Cardiol 1995;75(4):220–3.

58. Christian TF, Miller TD, Chareonthaitawee P, et al. Prevalence of normal resting left ventricular function with normal rest electrocardiograms. Am J Cardiol 1997;79(9):1295–8.

59. Talreja D, Gruver C, Sklenar J, et al. Efficient utilization of echocardiography for the assessment of left ventricular systolic function. Am Heart J 2000; 139(3):394–8.

60. Meyers DG, Bendon KA, Hankins JH, et al. The effect of baseline electrocardiographic abnormalities on the diagnostic accuracy of exercise-induced ST segment changes. Am Heart J 1990; 119:272–6.

61. Hlatky MA, Boineau RE, Higginbotham MB, et al. A brief self-administered questionnaire to determine functional capacity (the Duke Activity Status Index). Am J Cardiol 1989;64(10):651–4.

62. Geleijnse ML, Elhendy A, van Domburg RT, et al. Cardiac imaging for risk stratification with dobutamine-atropine stress testing in patients with chest pain: echocardiography, perfusion scintigraphy, or both? Circulation 1997;96(1):137–47.

63. Olmos LI, Dakik H, Gordon R, et al. Long-term prognostic value of exercise echocardiography compared with exercise 201Tl, ECG, and clinical variables in patients evaluated for coronary artery disease. Circulation 1998;98(24):2679–86.

64. Wolk MJ, Bailey SR, Doherty JU, et al. ACCF/AHA/ASE/ASNC/HFSA/HRS/SCAI/SCCT/SCMR/STS 2013 multimodality appropriate use criteria for the detection and risk assessment of stable ischemic heart

disease: a report of the American College of Cardiology Foundation Appropriate Use Criteria Task Force, American Heart Association, American Society of Echocardiography, American Society of Nuclear Cardiology, Heart Failure Society of America, Heart Rhythm Society, Society for Cardiovascular Angiography and Interventions, Society of Cardiovascular Computed Tomography, Society for Cardiovascular Magnetic Resonance, and Society of Thoracic Surgeons. J Card Fail 2014;20(2):65–90.

65. Poornima IG, Miller TD, Christian TF, et al. Utility of myocardial perfusion imaging in patients with low risk treadmill scores. J Am Coll Cardiol 2004;43: 194–9.

66. Fine NM, Pellikka PA, Scott CG, et al. Characteristics and outcomes of patients who achieve high workload (≥10 metabolic equivalents) during treadmill exercise echocardiography. Mayo Clin Proc 2013;88(12):1408–19.

67. Klodas E, Miller T, Christian T, et al. Prognostic significance of ischemic electrocardiographic changes during vasodilator stress testing in patients with normal SPECT images. J Nucl Cardiol 2003;10(1):4–8.

68. Abbott B, Afshar M, Berger A, et al. Prognostic significance of ischemic electrocardiographic changes during adenosine infusion in patients with normal myocardial perfusion imaging. J Nucl Cardiol 2003;10(1):9–16.

69. Tricoci P, Allen JM, Kramer JM, et al. Scientific evidence underlying the ACC/AHA clinical practice guidelines. JAMA 2009;301(8):831–41.

70. Wackers FJ, Young LH, Inzucchi SE, et al. Detection of silent myocardial ischemia in asymptomatic diabetic subjects: the DIAD study. Diabetes Care 2004;27(8):1954–61.

71. Young LH, Wackers FJ, Chyun DA, et al. Cardiac outcomes after screening for asymptomatic coronary artery disease in patients with type 2 diabetes: the DIAD study: a randomized controlled trial. J Am Med Assoc 2009;301:1547–55.

72. Shaw LJ, Mieres JH, Hendel RH, et al. Comparative effectiveness of exercise electrocardiography with or without myocardial perfusion single photon emission computed tomography in women with suspected coronary artery disease: results from the What is the Optimal Method for Ischemia Evaluation in Women (WOMEN) trial. Circulation 2011; 124(11):1239–49.

73. Boden WE, O'Rourke RA, Teo KK, et al. Optimal medical therapy with or without PCI for stable coronary disease. N Engl J Med 2007;356(15):1503–16.

74. Frye RL. A randomized trial of therapies for type 2 diabetes and coronary artery disease. N Engl J Med 2009;360(24):2503–15.

75. Velazquez EJ, Lee KL, Deja MA, et al. Coronary-artery bypass surgery in patients with left ventricular dysfunction. N Engl J Med 2011; 364(17):1607–16.

76. Shaw LJ, Berman DS, Maron DJ, et al. Optimal medical therapy with or without percutaneous coronary intervention to reduce ischemic burden: results from the Clinical Outcomes Utilizing Revascularization and Aggressive Drug Evaluation (COURAGE) trial nuclear substudy. Circulation 2008;117(10): 1283–91.

77. Shaw LJ, Weintraub WS, Maron DJ, et al. Baseline stress myocardial perfusion imaging results and outcomes in patients with stable ischemic heart disease randomized to optimal medical therapy with or without percutaneous coronary intervention. Am Heart J 2012;164(2):243–50.

78. Shaw L, Cerqueira M, Brooks M, et al. Impact of left ventricular function and the extent of ischemia and scar by stress myocardial perfusion imaging on prognosis and therapeutic risk reduction in diabetic patients with coronary artery disease: results from the Bypass Angioplasty Revascularization Investigation 2 Diabetes (BARI 2D) trial. J Nucl Cardiol 2012;19(4):658–69.

79. Panza JA, Holly TA, Asch FM, et al. Inducible myocardial ischemia and outcomes in patients with coronary artery disease and left ventricular dysfunction. J Am Coll Cardiol 2013;61(18): 1860–70.

80. Moir S, Shaw L, Haluska B, et al. Left ventricular opacification for the diagnosis of coronary artery disease with stress echocardiography: an angiographic study of incremental benefit and cost-effectiveness. Am Heart J 2007;154(3):510–8.

81. Ishii K, Imai M, Suyama T, et al. Exercise-induced post-ischemic left ventricular delayed relaxation or diastolic stunning: is it a reliable marker in detecting coronary artery disease? J Am Coll Cardiol 2009;53(8):698–705.

82. Ishii K, Miwa K, Sakurai T, et al. Detection of post-ischemic regional left ventricular delayed outward wall motion or diastolic stunning after exercise-induced ischemia in patients with stable effort angina by using color kinesis. J Am Soc Echocardiogr 2008;21(4):309–14.

83. Bjork Ingul C, Stoylen A, Slordahl SA, et al. Automated analysis of myocardial deformation at dobutamine stress echocardiography: an angiographic validation. J Am Coll Cardiol 2007; 49(15):1651–9.

84. Reant P, Labrousse L, Lafitte S, et al. Experimental validation of circumferential, longitudinal, and radial 2-fimensional strain during dobutamine stress echocardiography in ischemic conditions. J Am Coll Cardiol 2008;51(2):149–57.

85. Yang B, Daimon M, Ishii K, et al. Prediction of coronary artery stenosis at rest in patients with normal left ventricular wall motion. Segmental

analyses using strain imaging diastolic index. Int Heart J 2013;54(5):266–72.

86. Sharir T, Slomka P, Berman D. Solid-State SPECT technology: fast and furious. J Nucl Cardiol 2010; 17(5):890–6.

87. Miller TD, Askew JW, O'Connor MK. New toys for nuclear cardiologists. Circ Cardiovasc Imaging 2011;4(1):5–7.

88. Berman DS, Maddahi J, Tamarappoo BK, et al. Phase II safety and clinical comparison with single-photon emission computed tomography myocardial perfusion imaging for detection of coronary artery disease: flurpiridaz F 18 positron emission tomography. J Am Coll Cardiol 2013;61(4):469–77.

89. Flett AS, Westwood MA, Davies LC, et al. The prognostic implications of cardiovascular magnetic resonance. Circ Cardiovasc Imaging 2009;2(3): 243–50.

90. Available at: https://www.promisetrial.org. Accessed March 14, 2014.

Invasive Testing for Coronary Artery Disease
FFR, IVUS, OCT, NIRS

Elliott M. Groves, MD, MEng[a,b],
Arnold H. Seto, MD, MPH[a,c],*, Morton J. Kern, MD[a,c]

KEYWORDS

- Fractional flow reserve • Intravascular ultrasonography • Optical coherence tomography
- Near-infrared spectroscopy • Coronary artery disease

KEY POINTS

- Fractional flow reserve is a well-validated technique that can be used to characterize whether a coronary lesion is physiologically significant.
- Intravascular ultrasonography is a flexible technology that can be used to determine luminal area and the composition of a coronary lesion.
- Optical coherence tomography is an emerging technology that can help guide percutaneous coronary intervention and visualize deployed stent struts with high accuracy despite the presence of plaque or neointimal hyperplasia.
- At this time, the clinical applications of near-infrared spectroscopy remains unclear, but potential uses include determination of plaque composition to identify vulnerable plaques, and guidance of medical treatment strategies.

INTRODUCTION

Coronary angiography or cineangiography provides direct visualization of the coronary luminal anatomy and is the gold standard for the diagnosis of coronary artery disease.[1] However, since the development of angiography in the 1960s, the primary method for assessing the lesions that are of physiologic significance has been visual assessment by the operator,[2] which is prone to significant intraobserver and interobserver variability.[2–4] The significance of a given stenosis is not determined solely by the reduction in luminal diameter, because numerous additional factors such as lesion length, shape, and eccentricity affect the flow dynamics of the lesion and thus the physiologic significance.[5–9] Therefore, coronary angiography cannot solely be relied on to provide the physiologic or clinical significance of a stenosis, particularly when the vessel is narrowed to between 40% and 80% of its normal diameter.[10,11]

Because of the need for a more comprehensive method for determining the anatomic and functional characteristics of a coronary artery lesion, several techniques have been developed to augment standard cineangiography.[12,13] These novel techniques are centered on the physiologic assessment of lesions and advanced intravascular imaging to provide a more comprehensive anatomic assessment.

Disclosures: None.
[a] Division of Cardiology, Department of Internal Medicine, University of California, 333 City Blvd West, Suite 400, Orange, CA 92868-3298, USA; [b] Department of Biomedical Engineering, University of California, 3120 Natural Sciences II, Irvine, CA 92697-2715, USA; [c] Division of Cardiology, Department of Internal Medicine, Long Beach Veterans Administration Hospital, 5901 East Seventh Street, Long Beach, CA 90822, USA
* Corresponding author. 5901 East Seventh Street 111C, Long Beach, CA 90822.
E-mail address: aseto@uci.edu

This article discusses invasive testing for coronary artery disease. Fractional flow reserve (FFR), defined as the ratio of the distal pressure in the coronary artery to aortic pressure at a maximal hyperemic state, describes the physiologic significance of a coronary stenosis and can predict whether percutaneous coronary intervention (PCI) will be beneficial. Following FFR, the intravascular imaging modalities are reviewed: intravascular ultrasonography (IVUS), optical coherence tomography (OCT), and near-infrared spectroscopy (NIRS). These complementary imaging modalities can help overcome technical limitations in the ability to optimally visualize a particular lesion, and can provide information about the contour of the vascular lumen and the composition of the vascular wall.

FFR

FFR is an elegantly simple principle based on the fundamentals of fluid dynamics that was first derived and published by Pijls and colleagues[14,15] in the early 1990s. It has recently gained increased clinical traction because of several important long-term outcome studies that showed the usefulness of FFR in decision making with regard to lesion-specific treatment.[16–18] As previously discussed, it is critical that lesions with ischemic potential be evaluated in a manner that determines more than their appearance on arteriography.[19] A standard cineangiogram provides a two-dimensional representation of a three-dimensional structure, namely the lumen of the coronary artery. Because of the inherent limitations of these so-called lumenograms, standard clinical practice is to obtain numerous angiographic views of the epicardial coronary arteries, but two-dimensional imaging modalities inherently fail to accurately represent a three-dimensional structure.[6,13,20,21] Vasomotor tone, shape, length, eccentricity, collateral contribution, and several other factors of a lesion are critical in determining its clinical significance, but are lacking or absent in the assessment of lesions through the sole use of standard arteriography.[5–8]

FFR is defined as the ratio of distal coronary pressure in the coronary artery to aortic pressure at a maximal hyperemic state averaged over the cardiac cycle; this represents the maximum achievable blood flow in the presence of a stenosis divided by the maximum flow if there was no lesion.[14] FFR is particularly useful clinically in that it is independent of basal flow, changes in hemodynamics, and the microcirculation. For each coronary artery in a patient, a normal FFR is 1, because pressure in a normal epicardial coronary artery should equal aortic pressure throughout

the artery.[14] Alternative methods of hemodynamic assessment such as coronary flow reserve (CFR) are subject to changes in hemodynamic conditions and fluctuations in microvascular resistance.[22] Instantaneous wave-free ratio (iFR) is another alternative in which the distal/reference pressure ratio is measured during a wave-free period during diastole. CFR and iFR lack large well-validated studies showing that their use results in a clear clinical benefit.

FFR uses standard interventional techniques and can be performed safely at the time of angiography.[23,24] A standard guide catheter is engaged in the artery of interest, followed by advancement of a pressure wire to the tip of the guide catheter.[23] Antithrombins and intracoronary nitroglycerin are administered.[24] The wire pressure is then equalized to the guide catheter pressure, and the wire passed distal to the lesion being interrogated. Hyperemia is induced, typically with intravenous adenosine (140 µg/kg/min), or through the use of intracoronary adenosine, intravenous regadenoson, or rarely dopamine, papaverine, and nitroprusside.[23,24] An FFR of less than 0.80 is considered to represent hemodynamic significance. **Fig. 1** shows an example of a positive FFR. A useful feature of the commercially available pressure wires is that they can be used interchangeably as interventional wires.[24] Thus if a positive FFR is obtained, coronary dilation catheters and coronary stent systems can be passed over the FFR wire. Following the procedure a postintervention FFR can be calculated, which has been shown to predict outcomes.

When assessing lesions of obviously high severity (>80%) or lesions that are clearly nonobstructive (<40%) visual assessment is adequate.[19] FFR shows its maximal utility for intermediate stenoses, which account for nearly half of the lesions seen during arteriography.[18,25] **Fig. 2** provides an example of lesions categorized by severity and FFR to illustrate that angiographic significance is not a reliable predictor of physiologic significance.[26] When an intermediate lesion is present and the translesional FFR is normal, then intervention can be deferred. The ability to intervene based on FFR data is based primarily on 3 pivotal studies: DEFER (Fractional Flow Reserve to Determine the Appropriateness of Angioplasty in Moderate Coronary Stenosis), FAME (Fractional Flow Reserve Versus Angiography for Guiding Percutaneous Coronary Intervention), and FAME II (Fractional Flow Reserve Versus Angiography for Multivessel Evaluation 2).

The DEFER study was a multicenter prospective randomized trial of 325 patients referred for single-vessel PCI based on a visual assessment of a greater than 50% de novo stenosis in a native

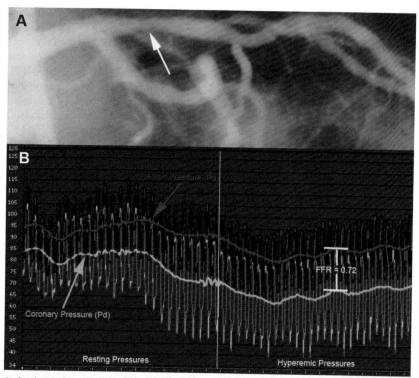

Fig. 1. (*A*) Digital subtraction angiography image of an epicardial coronary lesion (*white arrow*). (*B*) Pressure signals used to calculate FFR showing colored signals of aortic pressure (Pa; *red arrow*) and distal coronary pressure (Pd; *green arrow*) for FFR of 0.72. Mean, Pa and Pd, are recorded at rest and then during hyperemia induced by adenosine (in this case intracoronary). The nadir of distal pressure is used for the FFR calculation.

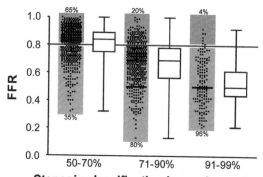

Stenosis classification by angiography

Fig. 2. Box and whisker plot showing the FFR values for 1129 coronary lesions based on angiographic severity (50%–70%, 71%–90%, and 91%–99%). The red line indicates an FFR of 0.8, which was used as the cutoff for physiologic significance. The blue boxes indicate the percentage of lesions that were not significant by FFR, and the red boxes the percentage of lesions that were significant by FFR. (*Adapted from* Tonino PA, Fearon WF, De Bruyne B, et al. Angiographic versus functional severity of coronary artery stenoses in the FAME study fractional flow reserve versus angiography in multivessel evaluation. J Am Coll Cardiol 2010;55:2818; with permission.)

coronary artery. Patients were excluded if any evidence of reversible ischemia was documented by noninvasive stress testing in the 2 months before enrollment. Patients were randomized to either a deferral or performance of PCI subset before FFR. In the deferral of PCI subset, 167 patients had FFR of their lesions, 91 had a negative FFR value, defined as greater than or equal to 0.75. Those 91 patients were classified as the Defer group and continued on medical therapy alone. If FFR was less than 0.75 then it was considered unethical to defer PCI and thus those 76 patients from the deferral subset received PCI. In the PCI subset, all 158 patients had a baseline FFR, but then received PCI regardless of the result. The 68 patients with an FFR less than 0.75 were grouped with the 76 patients from the deferral subset who had PCI, and were compared as the Reference group. In addition, the 90 patients with an FFR greater than or equal to 0.75 who underwent PCI were termed the Perform group, thus resulting in 3 groups.

In DEFER, the primary end point was freedom from cardiac events. At 5 years of follow-up, event-free survival was 80%, 73%, and 63% for Defer,

Perform, and Reference groups respectively.[17] The patients with FFR greater than or equal to 0.75 (Defer and Perform groups) showed no significant difference in the number of patients with chest pain regardless of PCI. If the FFR of a lesion was less than 0.75, there was a significant increase in events despite PCI, and if the FFR was greater than or equal to 0.75 then the patients did significantly better whether they had PCI or not. Therefore, if a lesion is nonsignificant by FFR (functionally nonsignificant) then PCI is of no benefit to the patient from a prognostic or symptom control standpoint. However, if a lesion is functionally significant by FFR then it is at an increased risk of causing myocardial infarction (MI) or cardiac death regardless of the visual severity.[17] Even if treated with PCI, a lesion that is functionally significant is 5 times more likely to cause an MI than a lesion of similar severity on arteriography that is nonsignificant by FFR.

The FAME study was a multicenter prospective randomized trial of 1005 patients with multivessel coronary artery disease, defined as a stenosis of at least 50% in at least 2 of the 3 major epicardial coronary arteries without left main coronary artery disease. Patients were randomized to 2 groups, the first having PCI guided solely by angiography and the second having FFR-guided PCI. In the FFR-guided group, all lesions underwent FFR and stents were only placed in lesions with an FFR of less than or equal to 0.80. The primary end point for the study was a composite of death, MI, and repeat revascularization. The angiography-guided group had an occurrence of the primary end point in 91 patients (18.3%) and the FFR-guided group had an occurrence in 67 (13.2%).[18] This difference was statistically significant (P = .02). Secondary end point analysis showed nonsignificant reductions in all-cause mortality, MI, repeat revascularization, and length of hospital stay through the use of FFR guidance.[18] Significant reductions in the cost of the procedure, contrast volume, and the number of stents per patient (2.7 ± 1.2 vs 1.9 ± 1.3; P<.001) were seen with the use of FFR guidance.[18] All of this was achieved without a significant increase in angina or an increase in procedure time. The FAME study shows that in patients with multivessel coronary artery disease the routine use of FFR significantly reduced the primary end point (death, MI, and repeat revascularization), and also reduced the cost and number of stents placed, without decreasing quality of life or increasing procedural time.

FAME 2 was a randomized all-comers trial of 888 patients with stable angina. Patients with angiographically assessed 1-vessel, 2-vessel, or 3-vessel coronary artery disease that was amenable to PCI were taken for FFR of each lesion. Those with at least 1 lesion with an FFR of less than or equal to 0.80 were either randomized to FFR-guided PCI plus optimal medical therapy (OMT) or OMT alone. All lesions with an FFR less than or equal to 0.80 in the FFR-guided PCI group were treated with drug-eluting stents. The primary end point was a composite of death, nonfatal MI, or unplanned hospitalization leading to revascularization during the first 2 years. Enrollment in the study was terminated after 19 months because of a highly significant difference in incidence rates between the groups. Of the patients with OMT, 12.7% reached the primary end point, whereas this occurred in only 4.3% of the FFR-guided PCI group (hazard ratio, 0.32; 95% confidence interval, 0.19 to 0.53; P<.001).[16] This result was primarily driven by an 8-fold increase in the need for urgent revascularization, which included unstable angina (52%) but also MI or unstable angina with electrocardiographic changes in 48%. A registry group of participants with documented coronary disease, but no functionally significant stenosis by FFR,[16] did not receive PCI and shared the low event rates seen in the PCI group. Therefore, not only does FFR-guided PCI greatly reduce the need for urgent revascularization but this study also confirms that deferring PCI based on the FFR is a safe and effective strategy. A summary of all discussed studies is given in **Table 1**.

Indications for FFR now extend beyond the assessment of appropriateness of PCI for simple lesions. Postprocedural FFR has been shown to predict outcomes after bare metal stenting.[27,28] If the postprocedural FFR is greater than 0.90 a given patient has a low 6-month event rate; however, if the FFR is less than 0.90 after PCI then the event rate is much higher.[27,28] Left main coronary artery lesions can also be accurately assessed by FFR by passing the wire into either the left circumflex or left anterior descending coronary artery when those vessels are free of disease. Five-year outcome data show that, in patients with angiographically equivocal left main stenosis, if the FFR is greater than or equal to 0.80 then the lesion can be treated medically with no significant change in outcome compared with those patients with a left main lesion with an FFR less than 0.80 who are treated surgically.[29] FFR can also be used to predict long-term saphenous vein graft patency rates: if a vessel with a nonsignificant lesion by FFR is grafted, the 1-year rate of occlusion is more than double that of grafts to vessels with significant lesions by FFR.[30] Because FFR depends on hyperemic flow and myocardial bed size, it is generally not considered to be useful in the first 24 to 48 hours after a diagnosis of acute coronary syndrome when assessing the causative lesion,

Table 1
Summary of FFR studies discussed

	DEFER		FAME I		FAME II	
Design	Randomized		Randomized		Randomized	
FFR cutoff	$\geq$0.75		>0.80		>0.80	
Mean follow-up (mo)	60		12		60	
Group	Defer	Perform	FFR	Angiography	PCI + Medical Therapy	Medical Therapy
Patients (n)	91	90	509	496	447	441
Clinical Outcomes						
Death, n (%)	—	—	9 (1.8)	15 (3.0)	—	—
Cardiac death	3 (3.3)	2 (2.3)	—	—	1 (0.2)	1 (0.2)
Noncardiac death	3 (3.3)	3 (3.4)	—	—	0 (0)	2 (0.4)
MI, n (%)	0 (0)	6 (5.6)	29 (5.7)	43 (8.7)	15 (3.4)	14 (3.2)
Revascularization, n (%)	14 (15.4)	14 (15.6)	33 (6.5)	47 (9.5)	14 (3.1)	86 (19.5)

but can be useful afterward or in assessing non-causative vessels.[31]

When assessing diffuse disease or serial lesions the operator needs to be aware that these disease states affect the FFR of each lesion. FFR depends on myocardial bed size, or the amount of myocardium that a specific artery is supplying.[32] It can be difficult to ascertain the functional significance of a lesion in the presence of significant collateral circulation or stenosis in series affecting the same epicardial vessel.[32] In order to examine serial lesions the pressure wire should first be passed distal to the final lesion; if the combined FFR is not significant, then the lesions are not significant individually.[33] If the series of lesions is significantly stenosed, the pressure gradient across each lesion in the series should be measured, the lesion that contributes the most significant pressure loss should undergo PCI, and the FFR measurement should be repeated to determine whether there are more functionally significant lesions in the series.[32] In diffuse disease a gradual, almost linear, increase in the FFR should be seen as the wire is pulled back, with no abrupt increase.[33]

FFR is thus a critical tool in the assessment of coronary artery lesions that can be used safely, quickly, and without any increase in procedural cost. Using FFR appropriately improves patient outcomes and symptoms.

IVUS

Although coronary arteriography is an invaluable tool for the detection and treatment of coronary artery lesions that result in myocardial ischemia, it has limitations, as discussed previously. Techniques such as FFR can assess the functional significance of a lesion but cannot augment the limited information the angiogram provides regarding the properties of the arterial wall. Because of positive remodeling (outward expansion of the vessel wall), angiography can underestimate the magnitude of atherosclerotic burden and fail to identify vulnerable plaques, which are a major substrate for acute coronary syndrome and sudden death.[34,35] Thin-cap fibroatheromas (TCFAs) consist of a lipid-laden necrotic core under a fibrous cap that measures less than 65 μg and contains scant smooth muscle cells and numerous macrophages.[34] These TCFAs are susceptible to plaque rupture, but are generally only mild to moderately obstructive on arteriography and may not be significant by FFR.[35] In addition, using only angiography as guidance for PCI is associated with lack of detection of edge complications and/or suboptimal stent expansion in 15% to 20% of cases, which is associated with adverse events.[36]

With the advent of intravascular imaging in the 1980s, clinicians were able to obtain in vivo information regarding the morphology of a given plaque. IVUS and angioscopy were the first imaging modalities that were able to provide information on the composition of a plaque.[37] Although angioscopy was never part of clinical practice outside Japan, IVUS is commonly used. IVUS currently has several incarnations that include the radiofrequency analysis of the IVUS backscatter (RF-IVUS), which can be used to produce Virtual Histology IVUS (VH-IVUS) and integrated backscatter IVUS (IB-IVUS).[38,39] RF-IVUS combines spectral (frequency) analysis with conventional amplitude data from the IVUS signal to generate an estimate of plaque composition that correlates with histologic samples.[38,39] The use of IVUS can help identify features of complex unstable plaques, facilitate optimal PCI by providing reference vessel diameter, identify landing zones, and confirm that stent struts are properly expanded.[40] When PCI is guided by IVUS in addition to angiography, reduced stent thrombosis and restenosis have been seen compared with PCI guidance solely by angiography.[41] In addition, IVUS can measure stenosis severity, calcification, remodeling, and plaque burden.[41]

At present there are 2 types of IVUS catheters: mechanical (rotational) and phased array. Mechanical catheters emit ultrasound in the range of 10 to 40 MHz, which can produce an overall resolution of 100 to 150 μm.[37] Phased array catheters are easier to use and can be pulled back manually, but have a lower resolution. The transducer is oriented at 90° to the catheter and thus the images produced are cross-sectional views of the artery, which is ideal for assessing plaque eccentricity and can provide a highly accurate assessment of the native vessel and plaque size.[42] After a guidewire is positioned in the artery to be imaged and antithrombins are given, an IVUS catheter is advanced until the transducer is in the most distal portion of the vessel that the operator intends to image. Intracoronary nitrates can be delivered for optimal imaging. Following placement, the imaging system is activated and an automatic motorized pullback device withdraws the IVUS catheter as the vessel is being imaged, the typical pullback speed being 0.5 to 1.0 mm/s.[43] A normal coronary artery appears as alternating bright and dark echo zones because the 3 coronary artery layers have distinct values of acoustic impedance.[44] When visualizing diseased coronary arteries, the appearance of the IVUS image depends on the composition of the plaque. For instance, a highly calcified plaque has a bright appearance with acoustic shadowing, whereas a lipid-rich plaque appears less echodense.[37] As previously mentioned, changes in the returning radiofrequency can be postprocessed to further elucidate plaque composition. The data are color coded and superimposed on the gray scale image (IB-IVUS, VH-IVUS).[45]

At this time the most common uses of IVUS clinically are to determine optimal stent placement and measure the minimal luminal area (MLA) of a lesion in a reference vessel to determine significance. As previously mentioned, IVUS can provide the operator with the ability to visualize reference vessel diameter, identify landing zones, quantitate the residual luminal diameter, and confirm that stent struts are properly expanded.[40,46,47] However, the clinical utility of this information is unclear. In the AVID (Angiography Versus Intravascular Ultrasound-Directed Stent Placement) trial, 800 patients undergoing elective bare metal stenting were randomized to placement by optimal angiographic result or IVUS-directed therapy. The primary end point was target lesion revascularization (TLR) at 1 year of follow-up. At 1 year the rate of TLR was decreased in the IVUS group, but not significantly (8.1% vs 12%; $P = .08$).[48] AVID did report secondary analysis that suggested a significant decrease in TLR when distal reference diameter is greater than or equal to 2.5 mm.[48] For PCI in long lesions (>20 mm), the TULIP (Thrombocyte Activity Evaluation and Effects of Ultrasound Guidance in Long Intracoronary Stent Placement) trial showed a significant reduction in greater than 50% angiographic restenosis (23% vs 45%; $P = .008$) and TLR (10% vs 23%; $P = .018$) at 1 year through the use of IVUS guidance.[49] IVUS guidance of PCI is most useful when underexpansion is suspected, with long lesions, when the reference vessel size is uncertain, or when stent expansion is expected to be difficult (calcified lesions or left main coronary artery).[50]

The use of IVUS to determine lesion significance has not been shown to have a strong correlation with FFR or perfusion imaging.[51–54] Most recently, the FIRST (Fractional Flow Reserve and Intravascular Ultrasound Relationship Study) showed that using IVUS-MLA to guide intervention in intermediate lesions was limited in accuracy (64% sensitivity and specificity) and highly variable based on reference vessel characteristics.[54] Previous work has varied greatly in defining an MLA that denotes functional significance, and the routine use of IVUS in place of FFR is not recommended.[50] Analysis of left main coronary artery stenosis by IVUS has a closer correlation (90%) with FFR, but the MLA cutoff to determine significance varies from 4.8 mm^2 to 5.9 mm^2 based on different studies.[55,56]

Several studies have examined the utility of IVUS in assessing the prognostic implications of different plaque compositions. Sano and colleagues[57] were the first to use RF-IVUS to examine patients with stable angina. Patients treated with PCI underwent IVUS of identified non–flow-limiting lesions. Within 30 ± 7 months, 10 of the studied plaques caused an acute event; these lesions were noted to have increased eccentricity, plaque burden, and lipid tissue.[57] More recently IB-IVUS was used to show that, in patients admitted for stable angina or acute coronary syndrome, a second nontarget event was more likely if the patient had lipid-rich nonobstructive plaques outside the causative lesion.[58] The largest prospective study using 3-vessel VH-IVUS was the PROSPECT

(Providing Regional Observations to Study Predictors of Events in the Coronary Tree) study.[45] The prognostic implications of atheroma burden and plaque composition in 697 patients treated for acute coronary syndrome was studied over 3 years. The primary end point was major adverse cardiovascular events (MACE), which occurred in 149 patients and of which 55 cases involved causative lesions that were previously studied with VH-IVUS. Through multivariate analysis it was determined that the independent predictors of future causative lesions were increased plaque burden ($\geq$70%), an MLA of less than 4 mm^2, and a TCFA phenotype.[45] Several other studies have confirmed the association between plaque composition and future MACE.[59,60] However, these studies fail to show a clinically useful predictive accuracy for VH-IVUS; for example, in the PROSPECT study only 18% of the plaques with plaque burden greater than or equal to 70%, MLA less than 4 mm^2, and a TCFA phenotype caused MACE.[45]

IVUS is useful for the guidance of PCI under certain conditions; however, its prognostic significance is yet to be determined. The inherent limitations of IVUS, such as moderate resolution, artifacts, and noise, along with the limited reliability of VH-IVUS need to be improved before its indications for use are expanded.[59]

OCT

OCT is a technique pioneered slightly more than a decade ago that uses the principles of pulse-echo ultrasonography imaging; however, instead of sound it uses light.[61] Near-infrared light is directed onto the vessel wall, reflected off the internal microstructure of the tissue, then the intensities of the returning waves are used to construct an image of the vessel wall. At present, available systems have axial resolutions of 10 to 15 μm with a lateral resolution of 20 to 40 μm and a maximal scan diameter of 7 mm, all of which continue to improve along with acquisition speeds.[62–64] Compared with IVUS, OCT provides an order of magnitude improvement in resolution; however, this is at the cost of a large decrease in the depth of imaging (from 10 mm with IVUS to 1–2.5 mm with OCT). An additional significant limitation of OCT is the need to clear blood from the arterial lumen because OCT cannot image through a blood field.[61] **Fig. 3** compares IVUS and OCT images from various disorders.

The procedure of OCT imaging is similar to that of IVUS, as is the imaging display. OCT imaging catheters have an imaging core at the distal tip of the catheter that is oriented at 90° to the catheter and the vessel. These small catheters are introduced over a standard coronary guidewire

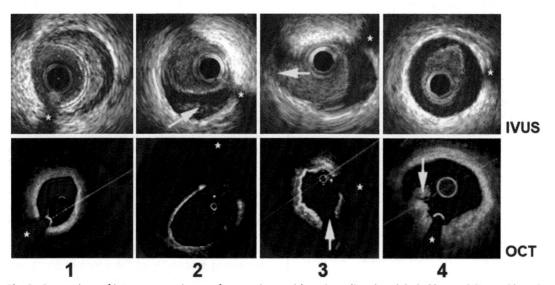

Fig. 3. Comparison of intracoronary images from patients with various disorders, labeled by modality and by columns 1 to 4. IVUS images from left to right: (1) crescent-shaped intramural hematoma, (2) double lumen with false-lumen thrombosis denoted by arrow, (3) double lumen with a side branch emerging from the true lumen at the site of the arrow, (4) elliptical, echogenic, true lumen fully detached from the outer vessel wall. OCT images from left to right: (1) double lumen with a thick and (2) thin intimal membrane, (3) intimal rupture denoted by the arrow, (4) intracoronary thrombus that is encroaching on the lumen, denoted by the arrow. Asterisk denotes wire artifact. (*Adapted from* Paulo M, Sandoval J, Lennie V, et al. Combined use of OCT and IVUS in spontaneous coronary artery dissection. JACC Cardiovasc Imaging 2013;6(7):832; with permission.)

distal to the region of interest after antithrombins and intracoronary nitroglycerin have been given. Blood is displaced from the region of interest by either an occlusive technique or flushing with contrast or saline.[61] An automated pullback system draws the catheter back at 1 to 25 mm/s as it images the vessel. OCT in a clinical setting has been found to be safe.[65,66] Normal OCT images are analogous to IVUS images with a 3-layer cross section with signal-rich layers of the external lamina and internal elastic membrane surrounding a dark layer representing the media.[67] **Table 2** shows the strengths of the various imaging modalities.

At present there are no established clinical indications for OCT and the 2011 ACCF/AHA/SCAI Guideline Update for Percutaneous Coronary Intervention states that "the appropriate role of optical coherence tomography in routine clinical decision making has not been established..."[50] However, there have been several studies assessing possible roles for OCT in clinical practice because of its high resolution and ability to identify TCFAs with a particularly high specificity.[68]

Examination of ex-vivo samples has yielded a 71% to 96% sensitivity and 90% to 98% specificity for plaque type detection, particularly TCFAs, in numerous studies.[68–72] One study of patients with non–ST segment elevation MI found that patients with no-reflow after PCI were more likely to have a significantly larger lipid arc (166° vs 44°; $P<.001$) and a TCFA (50% vs 16%; $P = .005$)[73] less than OCT compared with patients who did not have no-reflow. Additional potential applications for

OCT include assessment of stent placement and long-term stent outcome because OCT provides a high-resolution image of the stent-vessel interface and has the capacity to detect very thin layers of neointima.[74] Mechanical stent failure (incomplete stent expansion, stent fracture) can be differentiated from impaired healing (absence of strut coverage, absence of homogeneous coverage, or late strut malapposition) by OCT as well.[75] The LEADERS (Limus Eluted from a Durable Versus Erodable Stent Coating) study and the HORIZONS-AMI (Harmonizing Outcomes with Revascularization and Stents in Acute Myocardial Infarction) trial had OCT substudies that compared strut coverage and neointimal hyperplasia in differing types of stents.[76,77] The significance of this work is not yet clear because of the relative infancy of the technology.

NIRS

Long established as a technique used in analytical chemistry for the identification of unknown organic molecules, NIRS has only recently begun to be accepted in clinical practice. With NIRS, light from the near-infrared region of the electromagnetic spectrum ($\sim$1300 nm) can be projected toward the wall of the coronary artery and then, based on known NIRS signatures, the reflected light is collected and analyzed.[78] At present, NIRS is available as a combined imaging system with IVUS (True Vessel Characterization, InfraReDx Inc, Burlington, MA).[79]

At present the primary application of NIRS is to characterize lipid core plaques (LCPs). The procedure is similar to those detailed earlier for IVUS and OCT imaging, particularly in the setting of a combined catheter. An algorithm to detect LCPs has been developed that processes the NIRS spectra and produces a longitudinal image of the arterial segment of interest.[78] Postprocessing assigns a false color map known as a chemogram that ranges from yellow (high probability of LCP) to red (low probability of LCP). From the initial chemogram, another chemogram is created that represents the probability that each 2-mm interval of vessel contains an LCP, and this uses 4 discrete colors (red, orange, tan, and yellow) that represent increasing probability of the segment containing an LCP.[78] An additional metric is the lipid core burden index (LCBI), which quantifies the amount of LCP in a scanned arterial segment on a 1 to 1000 scale.[78] **Fig. 4** shows an example of NIRS images compared with the corresponding autopsy specimens.

The clinical utility of NIRS remains to be established. PCI of large LCP lesions has been

Table 2
Characteristics of the various imaging modalities

	Angiography	OCT	IVUS	NIRS
Plaque volume	—	—	++	—
Calcification	++	+	++	—
Cap thickness	—	++	+	+
Thrombus	+	++	+	+
Lipid core	—	+	+	++
Remodeling	—	—	++	—
Stent strut expansion	—	++	++	—
Neointimal hyperplasia	+	++	+	—
Requires blood-free field of view	No	Yes	No	No

++, Direct, robust and/or validated; +, indirect, inferred, and/or unvalidated; —, not applicable.

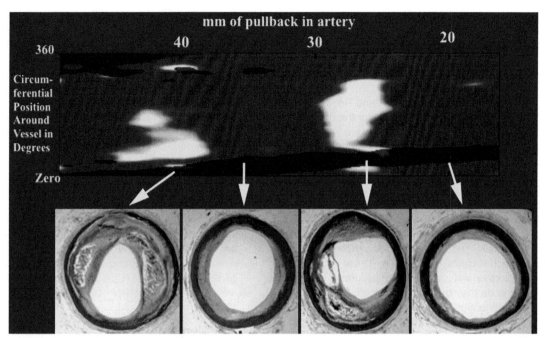

Fig. 4. An NIRS chemogram and the underlying coronary histologic features in a human coronary autopsy specimen. The X axis shows the millimeter in pullback within the artery, whereas the Y axis shows the degree of rotation within the artery from 0° to 360°. Sites with a high probability of the presence of a lipid-rich plaque are shown in yellow. Note the close correspondence between the yellow spots on the chemograms and lipid-rich plaques documented by histology. (*Adapted from* Rizik D, Goldstein JA. NIRS-IVUS imaging to characterize the composition and structure of coronary plaques. J Invasive Cardiol 2013;25:4A; with permission.)

associated with an increased rate of post-PCI MI, in part because of distal embolization, and stent thrombosis.[80–83] NIRS may be used in a predictive capacity to prompt interventions to prevent these complications, such as distal embolic protection devices and more aggressive anticoagulation or antiplatelet therapy.[84] In addition, NIRS can be used to assess coronary lesions over time and monitor the response to medical therapy. In the YELLOW (Reduction in Yellow Plaque by Aggressive Lipid Lowering Therapy) trial, a significant reduction in LCBI was found after patients were treated with 6 to 8 weeks of rosuvastatin 40 mg daily (**Table 3**).[85] NIRS can assist in detection

Table 3
Relevant study acronyms and titles

Study Acronym	Study Title
DEFER	Fractional Flow Reserve to Determine the Appropriateness of Angioplasty in Moderate Coronary Stenosis
FAME	Fractional Flow Reserve versus Angiography for Guiding Percutaneous Coronary Intervention
FAMEII	Fractional Flow Reserve versus Angiography for Multivessel Evaluation 2
AVID	Angiography Versus Intravascular ultrasound-Directed stent placement
TULIP	Thrombocyte activity evaluation and effects of Ultrasound guidance in Long Intracoronary stent Placement
FIRST	Fractional Flow Reserve and Intravascular Ultrasound Relationship Study
PROSPECT	Providing Regional Observations to Study Predictors of Events in the Coronary Tree
LEADERS	Limus Eluted from A Durable versus ERodable Stent coating
HORIZIONS-AMI	Harmonizing Outcomes With Revascularization and Stents in Acute Myocardial Infarction
YELLOW	Reduction in YELlow Plaque by Aggressive Lipid LOWering Therapy

and evaluation of LCPs for research and prognostic purposes. This evaluation may have an indication for augmentation of PCI in the future.

SUMMARY

Conventional angiography is, and is likely to continue to be, the gold standard for the diagnosis of coronary artery disease. However, arteriography is unable to assess the functional significance of lesions, provide ideal guidance for PCI, or assess the content of atherosclerotic plaques. Thus new technologies have emerged to augment coronary angiograms and aid in achieving these goals. This article reviews the scientific basis of FFR, IVUS, OCT, and NIRS, along with the procedural details and significant evidence to justify each technology's clinical use. These promising technologies will continue to progress and be analyzed as they become accepted in cardiovascular diagnostics, or become clinically irrelevant.

REFERENCES

1. Gould KL. Percent coronary stenosis: battered gold standard, pernicious relic or clinical practicality? J Am Coll Cardiol 1988;11:886–8.
2. DeRouen T, Murray J, Owen W. Variability in the analysis of coronary arteriograms. Circulation 1977;55:324–8.
3. Zir LM, Miller SW, Dinsmore RE, et al. Interobserver variability in coronary angiography. Circulation 1976;53:627–32.
4. Vas R, Eigler N, Miyazono C, et al. Digital quantification eliminates intraobserver and interobserver variability in the evaluation of coronary artery stenosis. Am J Cardiol 1985;56:718–23.
5. Fleming RM, Kirkeeide RL, Smalling RW, et al. Patterns in visual interpretation of coronary arteriograms as detected by quantitative coronary arteriography. J Am Coll Cardiol 1991;18:945–51.
6. Vlodaver Z, Neufeld HN, Edwards JE. Pathology of coronary disease. Semin Roentgenol 1972;7:376–94.
7. Epstein SE, Cannon RO, Watson RM, et al. Dynamic coronary obstruction as a cause of angina pectoris: Implications regarding therapy. Am J Cardiol 1985;55:B61–8.
8. Feldman RL, Nichols WW, Pepine CJ, et al. Hemodynamic significance of the length of a coronary arterial narrowing. Am J Cardiol 1978;41:865–71.
9. Feldman R, Nichols W, Pepine C, et al. The coronary hemodynamics of left main and branch coronary stenoses. The effects of reduction in stenosis diameter, stenosis length, and number of stenoses. J Thorac Cardiovasc Surg 1979;77:377–88.
10. White CW, Wright CB, Doty DB, et al. Does visual interpretation of the coronary arteriogram predict the physiologic importance of a coronary stenosis? N Engl J Med 1984;310:819–24.
11. Kern MJ, Samady H. Current concepts of integrated coronary physiology in the catheterization laboratory. J Am Coll Cardiol 2010;55:173–85.
12. Ambrose JA. Prognostic implications of lesion irregularity on coronary angiography. J Am Coll Cardiol 1991;18:675–6.
13. Haase J, Ozaki Y, Di Mario C, et al. Can intracoronary ultrasound correctly assess the luminal dimensions of coronary artery lesions? A comparison with quantitative angiography. Eur Heart J 1995;16:112–9.
14. Pijls N, Van Son J, Kirkeeide R, et al. Experimental basis of determining maximum coronary, myocardial, and collateral blood flow by pressure measurements for assessing functional stenosis severity before and after percutaneous transluminal coronary angioplasty. Circulation 1993;87:1354–67.
15. Pijls NH, Van Gelder B, Van der Voort P, et al. Fractional flow reserve a useful index to evaluate the influence of an epicardial coronary stenosis on myocardial blood flow. Circulation 1995;92:3183–93.
16. De Bruyne B, Pijls NH, Kalesan B, et al. Fractional flow reserve–guided PCI versus medical therapy in stable coronary disease. N Engl J Med 2012;367:991–1001.
17. Pijls N, van Schaardenburgh P, Manoharan G, et al. Percutaneous coronary intervention of functionally nonsignificant stenosis: 5-year follow-up of the DEFER study. J Am Coll Cardiol 2007;49:2105–11.
18. Tonino PA, De Bruyne B, Pijls NH, et al. Fractional flow reserve versus angiography for guiding percutaneous coronary intervention. N Engl J Med 2009;360:213–24.
19. Chamuleau SA, Meuwissen M, Koch KT, et al. Usefulness of fractional flow reserve for risk stratification of patients with multivessel coronary artery disease and an intermediate stenosis. Am J Cardiol 2002;89:377–80.
20. Stiel GM, Stiel L, Schofer J, et al. Impact of compensatory enlargement of atherosclerotic coronary arteries on angiographic assessment of coronary artery disease. Circulation 1989;80:1603–9.
21. Umans VA, Robert A, Foley D, et al. Clinical, histologic and quantitative angiographic predictors of restenosis after directional coronary atherectomy: a multivariate analysis of the renarrowing process and late outcome. J Am Coll Cardiol 1994;23:49–58.
22. Sen S, Asrress KN, Nijjer S, et al. Diagnostic classification of the instantaneous wave-free ratio is equivalent to fractional flow reserve and is not improved with adenosine administration. Results of CLARIFY (Classification Accuracy of Pressure-Only Ratios

Against Indices Using Flow Study). J Am Coll Cardiol 2013;61:1409–20.

23. Qian J, Ge J, Baumgart D, et al. Safety of intracoronary Doppler flow measurement. Am Heart J 2000; 140:502–10.

24. Pijls NH, Kern MJ, Yock PG, et al. Practice and potential pitfalls of coronary pressure measurement. Catheter Cardiovasc Interv 2000;49:1–16.

25. Tobis J, Azarbal B, Slavin L. Assessment of intermediate severity coronary lesions in the catheterization laboratory. J Am Coll Cardiol 2007;49:839–48.

26. Tonino PA, Fearon WF, De Bruyne B, et al. Angiographic versus functional severity of coronary artery stenoses in the FAME study fractional flow reserve versus angiography in multivessel evaluation. J Am Coll Cardiol 2010;55:2816–21.

27. Pijls NH, Klauss V, Siebert U, et al. Coronary pressure measurement after stenting predicts adverse events at follow-up a multicenter registry. Circulation 2002;105:2950–4.

28. Samady H, McDaniel M, Veledar E, et al. Baseline fractional flow reserve and stent diameter predict optimal post-stent fractional flow reserve and major adverse cardiac events after bare-metal stent deployment. JACC Cardiovasc Interv 2009;2: 357–63.

29. Hamilos M, Muller O, Cuisset T, et al. Long-term clinical outcome after fractional flow reserve–guided treatment in patients with angiographically equivocal left main coronary artery stenosis. Circulation 2009;120:1505–12.

30. Botman CJ, Schonberger J, Koolen S, et al. Does stenosis severity of native vessels influence bypass graft patency? A prospective fractional flow reserve–guided study. Ann Thorac Surg 2007;83: 2093–7.

31. De Bruyne B, Pijls NH, Bartunek J, et al. Fractional flow reserve in patients with prior myocardial infarction. Circulation 2001;104:157–62.

32. Pijls NH, De Bruyne B, Bech GJ, et al. Coronary pressure measurement to assess the hemodynamic significance of serial stenoses within one coronary artery validation in humans. Circulation 2000;102: 2371–7.

33. De Bruyne B, Hersbach F, Pijls NH, et al. Abnormal epicardial coronary resistance in patients with diffuse atherosclerosis but "normal" coronary angiography. Circulation 2001;104:2401–6.

34. Virmani R, Burke AP, Farb A, et al. Pathology of the vulnerable plaque. J Am Coll Cardiol 2006;47: C13–8.

35. Burke AP, Farb A, Malcom GT, et al. Plaque rupture and sudden death related to exertion in men with coronary artery disease. JAMA 1999; 281:921–6.

36. Witzenbichler B, Maehara A, Weisz G, et al. TCT-21 use of IVUS reduces stent thrombosis: results from

the prospective, multicenter ADAPT-DES study. J Am Coll Cardiol 2012;60(17 Suppl B):B6–7.

37. Yock M, Paul G, Fitzgerald M, et al. Intravascular ultrasound: State of the art and future directions. Am J Cardiol 1998;81:27E–32E.

38. Nair A, Kuban BD, Obuchowski N, et al. Assessing spectral algorithms to predict atherosclerotic plaque composition with normalized and raw intravascular ultrasound data. Ultrasound Med Biol 2001; 27:1319–31.

39. Bridal SL, Fornès P, Bruneval P, et al. Correlation of ultrasonic attenuation (30 to 50 MHz) and constituents of atherosclerotic plaque. Ultrasound Med Biol 1997;23:691–703.

40. Madder RD, Smith JL, Dixon SR, et al. Composition of target lesions by near-infrared spectroscopy in patients with acute coronary syndrome versus stable angina. Circ Cardiovasc Interv 2012;5:55–61.

41. Claessen BE, Mehran R, Mintz GS, et al. Impact of intravascular ultrasound imaging on early and late clinical outcomes following percutaneous coronary intervention with drug-eluting stents. JACC Cardiovasc Interv 2011;4:974–81.

42. Nishimura RA, Edwards WD, Warnes CA, et al. Intravascular ultrasound imaging: In vitro validation and pathologic correlation. J Am Coll Cardiol 1990; 16:145–54.

43. Jakabčin J, Špaček R, Bystroň M, et al. Long-term health outcome and mortality evaluation after invasive coronary treatment using drug eluting stents with or without the IVUS guidance. Randomized control trial. HOME DES IVUS. Catheter Cardiovasc Interv 2010;75:578–83.

44. Gussenhoven EJ, Essed CE, Lancée CT, et al. Arterial wall characteristics determined by intravascular ultrasound imaging: an in vitro study. J Am Coll Cardiol 1989;14:947–52.

45. Stone GW, Maehara A, Lansky AJ, et al. A prospective natural-history study of coronary atherosclerosis. N Engl J Med 2011;364:226–35.

46. Nakamura S, Colombo A, Gaglione A, et al. Intracoronary ultrasound observations during stent implantation. Circulation 1994;89:2026–34.

47. Goldberg SL, Colombo A, Nakamura S, et al. Benefit of intracoronary ultrasound in the deployment of Palmaz-Schatz stents. J Am Coll Cardiol 1994;24:996–1003.

48. Russo RJ, Silva PD, Teirstein PS, et al. A randomized controlled trial of angiography versus intravascular ultrasound-directed bare-metal coronary stent placement (the AVID trial). Circ Cardiovasc Interv 2009;2:113–23.

49. Oemrawsingh PV, Mintz GS, Schalij MJ, et al. Intravascular ultrasound guidance improves angiographic and clinical outcome of stent implantation for long coronary artery stenoses final results of a

randomized comparison with angiographic guidance (TULIP study). Circulation 2003;107:62–7.

50. Levine GN, Bates ER, Blankenship JC, et al. 2011 ACCF/AHA/SCAI guideline for percutaneous coronary intervention: Executive summary: A report of the American College of Cardiology Foundation/American Heart Association Task Force on Practice Guidelines and the Society for Cardiovascular Angiography and Interventions. J Am Coll Cardiol 2011;58:2550–83.

51. Abizaid AS, Mintz GS, Mehran R, et al. Long-term follow-up after percutaneous transluminal coronary angioplasty was not performed based on intravascular ultrasound findings: importance of lumen dimensions. Circulation 1999;100:256–61.

52. Takagi A, Tsurumi Y, Ishii Y, et al. Clinical potential of intravascular ultrasound for physiological assessment of coronary stenosis relationship between quantitative ultrasound tomography and pressure-derived fractional flow reserve. Circulation 1999;100:250–5.

53. Kang SJ, Lee JY, Ahn JM, et al. Validation of intravascular ultrasound–derived parameters with fractional flow reserve for assessment of coronary stenosis severity. Circ Cardiovasc Interv 2011;4:65–71.

54. Waksman R, Legutko J, Singh J, et al. FIRST: Fractional Flow Reserve and Intravascular Ultrasound Relationship Study. J Am Coll Cardiol 2013;61(9):917–23.

55. Jasti V, Ivan E, Yalamanchili V, et al. Correlations between fractional flow reserve and intravascular ultrasound in patients with an ambiguous left main coronary artery stenosis. Circulation 2004;110:2831–6.

56. Kang SJ, Lee JY, Ahn JM, et al. Intravascular ultrasound-derived predictors for fractional flow reserve in intermediate left main disease. JACC Cardiovasc Interv 2011;4:1168–74.

57. Sano K, Kawasaki M, Ishihara Y, et al. Assessment of vulnerable plaques causing acute coronary syndrome using integrated backscatter intravascular ultrasound. J Am Coll Cardiol 2006;47:734–41.

58. Amano T, Matsubara T, Uetani T, et al. Lipid-rich plaques predict non-target-lesion ischemic events in patients undergoing percutaneous coronary intervention. Circ J 2011;75:157.

59. Thim T, Hagensen MK, Wallace-Bradley D, et al. Unreliable assessment of necrotic core by virtual histology intravascular ultrasound in porcine coronary artery disease. Circ Cardiovasc Imaging 2010;3:384–91.

60. Surmely JF, Nasu K, Fujita H, et al. Coronary plaque composition of culprit/target lesions according to the clinical presentation: a virtual histology intravascular ultrasound analysis. Eur Heart J 2006;27:2939–44.

61. Prati F, Regar E, Mintz GS, et al. Expert review document on methodology, terminology, and clinical applications of optical coherence tomography: physical principles, methodology of image acquisition, and clinical application for assessment of coronary arteries and atherosclerosis. Eur Heart J 2010;31:401–15.

62. Yun SH, Tearney GJ, Vakoc BJ, et al. Comprehensive volumetric optical microscopy in vivo. Nat Med 2006;12:1429–33.

63. Schmitt JM, Huber R, Fujimoto JG. Limiting ischemia by fast Fourier-domain imaging. In: Regar E, Serruys PW, van Leeuwen TG, editors. Optical coherence tomography in cardiovascular research. London: Informa HealthCare; 2007. p. 257.

64. Swanson EA, Petersen CL. Methods and apparatus for high speed longitudinal scanning in imaging systems. US patent 6,191,862 B1. 2001.

65. Prati F, Cera M, Ramazzotti V, et al. Safety and feasibility of a new non-occlusive technique for facilitated intracoronary optical coherence tomography (OCT) acquisition in various clinical and anatomical scenarios. EuroIntervention 2007;3:365–70.

66. Yamaguchi T, Terashima M, Akasaka T, et al. Safety and feasibility of an intravascular optical coherence tomography image wire system in the clinical setting. Am J Cardiol 2008;101:562–7.

67. Kume T, Akasaka T, Kawamoto T, et al. Assessment of coronary intima–media thickness by optical coherence tomography. Circulation 2005;69:903–7.

68. Yabushita H, Bouma BE, Houser SL, et al. Characterization of human atherosclerosis by optical coherence tomography. Circulation 2002;106:1640–5.

69. Kawasaki M, Bouma BE, Bressner J, et al. Diagnostic accuracy of optical coherence tomography and integrated backscatter intravascular ultrasound images for tissue characterization of human coronary plaques. J Am Coll Cardiol 2006;48:81–8.

70. Kume T, Okura H, Yamada R, et al. Frequency and spatial distribution of thin-cap fibroatheroma assessed by 3-vessel intravascular ultrasound and optical coherence tomography: an ex vivo validation and an initial in vivo feasibility study. Circ J 2009;73:1086–91.

71. Rieber J, Meissner O, Babaryka G, et al. Diagnostic accuracy of optical coherence tomography and intravascular ultrasound for the detection and characterization of atherosclerotic plaque composition in ex-vivo coronary specimens: a comparison with histology. Coron Artery Dis 2006;17:425–30.

72. Meissner OA, Rieber J, Babaryka G, et al. Intravascular optical coherence tomography: Comparison with histopathology in atherosclerotic peripheral artery specimens. J Vasc Interv Radiol 2006;17:343–9.

73. Tanaka A, Imanishi T, Kitabata H, et al. Lipid-rich plaque and myocardial perfusion after successful stenting in patients with non-ST-segment elevation acute coronary syndrome: an optical coherence tomography study. Eur Heart J 2009;30:1348–55.

74. Gonzalo N, Garcia-Garcia HM, Serruys PW, et al. Reproducibility of quantitative optical coherence tomography for stent analysis. EuroIntervention 2009;5:224–32.

75. Gonzalo N, Serruys PW, Okamura T, et al. Optical coherence tomography patterns of stent restenosis. Am Heart J 2009;158:284–93.

76. Barlis P, Regar E, Serruys PW, et al. An optical coherence tomography study of a biodegradable vs. durable polymer-coated limus-eluting stent: a LEADERS trial sub-study. Eur Heart J 2010;31:165–76.

77. Guagliumi G, Costa MA, Sirbu V, et al. Strut coverage and late malapposition with paclitaxel-eluting stents compared with bare metal stents in acute myocardial infarction optical coherence tomography substudy of the harmonizing outcomes with revascularization and stents in acute myocardial infarction (HORIZONS-AMI) trial. Circulation 2011;123:274–81.

78. Gardner CM, Tan H, Hull EL, et al. Detection of lipid core coronary plaques in autopsy specimens with a novel catheter-based near-infrared spectroscopy system. JACC Cardiovasc Imaging 2008;1:638–48.

79. Garg S, Serruys PW, van der Ent M, et al. First use in patients of a combined near infra-red spectroscopy and intra-vascular ultrasound catheter to identify composition and structure of coronary plaque. EuroIntervention 2010;5:755.

80. Goldstein JA, Grines C, Fischell T, et al. Coronary embolization following balloon dilation of lipid-core plaques. JACC Cardiovasc Imaging 2009;2:1420–4.

81. Maini B, Brilakis ES, Kim M, et al. Association of large lipid core plaque detected by near infrared spectroscopy with post percutaneous coronary intervention myocardial infarction. J Am Coll Cardiol 2010;55:A179.E1672.

82. Goldstein JA, Maini B, Dixon SR, et al. Detection of lipid-core plaques by intracoronary near-infrared spectroscopy identifies high risk of periprocedural myocardial infarction. Circ Cardiovasc Interv 2011;4:429–37.

83. Sakhuja R, Suh WM, Jaffer FA, et al. Residual thrombogenic substrate after rupture of a lipid-rich plaque possible mechanism of acute stent thrombosis? Circulation 2010;122:2349–50.

84. Brilakis ES, Abdel-Karim AR, Papayannis AC, et al. Embolic protection device utilization during stenting of native coronary artery lesions with large lipid core plaques as detected by near-infrared spectroscopy. Catheter Cardiovasc Interv 2012;80:1157–62.

85. Kini AS, Baber U, Kovacic JC, et al. Changes in plaque lipid content after short-term, intensive versus standard statin therapy: the yellow trial. J Am Coll Cardiol 2013;62(1):21–9.

Calcium Scoring and Cardiac Computed Tomography in 2014

 CrossMark

Swapnesh Parikh, MD, Matthew J. Budoff, MD*

KEYWORDS

- Atherosclerosis • Angiography • Risk stratification • Outcomes • Cardiac computed tomography
- Calcium score

KEY POINTS

- Computed tomography (CT) angiography is now the most accurate noninvasive assessment tool for heart disease, with the highest concordance to invasive angiography.
- The use of CT angiography in the emergency department will undoubtedly become the dominant strategy, with emphasis on diagnosis, cost, and prognosis.
- Coronary artery calcium can be accurately depicted on nongated studies, such as those performed for lung cancer screening, and can help doctors identify patients at high risk for future cardiovascular disease.

INTRODUCTION

Accurate and efficient evaluation of acute chest pain remains clinically challenging because traditional diagnostic modalities have many limitations. Recent advances in noninvasive imaging technologies have potentially improved both diagnostic efficiency and clinical outcomes of patients with acute chest pain while reducing unnecessary hospitalizations. However, controversy remains regarding much of the evidence for these technologies. This article primarily reviews the role of coronary computed tomography (CT) angiography (CTA) in the assessment of an individual's coronary risk, and its usefulness in the emergency department (ED) in facilitating appropriate disposition decisions. Also discussed is coronary artery calcification (CAC) incidentally found on CT scans when done for indications such as evaluation of pulmonary embolism or lung cancer. The evidence base and clinical applications for both techniques are described, together with cost-effectiveness and radiation exposure considerations.

BACKGROUND

In the United States more than 6 million patients with chest pain present to the ED each year.[1] The limited predictive value of clinical history and physical examination complicates accurate risk stratification, particularly in patients with normal cardiac biomarkers and nondiagnostic electrocardiograms (ECG).[2] Consequently, more than 60% of patients admitted to the hospital for evaluation of acute coronary syndrome (ACS) are discharged with a noncardiac diagnosis.[3] Conversely, the rate of missed diagnosis of ACS in the ED remains unacceptably high, ranging from 2% to 8%, with missed diagnoses associated with a 2-fold increase in mortality.[4,5]

Effectively ruling out an acute myocardial infarction is difficult. The standard 12-lead ECG has inadequate sensitivity and negative predictive value (NPV) in ruling out any form of ACS.[6] Troponin measurement has a low sensitivity in excluding myocardial ischemia or early manifestations of ACS.[7] Rest echocardiography has limited

Internal Medicine Department, Los Angeles Biomedical Research Institute, 1124 West Carson Street, Torrance, CA 90502, USA
* Corresponding author.
E-mail address: budoff@ucla.edu

Cardiol Clin 32 (2014) 419–427
http://dx.doi.org/10.1016/j.ccl.2014.04.007
0733-8651/14/$ – see front matter © 2014 Elsevier Inc. All rights reserved.

sensitivity in detecting ACS, and is generally not relied on in this setting.[8] Exercise treadmill echocardiography is limited by moderate predictive accuracy in detecting coronary artery disease (CAD) and the frequent presence of baseline ECG abnormalities (eg, left bundle branch block) that preclude accurate interpretation.[9] Single-photon emission CT myocardial perfusion imaging (MPI) remains a cornerstone of evolving clinical care, with emerging and novel applications that will continue to improve the care of patients with cardiovascular disease in the future.[10] Multidetector CT now provides noninvasive coronary imaging, and patients with a low or intermediate probability of CAD can be imaged with radiation levels significantly lower than those of catheterization and nuclear imaging.[11]

CORONARY COMPUTED TOMOGRAPHIC ANGIOGRAPHY

In recent years, cardiac CT angiography (CCTA) has evolved significantly, with a reduction in radiation dose and improvement in diagnostic accuracy. Prospective electrocardiographic gating is becoming more frequently used, as it results in high-quality images at the lowest possible radiation dose, but requires adequate patient preparation and heart-rate control to avoid misregistration (misalignment) artifacts.[12] When appropriately applied, the doses for a CCT angiogram average 2 mSv, markedly lower than for invasive coronary angiography or nuclear imaging.

Diagnostic Accuracy of CT Angiography

The accuracy of CCTA for assessing the presence and severity of coronary stenosis (**Fig. 1**), relative to that of invasive angiography, has been extensively reported.[13] One of the first studies assessing this issue, reported by Sato and colleagues,[14] used 4- and 16-detector scanners, and found sensitivity of 95.5% and specificity of 88.9% for the detection of ACS. Gallagher and colleagues[15] compared CCTA with stress nuclear imaging for the diagnosis of ACS in 85 patients, and found that CCTA accuracy was at least comparable with that of nuclear imaging. A meta-analysis including 9 studies totaling 566 patients using scanners with 64 or fewer detectors revealed a per-patient pooled sensitivity of 95% (95% confidence interval [CI] 90%–98%) and specificity of 90% (95% CI 87%–93%) in detecting ACS in comparison with invasive coronary angiography.[16] A second meta-analysis including 16 studies, totaling 1119 patients, found sensitivity and specificity of 96% (95% CI 93%–98%) and 92% (95% CI 89%–94%), respectively.[17] Both studies

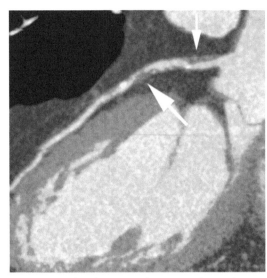

Fig. 1. Example of computed tomography angiogram demonstrating stenosis and atherosclerotic plaque in the left anterior descending artery (*white arrows*).

demonstrate higher diagnostic accuracy for ACS with CCTA than with other previously studied modalities, including exercise treadmill, stress magnetic resonance imaging, stress nuclear imaging, and stress echocardiography.

The ROMICAT trial,[18] which was an observational cohort study of patients with acute chest pain and normal initial ECG and troponins, found sensitivity and NPV of 100% for the absence of plaques on CCTA to detect ACS, and sensitivity and NPV for nonsignificant CAD of 77% and 98%, respectively.

Recently, Chow and colleagues[19] reported sensitivity of 98% (95% CI 87%–100%), specificity of 100% (95% CI 85%–100%), a positive predictive value of 100% (95% CI 90%–100%), and an NPV of 97% (95% CI 80%–100%) for 64-slice CCTA in comparison with invasive coronary angiography in 107 patients with acute chest pain.

Rubinshtein and colleagues[20] reported higher predictive values of CCTA in diagnosing ACS in comparison with standard diagnostic criteria. In a preliminary study, Hoffmann and colleagues[21] evaluated 40 patients with acute chest pain, normal cardiac biomarkers, and a nondiagnostic ECG who underwent CCTA in addition to the standard of care (SOC) diagnostic evaluation before hospital admission. The investigators found at least 1 significant coronary stenosis on CCTA in all patients with final diagnosis of ACS, whereas significant CAD was excluded in 26 of the 35 patients without a final diagnosis of ACS. In another study the same group, low-risk patients randomized to CCTA or SOC diagnostic evaluation were found to have similar accuracy and safety for

CCTA but a shorter time to diagnosis, potentially reducing costs.[22] In a study of 268 patients with acute chest pain randomized to either immediate 64-slice CCTA or conventional diagnostic strategy, the CCTA approach showed a decrease in length of stay in hospital and repeat hospital admissions.[23] In a study conducted by May and colleagues[5] in low-risk patients with acute chest pain, ED discharge based on negative CCTA resulted in significantly shorter length of stay and lower hospital charges when compared with the SOC. Four randomized studies have been performed to compare SOC with CCTA in the setting of low-risk ACS evaluations. The first was published by Goldstein and colleagues,[22] and included patients who were randomized to CCTA (n = 99) or SOC (n = 98) protocols. The CCTA patients with minimal disease were discharged; those with stenosis of greater than 70% underwent invasive coronary angiography, whereas patients with intermediate lesions or nondiagnostic scans underwent stress testing. Outcomes included: safety (freedom from major adverse events over 6 months); diagnostic efficacy (clinically correct and definitive diagnosis); time; and cost of care. Both approaches were completely (100%) safe. The CCTA alone immediately excluded or identified coronary disease as the source of chest pain in 75% of patients, including 67 with normal coronary arteries and 8 with severe disease referred for invasive evaluation. The remaining 25% of patients required stress testing, owing to intermediate severity lesions or nondiagnostic scans. During the index visit, CCTA evaluation reduced diagnostic time in comparison with SOC (3.4 vs 15.0 hours, P<.001) and lowered costs ($1586 vs $1872, P<.001). Of note, CCTA patients required fewer repeat evaluations for recurrent chest pain (multislice CT, 2 of 99 [2.0%] patients vs SOC, 7 of 99 [7%] patients; P = .10). A larger multicenter randomized trial was then undertaken. The Computed Tomographic Angiography for the Systematic Triage of Acute Chest Pain Patients to Treatment (CT-STAT) trial[24] is a prospective, randomized, multicenter, comparative effectiveness trial that compared a coronary CTA-based diagnostic strategy with the usual SOC, including MPI, in the triage of patients of low to intermediate risk with acute chest pain in the ED with a low thrombolysis in myocardial infarction (TIMI) risk score (<4). CT-STAT, covering 750 patients from 16 sites, found the coronary CTA-based strategy reduced the time to diagnosis by 54% compared with MPI (median 2.9 vs 6.3 hours; P<.0001) and lowered total costs of care by 38% (median, $2137 vs $3458; P<.0001). No differences were observed in major adverse coronary events

(0.8% in the CT arm vs 0.4% in the MPI arm; P = .29). In addition, the coronary CTA arm resulted in significantly lower effective radiation dose (11.5 vs 12.8 mSv; P = .02).

The ACRIN-PA trial is a multicenter, randomized, controlled study with the objective of comparing CCTA with standard care of low-risk patients in EDs who present with potential ACS.[25] In this study, 1392 low-risk potential ACS patients were randomly assigned to either standard triage or CCTA. Patients evaluated with CCTA had a shorter mean hospital stay (total length of stay 18 vs 25 hours; P<.0001), and were also discharged more rapidly and more frequently (50% vs 23%) than patients undergoing the standard care evaluation. A 3-fold greater rate of identification of CAD was observed in the coronary CCTA group, demonstrating the known higher sensitivity of CCTA over nuclear imaging in detecting obstructive CAD. None of the 640 subjects with a negative CCTA died or had a myocardial infarction, showing the safety of this approach.

ROMICAT II is a multicenter, randomized, comparative effectiveness trial of CCTA versus standard triage evaluation in patients in the ED with acute chest pain.[26] This study examined whether integrating CCTA improves the efficiency of the management of patients at low to intermediate risk. The trial involved 1000 patients who entered the ED with chest pain who, after initial evaluation, were randomly assigned to either a CCTA or standard triage evaluation. Patients in the CCTA group had more rapid ED disposition (mean average time spent in hospital, 7.6 hours), and 50% of patients in the CT group were safely discharged from the ED within 9 hours, compared with only 15% of the standard-care group. Costs in the ED were 19% lower in the CT group ($2101 vs $2566; P<.0001). However, the mean cost of care, including hospital stay, was similar between both groups ($4026 vs $3874; P not significant), as more patients undergoing CTA were found to have obstructive disease, again thought to be due to the higher sensitivity of CTA, most often 95% in studies, compared with lower sensitivity for obstructive CAD with functional testing. The researchers concluded that CTA significantly reduced the length of stay and time to diagnosis, and increased direct ED discharge rates without putting patients at greater risk for missed ACS. Long-term costs have not been reported.

Beyond Coronary Imaging: The Triple Rule-Out Scan

Numerous studies have demonstrated good to excellent diagnostic accuracy of dedicated CCTA for the evaluation of CAD, with excellent NPV, most commonly in the 99% range.[27–29] However, in the ED, 3 primary causes of chest pain are typically considered, including not only cardiac (for which CTA is excellent, as already outlined) but also pulmonary embolism and aortic dissection.[30] The mortality of each of these missed diagnoses is significant, and the additional ability of CT to simultaneously evaluate pulmonary arteries for embolism and the entire thoracic aorta for aneurysm/dissection makes this attractive to ED clinicians evaluating patients with acute chest pain syndromes of unclear etiology. A recent survey of radiology practices found that 33% used CT in the ED for the workup of chest pain, and that 18% were using a triple rule-out protocol.[30] One of the more recent CT advances, dual-source CT, maintains the high spatial resolution of previous single-source 64-slice CT systems while enabling ECG-gated imaging with an increased temporal resolution.[31] Alternatively, some manufacturers have developed systems with more detectors, thus increasing coverage and requiring less contrast, less breath-hold, and fewer scan times for systems with greater than 64 detectors per rotation. A third approach to improve CT resolution and diagnostic quality is to improve detectors, and high-resolution detector systems have been introduced over the last few years to better visualize coronary plaque, stenosis severity, coronary stents, and bypass grafts.

Clinical application of CCTA in the ED for evaluation of chest pain: selection of patients

Advances in triple rule-out protocols to improve image quality and radiation exposure have also been made. In the study conducted by Vrachliotis and colleagues,[32] a triphasic injection protocol with caudal-cranial scan acquisition resulted in consistent good opacification (>250 Hounsfield units [HU]) of the left main coronary artery, aorta, and main pulmonary artery. Recently, a high-pitch dual-spiral technique using dual-source coronary CT offers an alternative approach to reducing radiation in cases where a triple rule-out protocol is deemed necessary (mean dose 4.08 ± 0.81 mSv).[33]

Triple rule-out protocols should be performed only in cases where there is reasonable suspicion of at least 2 potentially lethal causes for the acute chest pain (ACS, aortic dissection, and pulmonary embolism).[34] Additional risk factors, such as age, diabetes, hypertension, history of CAD, and higher heart rate, have been reported to be independent predictors of poor-quality images in patients with acute chest pain undergoing 64-slice CCTA.[35]

Evaluating for Vulnerable Plaque

Typically the stenosis is usually graded as mild (<50% obstruction of luminal diameter), moderate (50%–69%), or severe (≥70%).[36] There is software available for automatic stenosis quantitation,[37] although most investigators use semiquantitative evaluations, similar to interpreting clinical invasive coronary angiography whereby quantitative coronary angiography measures are rarely used. However, CCTA also provides direct visualization of vessel walls, thus providing a good assessment of the atherosclerotic burden.[38] The goal of plaque characterization is to identify the vulnerable plaque, responsible for most ACS.[39] Many studies have demonstrated the correlation with histology,[40] intravascular ultrasonography,[41] and optical coherence.[42] Extent of plaque measured by wall components of stenosis is classified as soft or lipid-rich (30–60 HU), fibrous (70–120 HU), or calcified (>350 HU).[43] In a study of 1059 patients who underwent CCTA, the investigators found that those with plaques showing positive remodeling and low attenuation on CCTA were at higher risk for ACS during the 27-month mean follow-up compared with patients with plaques without these characteristics.[44] Another clinical study by Fernandez-Friera and colleagues[45] described that plaque characteristics assessed by various imaging modalities, including CCTA, intravascular ultrasonography, and near-infrared spectroscopy, may predict clinical outcomes.

Evaluating Incidentally Found Coronary Artery Calcification on CT Scans

In the aging and smoking population, CAC is a common finding. Given the increasing age and history of smoking in the population, a common concern alongside heart disease, pulmonary embolism, and/or aortic dissection is cancer.[46] In the typical evaluation of CT scans, concern over lung cancer becomes paramount, and while lung nodules are evaluated coronary calcification is a frequent finding.[47] Of note, heart disease is a leading cause of death in all patients with lung diseases, including chronic obstructive pulmonary disease and lung cancer.[47] As nontriggered CT (a scan for evaluation of lung disease or pulmonary embolism) can be used for calcium scoring, to stratify individuals in categories of cardiovascular risk, and to identify those at high cardiovascular risk, there may be an enormous unused primary prevention potential.[48] The calcium scores derived from nongated studies (ie, for lung cancer screening) are often semiquantitatively evaluated rather than by using the Agatston score (the most commonly used quantitative method).[47,48]

Moreover, deriving the calcium score from the same examination as is used in lung cancer screening may positively affect the cost-effectiveness of screening.[49] Testing for the principal (CAD) and second-ranked (lung cancer) cause of death with a single low-dose scan may prove insightful and cost-effective.[50–52] Younger patients (mean age, 43 years) were analyzed in the Prospective Army Coronary Calcium Project, which reported an 11-fold increased risk for hard coronary events.[53] In this study of young, asymptomatic men, the presence of CAC provided substantial, cost-effective, independent prognostic value in predicting incident cardiovascular heart disease that was incremental to measured coronary risk factors. In a properly selected population, coronary CT can provide a cost-effective evaluation,[54] with reduced diagnostic time, lower costs, and fewer repeat evaluations for recurrent chest pain in comparison with standard diagnostic evaluation.[22] Multiple studies have evaluated the use of CAC in addition to coronary risk factors in predicting the risk of future cardiovascular events (**Table 1**). Based upon the c-statistic, CAC provides incremental benefit compared to the use of coronary risk factors.

New technology has reduced both the required phase window for diagnostic imaging of the coronary arteries and the effects of variability in heart rhythm on coronary image quality.[55]

Because CAC on CT distinctly identifies atherosclerosis,[56] it may be advantageous to screen for the CAD and lung cancer simultaneously in a combined CT examination, thus leading to a broader diagnosis of these common and morbid diseases. CAC and thoracic aortic calcification (TAC) can be quantified on chest CT scans.[57,58] Kim and colleagues[59] have reported that, in comparisons of CAC between low-radiation-dose chest multidetector CT and ECG-triggered standard-dose CT, more than 90% of patients with CAC on ECG-triggered

scans can be visualized on ungated CT. Budoff and colleagues[57] showed high concordance between ungated and gated studies for both CAC and TAC.

TAC noted on gated studies has been independently associated with adverse cardiovascular events,[60] inflammation,[61] coronary calcium,[62] and cardiac risk factors.[63] Similarly, agreement was also excellent for CAC, although CAC scores were systematically overestimated on the ungated scan, potentially requiring transformation and/or a correction factor if compared directly with gated cardiac studies.[57]

A recent study of ungated thoracic CT scans performed for lung cancer screening in 8782 smokers, with a mean follow-up of 72 months, revealed significant ability of ungated studies to predict cardiovascular mortality.[63] There is a great potential to screen for cardiovascular disease among the 19 million ungated thoracic scans done annually in the United States, without additional radiation, cost, or participant burden. Because in the United States cardiovascular disease is the leading cause of death and lung cancer is the second leading cause,[64] evaluating for both with one scan may prove an effective addition to standard evaluation.

The radiation dose for low-dose chest CT is 0.6 to 1.1 mSv, compared with 7.0 mSv for conventional CT.[65] In low-dose chest CT screening for lung cancer, Brenner[66] reported an estimated upper limit of a 5.5% increase in the risk for lung cancer attributable to annual CT-related radiation exposure. To minimize the risk of radiation-induced lung cancer or CAD, one should choose a CT examination with a lower radiation dose for a screening study, and minimize the number of CT examinations.[66] A previous study has determined the frequency of calcification of the thoracic aorta and its relationship to risk factors and CAD using a CT examination for lung cancer and tuberculosis.[67] In another study, although a negative or extremely low calcium score ($\leq$10) could not

Table 1
C-statistic with risk factors and with the addition (or substitution) of coronary artery calcium

Study, Year	No. of Participants	Follow-Up (y)	C-Statistic with Risk Factors	C-Statistic with Coronary Artery Calcium	P Value
St Francis Heart Study,[69] 2005	4903	4.3	0.69	0.79	.0006
Budoff et al,[50] 2007	25,253	6.8	0.611	0.813	<.0001
Anand et al,[71] 2006	510	2.3	0.60	0.92	<.0001
Becker et al,[70] 2008	716	8.1	0.68	0.77	<.01
Multi-Ethnic Study of Atherosclerosis,[52] 2012	6722	3.8	0.623	0.784	<.001
Recall,[52] 2009	4814	5.0	0.667	0.754	.0001

Data from Refs.[50,52,69–71]

totally exclude the presence of coronary atherosclerosis, it was consonant with the absence of a fixed (significant) coronary obstructive lesion, regardless of age and sex.[68]

SUMMARY

CCTA is now the most accurate noninvasive tool for the assessment of heart disease, with the highest concordance to invasive coronary angiography. The use CCTA in the ED for patients presenting with chest pain will likely become a dominant strategy, with emphasis on diagnosis, cost, and prognosis. The ability to evaluate CAC, pulmonary embolism, and aortic dissection, in addition to angiographic disease, favors CT imaging. Accurate assessment using CCTA has allowed for rapid triage within the ED, lower costs, and improved diagnosis over other ED-based strategies in 4 large-scale randomized trials. The visualization of subclinical atherosclerosis (on either coronary calcium scanning or seeing nonobstructive plaques on CCTA), not possible with functional imaging, allows for targeted antiatherosclerotic treatment strategies and improved adherence to these treatments. Furthermore, a large number of nontriggered CT examinations are performed annually worldwide. Age and smoking, the current selection criteria for lung cancer screening, are also correlated with coronary calcification and coronary heart disease, potentially allowing simultaneous screening for both heart and lung disease.

REFERENCES

1. Fernandez-Friera L, Garcia-Alvarez A, Guzman G, et al. Coronary CT and the coronary calcium score, the future of ED risk stratification? Curr Cardiol Rev 2012;8(2):86–97.
2. Kumar A, Cannon CP. Acute coronary syndromes: diagnosis and management, part I. Mayo Clin Proc 2009;84(10):917–38.
3. Hoffmann U, Nagurney JT, Moselewski F, et al. Coronary multidetector computed tomography in the assessment of patients with acute chest pain. Circulation 2006;114:2251–60.
4. Pope JH, Aufderheide TP, Ruthazer R, et al. Missed diagnoses of acute cardiac ischemia in the emergency department. N Engl J Med 2000;342(16):1163–70.
5. May JM, Shuman WP, Strote JN, et al. Low-risk patients with chest pain in the emergency department: negative 64-MDCT coronary angiography may reduce length of stay and hospital charges. AJR Am J Roentgenol 2009;193(1):150–4.
6. Zimetbaum PJ, Josephson ME. Use of the electrocardiogram in acute myocardial infarction. N Engl J Med 2003;348:933–40.
7. Daubert MA, Jeremias A. The utility of troponin measurement to detect myocardial infarction: review of the current findings. Vasc Health Risk Manag 2010;6:691–9.
8. Lim SH, Sayre MR, Gibler WB. 2-D echocardiography prediction of adverse events in ED patients with chest pain. Am J Emerg Med 2003;21:106–10.
9. Heng MK, Simard M, Lake R, et al. Exercise two-dimensional echocardiography for diagnosis of coronary artery disease. Am J Cardiol 1984;54(6):502–7.
10. Driver KA, Atchley AE, Kaul P, et al. Single photon emission computed tomography myocardial imaging: clinical applications and future directions. Minerva Cardioangiol 2009;57(3):333–47.
11. Otero HJ, Steigner ML, Rybicki FJ. The "post-64" era of coronary CT angiography: understanding new technology from physical principles. Radiol Clin North Am 2009;47(1):79–90.
12. Choi TY, Malpeso J, Li D, et al. Radiation dose reduction with increasing utilization of prospective gating in 64-multidetector cardiac computed tomography angiography. J Cardiovasc Comput Tomogr 2011;5:264–70.
13. Hamon M, Biondi-Zoccai GG, Malagutti P, et al. Diagnostic performance of multislice spiral computed tomography of coronary arteries as compared with conventional invasive coronary angiography: a meta-analysis. J Am Coll Cardiol 2006;48:1896–910.
14. Sato Y, Matsumoto N, Ichikawa M, et al. Efficacy of multislice computed tomography for the detection of acute coronary syndrome in the emergency department. Circ J 2005;69:1047–51.
15. Gallagher MJ, Ross MA, Raff GL, et al. The diagnostic accuracy of 64-slice computed tomography coronary angiography compared with stress nuclear imaging in emergency department low-risk chest pain patients. Ann Emerg Med 2007;49:125–36.
16. Vanhoenacker PK, Decramer I, Bladt O, et al. Detection of non-ST-elevation myocardial infarction and unstable angina in the acute setting: meta-analysis of diagnostic performance of multi-detector computed tomographic angiography. BMC Cardiovasc Disord 2007;7:39.
17. Athappan G, Habib M, Ponniah T, et al. Multi-detector computerized tomography angiography for evaluation of acute chest pain–a meta-analysis and systematic review of literature. Int J Cardiol 2010;141:132–40.
18. Hoffmann U, Bamberg F, Chae CU, et al. Coronary computed tomography angiography for early triage of patients with acute chest pain: the ROMICAT

(Rule Out Myocardial Infarction using Computer Assisted Tomography) trial. J Am Coll Cardiol 2009;53:1642–50.

19. Chow BJ, Joseph P, Yam Y, et al. Usefulness of computed tomographic coronary angiography in patients with acute chest pain with and without high-risk features. Am J Cardiol 2010;106:463–9.

20. Rubinshtein R, Halon DA, Gaspar T, et al. Usefulness of 64-slice cardiac computed tomographic angiography for diagnosing acute coronary syndromes and predicting clinical outcome in emergency department patients with chest pain of uncertain origin. Circulation 2007;115:1762–8.

21. Hoffmann U, Pena AJ, Moselewski F, et al. MDCT in early triage of patients with acute chest pain. Am J Roentgenol 2006;187:1240–7.

22. Goldstein JA, Gallagher MJ, O'Neill WW, et al. A randomized controlled trial of multi-slice coronary computed tomography for evaluation of acute chest pain. J Am Coll Cardiol 2007;49(8):863–71.

23. Chang SA, Choi SI, Choi EK, et al. Usefulness of 64-slice multidetector computed tomography as an initial diagnostic approach in patients with acute chest pain. Am Heart J 2008;156:375–83.

24. Goldstein JA, Chinnaiyan KM, Abidov A, et al. The CT-STAT (Coronary Computed Tomographic Angiography for Systematic Triage of Acute Chest Pain Patients to Treatment) trial. J Am Coll Cardiol 2011;58:1414–22.

25. Litt HI, Gatsonis C, Snyder B, et al. CT angiography for safe discharge of patients with possible acute coronary syndromes. N Engl J Med 2012;366:1393–403.

26. Hoffmann U, Truong QA, Schoenfeld DA, et al. Coronary CT angiography versus standard evaluation in acute chest pain. N Engl J Med 2012;367:299–308.

27. Halpern EJ. Clinical applications of cardiac CT angiography. Insights Imaging 2010;1(4):205–22.

28. Miller JM, Rochitte CE, Dewey M, et al. Diagnostic performance of coronary angiography by 64-row CT. N Engl J Med 2008;359:2324–36.

29. Arbab-Zadeh A, Miller JM, Rochitte CE, et al. Diagnostic accuracy of computed tomography coronary angiography according to pre-test probability of coronary artery disease and severity of coronary arterial calcification. J Am Coll Cardiol 2012;59(4):379–87.

30. Thomas J, Rideau AM, Paulson EK, et al. Emergency department imaging: current practice. J Am Coll Radiol 2008;5(7):811–6.

31. Frauenfelder T, Appenzeller P, Karlo C, et al. Triple rule-out CT in the emergency department: protocols and spectrum of imaging findings. Eur Radiol 2009;19(4):789–99.

32. Vrachliotis TG, Bis KG, Haidary A, et al. Atypical chest pain: coronary, aortic, and pulmonary vasculature enhancement at biphasic single-injection 64-section CT angiography. Radiology 2007;243:368–76.

33. Sommer WH, Schenzle JC, Becker CR, et al. Saving dose in triple-rule-out computed tomography examination using a high-pitch dual spiral technique. Invest Radiol 2010;45:64–71.

34. Taylor AJ, Cerqueira M, Hodgson JM, et al. ACCF/SCCT/ACR/AHA/ASE/ASNC/SCAI/SCMR appropriate use criteria for cardiac computed tomography. A report of the American College of Cardiology Foundation Appropriate Use Criteria Task Force, the Society of Cardiovascular Computed Tomography, the American College of Radiology, the American Heart Association, the American Society of Echocardiography, the American Society of Nuclear Cardiology, the Society for Cardiovascular Angiography and Interventions, and the Society for Cardiovascular Magnetic Resonance. Circulation 2010;122(21):e525–55.

35. Bamberg F, Abbara S, Schlett CL, et al. Predictors of image quality of coronary computed tomography in the acute care setting of patients with chest pain. Eur J Radiol 2010;74(1):182–8.

36. Busch S, Johnson TR, Nikolaou K, et al. Visual and automatic grading of coronary artery stenoses with 64-slice CT angiography in reference to invasive angiography. Eur Radiol 2007;17(6):1445–51.

37. Boogers MJ, Schuijf JD, Kitslaar PH, et al. Automated quantification of stenosis severity on 64-slice CT: a comparison with quantitative coronary angiography. JACC Cardiovasc Imaging 2010;3(7):699–709.

38. Schuijf JD, Shaw LJ, Wijns W, et al. Cardiac imaging in coronary artery disease: differing modalities. Heart 2005;91(8):1110–7.

39. Motoyama S, Kondo T, Sarai M, et al. Multislice computed tomographic characteristics of coronary lesions in acute coronary syndromes. Heart 2005;91(8):1110–7.

40. Dettmer M, Glaser-Gallion N, Stolzmann P, et al. Quantification of coronary artery stenosis with high-resolution CT in comparison with histopathology in an ex vivo study. Eur J Radiol 2013;82(2):264–9.

41. Pundziute G, Schuijf JD, Jukema JW, et al. Evaluation of plaque characteristics in acute coronary syndromes: non-invasive assessment with multi-slice computed tomography and invasive evaluation with intravascular ultrasound radiofrequency data analysis. Eur Heart J 2008;29:2373–81.

42. Soeda T, Uemura S, Morikawa Y, et al. Diagnostic accuracy of dual-source computed tomography in the characterization of coronary atherosclerotic plaques: comparison with intravascular optical coherence tomography. Int J Cardiol 2011;148(3):313–8.

43. Falk E, Shah PK, Fuster V. Coronary plaque disruption. Circulation 1995;92:657–71.

44. Motoyama S, Sarai M, Harigaya H, et al. Computed tomographic angiography characteristics of atherosclerotic plaques subsequently resulting in acute coronary syndrome. J Am Coll Cardiol 2009;54:49–57.

45. Fernandez-Friera L, Garcia-Alvarez A, Romero A, et al. Lipid-rich obstructive coronary lesions is plaque characterization any important? JACC Cardiovasc Imaging 2010;3:893–5.

46. Oei HH, Vliegenthart R, Hofman A, et al. Risk factors for coronary calcification in older subjects. The Rotterdam Coronary Calcification Study. Eur Heart J 2004;25:48–55.

47. Jacobs PC, Gondrie MJ, van der Graaf Y, et al. Coronary artery calcium can predict all-cause mortality and cardiovascular events on low-dose CT screening for lung cancer. AJR Am J Roentgenol 2012;198:505–11.

48. Mets OM, de Jong PA, Prokop M, et al. Computed tomographic screening for lung cancer: an opportunity to evaluate other diseases. JAMA 2012;308:1433–4.

49. National Lung Screening Trial Research Team, Church TR, Black WC, Aberle DR, et al. Results of initial low-dose computed tomographic screening for lung cancer. N Engl J Med 2013;368(21):1980–91.

50. Budoff MJ, Shaw LJ, Liu ST, et al. Long-term prognosis associated with coronary calcification: observations from a registry of 25,253 patients. J Am Coll Cardiol 2007;49:1860–70.

51. Shaw LJ, Raggi P, Schisterman E, et al. Prognostic value of cardiac risk factors and coronary artery calcium screening for all-cause mortality. Radiology 2003;228:826–33.

52. Budoff MJ, Möhlenkamp S, McClelland R, et al, Multi-Ethnic Study of Atherosclerosis and the Investigator Group of the Heinz Nixdorf RECALL Study. A comparison of outcomes with coronary artery calcium scanning in unselected populations: The Multi-Ethnic Study of Atherosclerosis (MESA) and Heinz Nixdorf RECALL study (HNR). J Cardiovasc Comput Tomogr 2013;7(3):182–91. http://dx.doi.org/10.1016/j.jcct.2013.05.009.

53. Taylor AJ, Bindeman J, Feuerstein I, et al. Coronary calcium independently predicts incident premature coronary heart disease over measured cardiovascular risk factors: mean three-year outcomes in the Prospective Army Coronary Calcium (PACC) project. J Am Coll Cardiol 2005;46:807–14.

54. Ladapo JA, Hoffmann U, Bamberg F, et al. Cost-effectiveness of coronary MDCT in the triage of patients with acute chest pain. AJR Am J Roentgenol 2008;191(2):455–63.

55. Steigner ML, Otero HJ, Cai T, et al. Narrowing the phase window width in prospectively ECG-gated single heart beat 320-detector row coronary CT angiography. Int J Cardiovasc Imaging 2009;25(1):85–90.

56. Greenland P, Bonow RO, Brundage BH, et al. Coronary artery calcium scoring: ACCF/AHA 2007 clinical expert consensus document on coronary artery calcium scoring by computed tomography in global cardiovascular risk assessment and in evaluation of patients with chest pain. J Am Coll Cardiol 2007;49:378–402.

57. Budoff MJ, Nasir K, Kinney GL, et al. Coronary artery and thoracic calcium on noncontrast thoracic CT scans: comparison of ungated and gated examinations in patients from the COPD Gene cohort. J Cardiovasc Comput Tomogr 2011;5(2):113–8.

58. Kim J, Bravo PE, Gholamrezanezhad A, et al. Coronary artery and thoracic aorta calcification is inversely related to coronary flow reserve as measured by [82]Rb PET/CT in intermediate risk patients. J Nucl Cardiol 2013;20(3):375–84.

59. Kim SM, Chung MJ, Lee KS, et al. Coronary calcium screening using low-dose lung cancer screening: effectiveness of MDCT with retrospective reconstruction. AJR Am J Roentgenol 2008;190:917–22.

60. Santos RD, Rumberger JA, Budoff MJ, et al. Thoracic aorta calcification detected by electron beam tomography predicts all-cause mortality. Atherosclerosis 2010;209(1):131–5.

61. Takasu J, Katz R, Shavelle DM, et al. Inflammation and descending thoracic aortic calcification as detected by computed tomography: the Multi-Ethnic Study of Atherosclerosis. Atherosclerosis 2008;199:201–6.

62. Takasu J, Budoff MJ, O'Brien KD, et al. Relationship between coronary artery and descending thoracic aortic calcification as detected by computed tomography: the Multi-Ethnic Study of Atherosclerosis. Atherosclerosis 2009;204(2):440–6.

63. Takasu J, Katz R, Nasir K, et al. Relationships of thoracic aortic wall calcification to cardiovascular risk factors: the Multi-Ethnic Study of Atherosclerosis. Am Heart J 2008;155:765–71.

64. Manser R, Dalton A, Carter R, et al. Cost-effectiveness analysis of screening for lung cancer with low dose spiral CT (computed tomography) in the Australian setting. Lung Cancer 2005;48:171–85.

65. Diederich S, Wormanns D, Semik M, et al. Screening for early lung cancer with low-dose spiral CT: prevalence in 817 asymptomatic smokers. Radiology 2003;222:773–81.

66. Brenner DJ. Radiation risks potentially associated with low-dose CT screening of adult smokers for lung cancer. Radiology 2004;231:440–5.

67. Itani Y, Watanabe S, Masuda Y. Aortic calcification detected in a mass chest screening program

using a mobile helical computed tomography unit: relationship to risk factors and coronary artery disease. Circ J 2004;68:538–41.

68. Rumberger JA, Brundage BH, Rader DJ. Electron beam computed tomographic coronary calcium scanning: a review and guidelines for use in asymptomatic persons. Mayo Clin Proc 1999;74: 243–52.

69. Arad Y, Goodman KJ, Roth M, et al. Coronary calcification, coronary disease risk factors, C-reactive protein, and atherosclerotic cardiovascular

disease events: the St. Francis Heart Study. J Am Coll Cardiol 2005;46:158–65.

70. Becker A, Leber A, Becker C, et al. Predictive value of coronary calcifications for future cardiac events in asymptomatic individuals. Am Heart J 2008; 155:154–60.

71. Anand DV, Lim E, Hopkins D, et al. Risk stratification in uncomplicated type 2 diabetes: prospective evaluation of the combined use of coronary artery calcium imaging and selective myocardial perfusion scintigraphy. Eur Heart J 2006;27:713–21.

Alternative Therapy for Medically Refractory Angina

Enhanced External Counterpulsation and Transmyocardial Laser Revascularization

Ozlem Soran, MD, MPH, FACC, FESC

KEYWORDS

- Medically refractory angina • Enhanced external counterpulsation therapy • Coronary artery disease
- Transmyocardial laser revascularization

KEY POINTS

- Numerous clinical trials in the past 2 decades have shown enhanced external counterpulsation (EECP) therapy to be safe and effective for patients with coronary artery disease (CAD), with a clinical response rate averaging 70% to 80%, which is sustained up to 5 years.
- Benefits associated with EECP therapy include reduction in angina and nitrate use, increased exercise tolerance, favorable psychosocial effects, and enhanced quality of life as well as prolongation of the time to exercise-induced ST-segment depression and an accompanying resolution of myocardial perfusion defects.
- In transmyocardial revascularization (TMR), 20 to 40 transmural channels are created using a high-energy carbon dioxide laser with brief manual compression of the epicardial surface to allow for closure of the epicardial opening sites.
- Studies with TMR have shown an improvement in subjective outcome measures that was counterbalanced by a higher risk of postoperative mortality and morbidity.
- Like TMR, studies with percutaneous transmyocardial laser revascularization (PTMLR) have shown improvement in subjective outcome measures that was counterbalanced by a higher risk of peri- and postmortality and morbidity.

INTRODUCTION

Medically refractory angina pectoris (RAP) is a significant health problem in the United States and worldwide and is defined by presence of severe angina with objective evidence of ischemia and failure to relieve symptoms with coronary revascularization. Before diagnosing a patient with RAP, repeated attempts at "maximizing" medical treatment and lifestyle modification (initiation an exercise program and discontinuation of tobacco) should be made. Additionally, all secondary causes of angina, such as anemia and uncontrolled hypertension, should be excluded.[1]

Based on the 2013 American Heart Association (AHA) statistical update, an estimated 15.4 million Americans greater than or equal to 20 years of age have CAD. Total CAD prevalence is 6.4% in US adults greater than or equal to 20 years of age. CAD makes up more than half of all cardiovascular events in men and women less than 75 years of age. The angina prevalence is 7,800,000 in US adults greater than or equal to 20 years of age.[2] Although not included in the 2013 AHA statistical

Heart and Vascular Institute, University of Pittsburgh, 200 Lothrop Street, Scaife Hall S-623, Pittsburgh, PA 15213, USA
E-mail address: soranzo@upmc.edu

Cardiol Clin 32 (2014) 429–438
http://dx.doi.org/10.1016/j.ccl.2014.04.009
0733-8651/14/$ – see front matter © 2014 Elsevier Inc. All rights reserved.

cardiology.theclinics.com

update, it is estimated that between 600,000 and 1.8 million patients in the United States have RAP, with as many as 75,000 new cases diagnosed each year.[3]

Medication and invasive revascularization are the most common approaches for treating CAD. Invasive revascularization includes percutaneous coronary interventions (PCIs)—coronary stent implantation and balloon angioplasty—and coronary artery bypass surgery (CABG). Even though both treatment options are commonly used, neither of these approaches provides a cure. Although the symptoms are eliminated or alleviated, the disease and its causes are still present after treatment. Both treatments target lesions that cause the obstructions; however, CAD is a progressive disease. New treatment approaches are in need to prevent the disease from progressing and the symptoms from recurring.

Current nonpharmacologic options for patients with RAP include neurostimulation (transcutaneous electrical nerve stimulation and spinal cord stimulation), EECP therapy, and laser revascularization. Extracorporeal shockwave myocardial revascularization, gene therapy, and percutaneous in situ coronary venous arterialization are still under investigation. This article summarizes the current evidence for using EECP therapy and TMR in RAP management.[4]

EECP THERAPY

EECP therapy with its different mode of action provides a new treatment modality in the management of CAD and can complement invasive revascularization procedures (**Fig. 1**).[4]

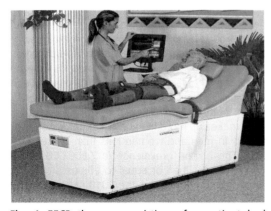

Fig. 1. EECP therapy, consisting of a patient bed attached to an air compressor unit, computerized control console, and 3 sets of cuffs wrapped around the lower legs and the buttocks of the patient. (*Courtesy of* Vasomedical Inc, Westbury, NY; with permission.)

EECP therapy consists of a treatment bed attached to an air compressor unit that is attached to a computerized control console. Three sets of cuffs are wrapped around the lower legs and the buttocks of the patient. It is a noninvasive outpatient therapy consisting of ECG-gated sequential leg compression, which produces hemodynamic effects similar to those of an intra-aortic balloon pump (IABP) (**Fig. 2**).[4]

Unlike IABP therapy, however, EECP therapy also increases venous return. Cuffs resembling oversized blood pressure cuffs—on the calves and lower and upper thighs, including the buttocks—inflate rapidly and sequentially via computer-interpreted ECG signals, starting from the calves and proceeding upward to the buttocks during the resting phase of each heartbeat (diastole). This creates a strong retrograde counterpulse in the arterial system, forcing freshly oxygenated blood toward the heart and coronary arteries while increasing the volume of venous blood return to the heart under increased pressure. Just before the next heartbeat, before systole, all 3 cuffs deflate simultaneously, significantly reducing the heart's workload. This is achieved because the vascular beds in the lower extremities are relatively empty when the cuffs are deflated, significantly lowering the resistance to blood ejected by the heart and reducing the amount of work the heart must do to pump oxygenated blood to the rest of the body. A finger plethysmogram is used throughout treatment to monitor diastolic and systolic pressure waveforms. The current EECP device can generate external cuff pressures as high as 220 to 300 mm Hg. A typical therapy course consists of 35 treatments administered for 1 hour a day over 7 weeks.[4]

Acute hemodynamic effects of EECP have been shown through both noninvasive and invasive studies.[5–10]

Acute hemodynamic effects of EECP are summarized (**Fig. 3**)[4]:
1. Increased retrograde aortic blood flow; diastolic augmentation
2. Increased coronary blood flow; increased perfusion pressure
3. Increased venous return
4. Increased cardiac output
5. Systolic unloading
6. Decreased left ventricular workload

EECP THERAPY IN RAP MANAGEMENT

Numerous clinical trials over the past decade have shown EECP therapy safe and effective for patients with RAP, with a clinical response

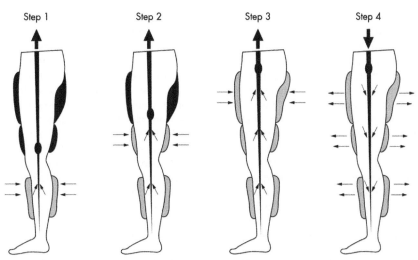

Fig. 2. Technique of EECP therapy. Three pairs of pneumatic cuffs are applied to the calves, lower thighs, and upper thighs. The cuffs are inflated sequentially during diastole, distal to proximal. The compression of the lower extremity vascular bed increases diastolic pressure and flow and increases venous return. The pressure is then released at the onset of systole. Inflation and deflation are timed according to the R wave on the patient's cardiac monitor. The pressures applied and the inflation–deflation timing can be altered by using the pressure waveforms and ECG on the EECP therapy monitor. (*From* Soran O. The role of enhanced external counterpulsation therapy in the management of coronary artery disease. In: Piscione F, editor. Angina pectoris. 1st edition. (Croatia): InTech; 2011.)

(reduction in angina and improvement in exercise capacity and quality of life) rate averaging 70% to 80%, which is sustained for up to 5 years.[11–18] It not only is safe in patients with coexisting heart failure but has also been shown to improve quality of life and exercise capacity and to improve long-term left ventricular function.[5,15,19–23]

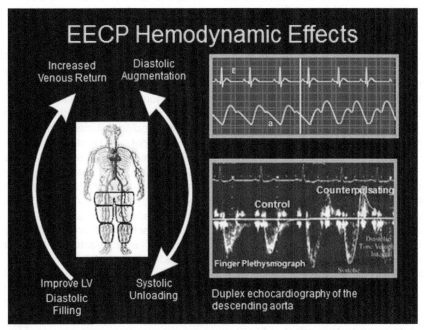

Fig. 3. Acute hemodynamic effects of EECP therapy. Right upper corner: showing the ECG tracing and finger pletysmogram. As soon as the device turned on (*yellow line*) diastolic augmentation starts. Right lower corner: showing the diastolic augmentation by echocardiography. a, aortic notch. (*Courtesy of* Drs Soran and Katz, Pittsburgh, PA.)

The Multicenter Study of EECP (MUST-EECP) was the first randomized double-blinded placebo-controlled trial, conducted in 7 university hospitals in 139 patients, to document a clinical benefit from EECP therapy in patients with stable angina and positive exercise stress tests. In this study, patients (mean age 63 years, range 35–81 years) with angina pectoris and documented coronary ischemia were equally randomized to hemodynamically inactive counterpulsation with EECP versus active counterpulsation. Patients in the active EECP therapy group showed a statistically significant increase in time to exercise-induced ST-segment depression compared with sham and baseline and reported a statistically significant decrease in the frequency of angina episodes compared with sham and baseline. Exercise duration increased significantly in both groups; however, the increase was greater in the active EECP group. Moreover, a MUST-EECP substudy demonstrated a significant improvement in quality-of-life parameters in patients assigned to active treatment, and this improvement was sustained during a 12-month follow-up.[12]

Tartaglia and colleagues[18] assessed the effect of EECP on exercise capacity and myocardial perfusion by comparing results of maximal exercise radionuclide testing pre- and post-EECP treatment in patients with angina who had performed maximal symptom-limited exercise tolerance tests with Bruce protocol and radionuclide perfusion single-photon emission CT study prior to and at completion of EECP treatment. After EECP therapy, 93% of patients improved by at least 1 functional angina class and 80% either no longer had ST depression or had a significant increase in their time to ST depression. The radionuclide perfusion scores also showed a significant reduction in ischemic segments. In this study, patients treated with EECP demonstrated a reduction in angina symptoms, improvement in exercise capacity, increase in time to ST-segment depression, and decrease in perfusion defects despite performing at a higher workload.[4,18]

In another prospective study, the effects of EECP therapy on dobutamine stress-induced wall motion score among patients with angina pectoris were assessed. In this study, 43% of patients with severe chronic angina pectoris who had a positive dobutamine stress echocardiogram had normal or reduced dobutamine-induced wall motion abnormalities after EECP therapy.[24]

The immediate and long-term effect of EECP in treatment of RAP was assessed by British investigators.[25] In this study, investigators enrolled 61 patients, and 58 completed a course of EECP treatment. Approximately 52% of patients suffered from CCS class III and IV angina prior to EECP. Immediately post-EECP, angina improved by at least 1 CCS class in 86% and by 2 classes in 59%. At 1-year follow-up, sustained improvement in CCS was observed in 78% of the patients. The median weekly angina frequency and nitroglycerin use were significantly reduced immediately after EECP. In 48 patients, their mean exercise time improved significantly after EECP. Major adverse events were rare. This study showed that for patients who fail to respond to conventional measures, a high proportion gain symptomatic benefit from EECP.[4,25]

In 2006, Swedish investigators assessed the long-term outcome of EECP treatment, at a Scandinavian center, in relieving angina in patients with chronic RAP; 55 patients were treated with EECP. CCS class, antianginal medication, and adverse clinical events were collected prior to EECP, at the end of the treatment, and at 6 and 12 months after EECP treatment. Clinical signs and symptoms were recorded. EECP treatment significantly improved the CCS class in 79% of the patients with chronic angina pectoris. The reduction in CCS angina class was seen in patients with CCS class III and IV and persisted 12 months after EECP treatment. In accordance with the reduction in CCS classes, there was a significant decrease in the weekly sublingual nitroglycerin usage. The results showed that EECP was a safe and effective treatment in CAD patients and the beneficial effects were sustained during a 12-month follow-up period.[4,26]

In the same year, Italian investigators[27] tested the efficacy of EECP to relieve symptoms to decrease myocardial ischemia and to improve cardiac performance in patients with RAP; 25 patients (mean age 65 years) with persistent ischemia, notwithstanding optimal medical therapy or after interventional or surgical procedure, received EECP sessions for 35 hours. Each patient underwent dobutamine stress echocardiography before and after treatment; 84% of patients showed an increase in at least 1 functional angina class and 36% of patients had a reduction in the area of inducible ischemia at dobutamine stress echocardiography after treatment. The investigators concluded that EECP therapy was effective in relieving symptoms in patients with refractory angina and may reduce inducible ischemia at dobutamine stress echocardiography, especially in patients with reduced systolic function and compromised segmental kinesis.[4,27]

Although randomized (including placebo-controlled) and nonrandomized studies have shown beneficial effects of EECP therapy, investigators saw the need to assess EECP's effectiveness in real-world settings, leading them to develop the International EECP Patient Registry (IEPR) under the management of the University of Pittsburgh.[13,15] More than 5000 patients were enrolled in phase I and another 2500 patients enrolled in phase II of the study, and more than 90 centers participated. Results from the IEPR and the EECP Clinical Consortium[28] have demonstrated that the symptomatic benefit observed in controlled studies translates to the heterogeneous patient population seen in clinical practice. Moreover, follow-up data indicate that the clinical benefit may be maintained for up to 5 years in patients with a favorable initial clinical response.[28,29]

Soran and colleagues[23] compared the repeat EECP and 6-months' major adverse cardiovascular event (MACE) (death/CABG/PCI/MI)–free survival rates for patients treated with EECP for RAP in the European Union (EU) with the United States (US); 4658 patients were treated and followed in US and 262 patients were treated and followed in the EU. EU patients were younger (P<.001) with a higher proportion of men. Previous revascularization rate was higher in US (P<.001). EU had less diabetes, hypertension, hyperlipidemia, multivessel disease, and class IV angina and higher rates of nitroglycerin usage (P<.001). After a mean treatment course of 34 hours, both groups showed a significant reduction in the severity of angina (78% vs 76%). Discontinuation of sublingual nitroglycerin usage was similar in both groups (50%). MACEs during the treatment period were low in both groups (<3%). Compliance with the treatment course was better in EU (P<.001). At 6-month follow-up, 66% of EU and 76% of US had maintained the improvement in angina class; survival rate was 99% in EU and 97% in US. MACE-free survival rate was 92% in EU versus 90% in US. Repeat EECP rates at 6-month follow-up were significantly lower in EU (0.5% vs 4%; P<.01). Patients presenting for EECP treatment from EU and US populations showed very different baseline profiles. Both cohorts, however, achieved substantial reduction in angina with high event-free survival rates at 6 months.[4,23]

EECP was suggested as a safe treatment option for selected symptomatic PCI candidates with obstructive CAD. Baseline characteristics and 1-year outcome in 2 cohorts of PCI candidates presenting with stable symptoms were compared: 323 patients treated with EECP in the IEPR versus 448 National Heart, Lung, and Blood Institute Dynamic Registry patients treated with elective PCIs. Compared with patients receiving PCIs, IEPR patients had a higher prevalence of many risk factors, including prior PCIs, prior coronary artery bypass grafting, prior myocardial infarction (MI), history of congestive heart failure, and history of diabetes. Left ventricular ejection fraction was lower among IEPR patients (mean 50.3% vs 59.2%; P<.001). At 1 year, survival was comparable in the 2 cohorts (98.7% IEPR vs 96.8% PCI; P = NS), as were rates of coronary artery bypass grafting during follow-up (4.5% IEPR vs 5.7% PCI; P = NS). At 1 year, 43.7% of IEPR patients reported no anginal symptoms compared with 73.4% of Dynamic Registry patients (P<.001). Rates of severe symptoms (CCS class III or IV or unstable) at 1 year were 15.5% among IEPR patients and 9.5% in the Dynamic Registry (P = .02). PCI candidates suitable for and treated with EECP had 1-year major event rates comparable to patients receiving elective PCIs. These results suggested that EECP, as a noninvasive treatment, could be used as a first-line treatment with invasive revascularization reserved for EECP failures, or high-risk patients.[4,30,31]

In a recently published study from Sweden, investigators evaluated the effects of EECP on physical capacity and health-related quality of life (HRQOL) at 6-months in patients with refractory AP. Six-minute walk test, functional class with Canadian Cardiovascular Society (CCS) classification, and self-reported HRQOL questionnaires as Short Form 36 (SF-36) were collected at baseline and after treatment in 34 patients. CCS class and SF-36 were repeated at 6-month follow-up. Patients enhanced walk distance an average of 29 meters after EECP (P<.01). CCS class also improved (P<.001) and persisted at 6-follow-up (P<.001). HRQOL improved significantly and the effects were maintained at follow-up after the treatment.

Patients with RAP and left ventricular dysfunction exert an enormous burden on health care resources, primarily because of the number of recurrent emergency department visits and hospitalizations. Improvements in symptoms and laboratory assessments in these patients may not correlate with a reduction in emergency room visits and hospitalizations. Soran and colleagues[22] assessed the impact of EECP therapy on emergency department visits and hospitalization rates at 6-month follow-up in patients with RAP and left ventricular dysfunction. In this prospective cohort study, clinical outcomes, number of all-cause emergency department visits, and hospitalizations within the 6 months before EECP therapy were compared with those at 6-month follow-up. After completion of EECP treatment, angina class decreased by at least 1 CCS class in 72% of the patients, 19% reported no angina, and 2% had an increase in angina class. Mean angina frequency decreased by 7 ± 14 episodes per week, from 11.4 ± 16.9 to 3.8 ± 10.9 ($P<.001$). MACEs occurring during EECP treatment were 0.7% MI, 0.2% CABG, 1.2% PCI, and no death for a total MACE rate of 1.8%. Heart failure exacerbation was reported in 2.6% of patients. Six months after completion of EECP treatment, cumulative mortality was 5.3% and MI was 1.9%. The mean number of emergency department visits per patient decreased from 0.9 ± 2.0 before EECP to 0.2 ± 0.7 at 6 months ($P<.001$), and hospitalizations were reduced from 1.1 ± 1.7 to 0.3 ± 0.7 ($P<.001$).[4,22]

Scientific data indicate that EECP provides a safe and effective treatment option for patients with RAP. Its different mode of action complements invasive revascularization treatment, including CABG and PCI. Currently, American College of Cardiology (ACC)/AHA guidelines recommend EECP therapy as a class IIb (level of evidence: B) intervention for treatment of CAD. The section about EECP is outdated, however, and refers only to the 1999 MUST-EECP study and a rather poor Cochrane review published in 2010, but with references only up to 2008. Due to the volume and quality of scientific data now available and the descriptions of the rating and evidence levels as defined by ACC and AHA guidelines, it is thought that EECP therapy has earned a class IIa treatment recommendation with level of evidence A. EECP therapy has been given a IIa class of recommendation in the 2013 European Society of Cardiology (ESC) Guidelines on the Management of Stable Coronary Artery Disease, indicating that physicians should consider EECP therapy as a treatment option for patients suffering from RAP.

Significant benefits associated with EECP therapy include
- Angina reduction
- Improvement in quality of life
- Prolongation of the time to exercise-induced ST-segment depression
- Resolution of myocardial perfusion defects
- Reduction of nitrate use
- Reduction in hospitalization
- Low MACE rates at long-term follow-up

Several placebo-controlled randomized trials have evaluated the mechanism of action of EECP therapy; these studies suggest that benefits are related to improved left ventricular diastolic filling and endothelial function, collateral development, neurohormonal and cytokine changes, and a peripheral training effect.[32–38]

Contraindications and side effects[4]

Contraindications to EECP include
- Arrhythmias that may interfere with EECP system triggering (uncontrolled atrial fibrillation or flutter or very frequent premature ventricular contractions)
- Coagulopathy with an international normalized ratio (INR) of prothrombin time greater than 2.5
- Severe hypertension: greater than 180/110 mm Hg (the augmented diastolic pressure may exceed safe limits)
- Cardiac catheterization or arterial puncture (risk of bleeding at femoral puncture site) within the past 2 weeks
- Moderate to severe aortic insufficiency (regurgitation would prevent diastolic augmentation)
- Decompensated heart failure
- Severe peripheral arterial disease (reduced vascular volume and muscle mass may prevent active counterpulsation)
- Aortic aneurysm (≥ 5 mm) or dissection (diastolic pressure augmentation may be deleterious)
- Severe chronic obstructive pulmonary disease (no safety data in pulmonary hypertension)
- Pregnancy or being of childbearing age (effects of EECP therapy on the fetus have not been studied)
- Venous disease (phlebitis, varicose veins, stasis ulcers, prior or current deep vein thrombosis, or pulmonary embolism)

Side effects from EECP include
- Paresthesias
- Skin abrasion or ecchymoses
- Bruises
- Worsening of heart failure in patients with severe arrhythmias
- Leg or waist pain

TRANSMYOCARDIAL LASER REVASCULARIZATION

Over the past 2 decades, several investigators have conducted research on TMR/transmyocardial laser revascularization (TMLR).[39–49] In this procedure, 20 to 40 transmural channels are created using a high-energy carbon dioxide laser with brief manual compression of the epicardial surface to allow for closure of the epicardial opening sites. Various energy sources have been used, including carbon dioxide XeCl excimer and holmium:YAG lasers.[50–52] There is no convincing evidence that one energy source is superior to the others. Its mechanism of action was initially thought to be direct perfusion of the myocardium with the left ventricular blood entering the ischemic myocardium via these endocardial channels, thus replicating the reptilian circulation. Early closure of these channels, however, and histopathologic studies demonstrating the absence of true communication between the epicardial channels and the endocardial cavity suggest that this hypothesis was wrong. It was then thought that the laser may stimulate angiogenesis and may destroy nerve fibers to the heart, making patients numb to their chest pain. Multiple randomized prospective controlled surgical trials have assessed the safety and efficacy of TMLR in patients with RAP. Although found efficacious in 80% of patients short term, there are few follow-up data to assess long-term efficacy and freedom from angina.[53–55]

A meta-analysis of 7 randomized clinical trials involving 1053 patients evaluated the effect of TMR on survival and angina relief.[56] The conclusion was that at 1 year, TMR improved angina class but not survival when used as the sole procedural intervention compared with medical therapy alone.

Although investigated initially as a sole therapy for RAP, TMR is now mainly used in conjunction with CABG. A single randomized multicenter comparison of TMR (with a holmium:YAG laser) plus CABG versus CABG alone in patients in whom some myocardial segments were perfused by arteries considered not amenable to grafting showed a significant reduction in perioperative mortality (1.5% vs 7.6%, respectively), with the survival benefit of the TMR–CABG combination present after 1 year of follow-up.[57] At the same time, a large retrospective analysis of data from the Society of Thoracic Surgeons National Cardiac Database, as well as a study of 169 patients from the Washington Hospital Center who underwent combined TMR–CABG, showed no difference in adjusted mortality compared with CABG alone.[58,59]

In summary, a TMR–CABG combination does not seem to improve survival compared with CABG alone. In selected patients, however, such a combination may be superior to CABG alone in relieving angina.

PERCUTANEOUS TRANSMYOCARDIAL LASER REVASCULARIZATION

TMR has also been performed percutaneously, using a less-invasive catheter-based approach that is referred to as PTMLR. The Potential Angina Class Improvement From Intramyocardial Channels (PACIFIC) trial was a multicenter, randomized study comparing PTMLR in addition to medical therapy with medical therapy alone in patients with CCS class III or IV RAP. At 12 months, exercise tolerance significantly increased in the PTMLR group, as did anginal class scores and quality-of-life measurements. There was no significant difference, however, in overall mortality.[60]

A similar study conducted by Whitlow and colleagues[61] compared PTMLR plus medical therapy to medical therapy alone in 330 patients with CCS class II, III, or IV RAP. After 12 months, there was a significant improvement in anginal class scores, exercise tolerance, and quality-of-life measures. Again, there was no difference in 1-year survival between the groups.

The results of the direct myocardial revascularization in the Regeneration of Endomyocardial Channels Trial (DIRECT) tempered the initial enthusiasm surrounding PTMLR. This randomized, placebo-controlled, prospective trial enrolled 298 patients into 3 treatment arms: placebo PTMLR procedure, low-dose PTMLR (10–15 channels created), or high-dose PTMLR (20–25 channels created). The results were similar for treatment arms, representing a large placebo effect.[62] Early studies of the percutaneous approach demonstrated no therapeutic benefit, and this therapy was thus promptly abandoned.[63]

TMR and PTMLR have been recently evaluated by Schofield and McNab.[64] Although there was an improvement in the more subjective outcome measures (including exercise tolerance testing, angina score, and quality of life), this was counterbalanced by a higher risk of postoperative mortality and morbidity (including MI, heart failure, thromboembolic events, pericarditis, acute mitral insufficiency, and neurologic events). In the same way, the evaluation of PTMLR includes 5 randomized trials. In evaluating all of these trials a group, overall mortality was not increased. Various measures of morbidity, however, including MI, ventricular perforation and tamponade, cerebrovascular events, and vascular complications, were increased by PTMLR.

ACC/AHA AND ESC GUIDELINES

On the basis of current evidence on both TMR and PTMLR for RAP, ESC 2013 guidelines state that these procedures show no efficacy and may pose unacceptable procedural-related risks; therefore, these procedures should not be used in RAP management (class III indication).[65] The ACC/AHA 2012 guidelines committee, however, classifies TMR as class IIB, in which usefulness/efficacy is less well established by evidence/opinion (**Table 1**).[66]

Table 1
Guidelines for the diagnosis and management of patients with stable ischemic heart disease

	ESC 2013 CAD Guidelines	ACC/AHA 2012 CAD Guidelines
EECP therapy	Class IIA	Class IIB
TMR	Class III	Class IIB

Class IIA: weight of evidence/opinion is in favor of usefulness/efficacy; Class IIB: usefulness/efficacy is less well established by evidence/opinion; and Class III: conditions for which there is evidence and/or general agreement that the procedure/treatment is not useful/effective and in some cases may be harmful.

The ACC/AHA 2012 guidelines recommend EECP therapy as class IIB.[66] The results of recent studies proving the concept and clinical effects of EECP treatment, however, led the ESC guidelines 2013 committee to the recommendation that EECP therapy should be considered for symptomatic treatment in patients with refractory angina (class IIA).[65]

In summary, EECP provides a noninvasive effective treatment option in patients with RAP, and currently available scientific data support that it should be considered as a first-line treatment in patients with RAP. On the other hand, the published literature shows that the benefit/risk ratio does not favor the routine use of TMR/PTMLR in the RAP management.

REFERENCES

1. Soran O. Treatment options for refractory angina pectoris: enhanced external counterpulsation therapy. Curr Treat Options Cardiovasc Med 2009;11:54–60.
2. Go AS, Mozaffarian D, Roger VL, et al. Heart disease and stroke statistics—2013 update: a report from the American Heart Association. Circulation 2013;127:e6–245.
3. Manchanda A, Soran O. Enhanced external counterpulsation and future directions: step beyond medical management for patients with angina and heart failure. J Am Coll Cardiol 2007;50:1523–31.
4. Soran O. The role of enhanced external counterpulsation therapy in the management of coronary artery disease. In: Piscione F, editor. Angina pectoris. 1st edition. (Croatia): InTech; 2011. Available at: http://www.intechopen.com/books/angina-pectoris/the-role-of-enhanced-external-counterpulsation-therapy-in-the-management-of-coronary-artery-disease.
5. Soran O, Michaels AD, Kennard ED, et al. Is diastolic augmentation an important predictor of treatment completion for patients with left ventricular dysfunction undergoing enhanced external counterpulsation for angina. J Card Fail 2001;7(Suppl 2):99.
6. Stys TP, Lawson WE, Hui JC, et al. Effects of enhanced external counterpulsation on stress radionuclide coronary perfusion and exercise capacity in chronic stable angina pectoris. Am J Cardiol 2002;89:822–82.
7. Michaels AD, Accad M, Ports TA, et al. Left ventricular systolic unloading and augmentation of intracoronary pressure and Doppler flow during enhanced external counterpulsation. Circulation 2002;106:1237–42.
8. Taguchi I, Ogawa K, Kanaya T, et al. Effects of enhanced external counterpulsation on hemodynamics and its mechanism. Circ J 2004;68(11):1030–4.
9. Michaels AD, Tacy T, Teitel D, et al. Invasive left ventricular energetics during enhanced external counterpulsation. Am J Ther 2009;16(3):239–46.
10. Lawson WE, Hui JC, Soroff HS, et al. Efficacy of enhanced external counterpulsation in the treatment of angina pectoris. Am J Cardiol 1992;70:859–62.
11. Lawson WE, Hui JC, Zheng ZS, et al. Improved exercise tolerance following enhanced external counterpulsation: cardiac or peripheral effect? Cardiology 1996;87:271–5.
12. Arora RR, Chou TM, Jain D, et al. The multicenter study of enhanced external counterpulsation (MUST - EECP): effect of EECP on exercise-induced myocardial ischemia and anginal episodes. J Am Coll Cardiol 1999;33:1833–40.
13. Barsness G, Feldman AM, Holmes DR Jr, et al, International EECP Patient Registry Investigators. The International EECP Patient Registry (IE PR): Design, methods, baseline characteristics, and acute results. Clin Cardiol 2001;24:435–42.
14. Fitzgerald CP, Lawson WE, Hui JC, et al, International EECP Patient Registry Investigators. Enhanced external counterpulsation as initial revascularization treatment for angina refractory to medical therapy. Cardiology 2003;100:129–35.
15. Soran O, Kennard ED, Kfoury AG, et al, International EECP Patient Registry Investigators. Two-year clinical outcomes after enhanced external counterpulsation (EECP) therapy in patients with refractory angina pectoris and left ventricular dysfunction (report from the International EECP Patient Registry). Am J Cardiol 2006;97:17–20.
16. Lawson WE, Hui JC, Kennard ED, et al, International Enhanced External Counterpulsation Patient Registry Investigators. Two-year outcomes in patients with mild refractory angina treated with enhanced external counterpulsation. Clin Cardiol 2006;29:69–73.

17. Soran O, Ikizler C, Sengül A, et al. Comparison of long term clinical outcomes, event free survival rates of patients undergoing enhanced external counterpulsation for coronary artery disease in the United States and Turkey. Turk Kardiyol Dern Ars 2012;40(4):323–30.

18. Tartaglia J, Stenerson J Jr, Charney R, et al. Exercise capability and myocardial perfusion in chronic angina patients treated with enhanced external counterpulsation. Clin Cardiol 2003;26(6):287–90.

19. Soran O, De Lame PA, Fleishman B, et al. Enhanced external counterpulsation in patients with heart failure: a multi-center feasibility study. Congest Heart Fail 2002;8:204–8.

20. Soran O, Kennard ED, Kelsey SF, et al. Enhanced external counterpulsation as treatment for chronic angina in patients with left ventricular dysfunction: a report from the International EECP Patient Registry (IEPR). Congest Heart Fail 2002;8:297–302.

21. Feldman AM, Silver MA, Francis GS, et al, PEECH Investigators. Enhanced external counterpulsation improves exercise tolerance in patients with chronic heart failure. J Am Coll Cardiol 2006; 48(6):1198–205.

22. Soran O, Kennard ED, Bart BA, et al, IEPR Investigators. Impact of external counterpulsation treatment on emergency department visits and hospitalizations in refractory angina patients with left ventricular dysfunction. Congest Heart Fail 2007;13:36–40.

23. Soran O, Kennard L, Kelsey SF, On behalf of IEPR Investigators. Comparison of six month clinical outcomes, event free survival rates of patients undergoing enhanced external counterpulsation (EECP) for coronary artery disease in the United States and Europe. Eur Heart J 2010;24(Suppl 31):353.

24. Bagger JP, Hall RJ, Koutroulis G, et al. Effect of enhanced external counterpulsation on dobutamine-induced left ventricular wall motion abnormalities in severe chronic angina pectoris. Am J Cardiol 2004;93(4):465–7.

25. Loh PH, Louis AA, Windram J, et al. The immediate and long-term outcome of enhanced external counterpulsation in treatment of chronic stable refractory angina. J Intern Med 2006;259(3):276–84.

26. Pettersson T, Bondesson S, Cojocaru D, et al. One year follow-up of patients with refractory angina pectoris treated with enhanced external counterpulsation. BMC Cardiovasc Disord 2006;6:28.

27. Novo G, Bagger JP, Carta R, et al. Enhanced external counterpulsation for treatment of refractory angina pectoris. J Cardiovasc Med (Hagerstown) 2006;7(5):335–9.

28. Lawson WE, Hui JC, Cohn PF. Long-term prognosis of patients with angina treated with enhanced external counterpulsation: five-year follow-up study. Clin Cardiol 2000;23:254–8.

29. Loh PH, Cleland JG, Louis AA, et al. Enhanced external counterpulsation in the treatment of chronic refractory angina: a long-term follow-up outcome from the International Enhanced External Counterpulsation Patient Registry. Clin Cardiol 2008;31:159–64.

30. Holubkov R, Kennard ED, Foris JM, et al. Comparison of patients undergoing enhanced external counterpulsation and percutaneous coronary intervention for stable angina pectoris. Am J Cardiol 2002;89:1182–6.

31. Wu E, Mårtensson J, Broström A. Enhanced external counterpulsation in patients with refractory angina pectoris: a pilot study with six months follow-up regarding physical capacity and health-related quality of life. Eur J Cardiovasc Nurs 2013;12(5):437–45.

32. Braith RW, Conti CR, Nichols WW, et al. Enhanced external counterpulsation improves peripheral artery flow-mediated dilation in patients with chronic angina: a randomized sham-controlled study. Circulation 2010;122(16):1612–20. American Heart Association.

33. Casey DP, Beck DT, Nichols WW, et al. Effects of enhanced external counterpulsation on arterial stiffness and myocardial oxygen demand in patients with chronic Angina Pectoris. Am J Cardiol 2011;107(10):1466–72.

34. Gloekler S, Meier P, de Marchi SF, et al. Coronary collateral growth by external counterpulsation: a randomised controlled trial. Heart 2010;96(3):202–7.

35. Buschmann EE, Utz W, Pagonas N, et al. Art.Net.-2 Trial: improvement of fractional flow reserve and collateral flow by treatment with EECP. Eur J Clin Invest 2009;39(10):866–75.

36. Levenson J, Simon A, Megnien JL, et al. Effects of enhanced external counterpulsation on carotid circulation in patients with coronary artery disease. Cardiology 2007;108:104–10.

37. Casey DP, Conti CR, Nichols WW, et al. Effect of enhanced external counterpulsation on inflammatory cytokines and adhesion molecules in patients with angina pectoris and angiographic coronary artery disease. Am J Cardiol 2008;10:300–2.

38. Levenson J, Pernollet MG, Iliou MC, et al. Cyclic GMP release by acute enhanced external counterpulsation: a randomized sham-controlled study. Am J Hypertens 2006;19:867–72.

39. Van der Sloot JA, Huikeshoven M, Tukkie R, et al. Transmyocardial revascularization using an XeCl excimer laser: results of a randomized trial. Ann Thorac Surg 2004;78:875–81.

40. Guleserian KJ, Maniar HS, Camillo CJ, et al. Quality of life and survival after transmyocardial laser revascularization with the holmium:YAG laser. Ann Thorac Surg 2003;75:1842–7.

41. Myers J, Oesterle SN, Jones J, et al. Do transmyocardial and percutaneous laser revascularization induce silent ischemia? An assessment by exercise testing. Am Heart J 2002;143:1052–7.

42. Ballegaard S, Pedersen F, Pietersen A, et al. Effects of acupuncture in moderate, stable angina pectoris: a controlled study. J Intern Med 1990;227:25–30.

43. Ballegaard S, Jensen G, Pedersen F, et al. Acupuncture in severe, stable angina pectoris: a randomized trial. Acta Med Scand 1986;220:307–13.

44. Spertus JA, Jones PG, Coen M, et al. Transmyocardial CO(2) laser revascularization improves symptoms, function, and quality of life:1–month results from a randomized controlled trial. Am J Med 2001;111:341–8.

45. Bridges CR, Horvath KA, Nugent WC, et al. The Society of Thoracic Surgeons practice guideline series: transmyocardial laser revascularization. Ann Thorac Surg 2004;77:1494–502.

46. Vineberg AM. Development of an anastomosis between the coronary vessels and a transplanted internal mammary artery. Can Med Assoc J 1946;55:117–9.

47. Galinanes M, Loubani M, Sensky PR, et al. Efficacy of transmyocardial laser revascularization and thoracic sympathectomy for the treatment of refractory angina. Ann Thorac Surg 2004;78:122–8.

48. Dowling RD, Petracek MR, Selinger SL, et al. Transmyocardial revascularization in patients with refractory, unstable angina. Circulation 1998;98:II73–5.

49. Allen KB, Dowling RD, Angell WW, et al. Transmyocardial revascularization: 5-year follow-up of a prospective, randomized multicenter trial. Ann Thorac Surg 2004;77:1228–34.

50. Aaberge L, Nordstrand K, Dragsund M, et al. Transmyocardial revascularization with CO2 laser in patients with refractory angina pectoris. Clinical results from the Norwegian randomized trial. J Am Coll Cardiol 2000;35:1170–7.

51. Frazier OH, March RJ, Horvath KA. Transmyocardial revascularization with a carbon dioxide laser in patients with end-stagecoronary artery disease. N Engl J Med 1999;341:1021–8.

52. Jones JW, Schmidt SE, Richman BW, et al. Holmium:YAG laser transmyocardial revascularization relieves angina and improves functional status. Ann Thorac Surg 1999;67:1596–601.

53. Schofield PM, Sharples LD, Caine N, et al. Transmyocardial laser revascularisation in patients with refractory angina: a randomized controlled trial. Lancet 1999;353:519–24.

54. Allen KB, Dowling RD, Fudge TL, et al. Comparison of transmyocardial revascularization with medical therapy in patients with refractory angina. N Engl J Med 1999;341:1029–36.

55. Burkhoff D, Schmidt S, Schulman SP, et al. Transmyocardiallaser revascularisation compared with continued medical therapy for treatment of refractory angina pectoris: a prospective randomised trial. ATLANTIC Investigators. Angina Treatments–Lasers and Normal Therapies in Comparison. Lancet 1999;354:885–90.

56. Liao L, Sarria-Santamera A, Matchar DB, et al. Meta-analysis of survival and relief of angina pectoris after transmyocardial revascularization. Am J Cardiol 2005;95:1243–5.

57. Allen KB, Dowling RD, DelRossi AJ, et al. Transmyocardial laser revascularization combined with coronary artery bypass grafting: a multicenter, blinded, prospective, randomized, controlled trial. J Thorac Cardiovasc Surg 2000;119:540–9.

58. Stamou SC, Boyce SW, Cooke RH, et al. One-year outcome after combined coronary artery bypass grafting and transmyocardial laser revascularization for refractory angina pectoris. Am J Cardiol 2002;89:1365–8.

59. Peterson ED, Kaul P, Kaczmarek RG, et al. From controlled trials to clinical practice: monitoring transmyocardial revascularization use and outcomes. J Am Coll Cardiol 2003;42:1611–6.

60. Oesterle SN, Sanborn TA, Ali N, et al. Percutaneous transmyocardial laser revascularisation for severe angina: the PACIFIC randomised trial. Potential class improvement from Intramyocardial channels. Lancet 2000;356:1705–10.

61. Whitlow PL, DeMaio SJ, Perin EC, et al. One-year results of percutaneous myocardial revascularization for refractory angina pectoris. Am J Cardiol 2003;91:1342–6.

62. Leon M. DIRECT trial: Late breaking trials. Presented at: Transcatheter Therapeutics. Washington, DC, October 20, 2000.

63. Stone GW, Teirstein PS, Rubenstein R, et al. A prospective, multicenter, randomized trial of percutaneous transmyocardial laser revascularization in patients with nonrecanalizable chronic total occlusions. J Am Coll Cardiol 2002;39:1581–7.

64. Schofield PM, McNab D. NICE evaluation of transmyocardial laser revascularization and percutaneous laser revascularisation for refractory angina. Heart 2010;96:312–3.

65. Task Force Members, Montalescot G, Sechtem U, Achenbach S. 2013 ESC guidelines on the management of stable coronary artery disease. The Task Force on the management of stable coronary artery disease of the European Society of Cardiology. Eur Heart J 2013;34(38):2949–3003.

66. Fihn SD, Gardin JM, Abrams J, et al. 2012 ACCF/AHA/ACP/AATS/PCNA/SCAI/STS Guideline for the Diagnosis and Management of Patients With Stable Ischemic Heart Disease: a report of the American College of Cardiology Foundation/American Heart Association Task Force on Practice Guidelines, and the American College of Physicians, American Association for Thoracic Surgery, Preventive Cardiovascular Nurses Association, Society for Cardiovascular Angiography and Interventions, and Society of Thoracic Surgeons. J Am Coll Cardiol 2012;60(No. 24):e44–164.

Coronary Artery Disease and Diabetes Mellitus

Doron Aronson, MD[a],*, Elazer R. Edelman, MD, PhD[b]

KEYWORDS

- Blood glucose • Coronary disease • Diabetes mellitus • Hypoglycemic agents • Revascularization
- Statins

KEY POINTS

- Large clinical trials have shown that a near-normal glycemic control does not reduce cardiovascular events in patients with diabetes mellitus.
- Recent studies indicate that statin use may be associated with the development of diabetes mellitus; however, the overall excess risk is low.
- There is a concern that some antidiabetes agents may impart greater cardiovascular risk but there is no sufficient evidence to support one drug or combination of drugs over another for the reduction of cardiovascular events.
- Optimal medical therapy is an appropriate initial strategy in patients with diabetes mellitus, mild symptoms, and moderate coronary artery disease.
- Bypass surgery is superior to percutaneous intervention in most diabetic patients with multivessel coronary disease; however, selection of the optimal myocardial revascularization strategy must take into account multiple factors and requires a multidisciplinary team approach ("heart team").

INTRODUCTION

Diabetes mellitus (DM) has reached epidemic proportions worldwide, and its prevalence is rising.[1,2] The implications of a diagnosis of DM are as severe as a diagnosis of coronary artery disease (CAD). Cardiovascular mortality in all age groups and for both sexes rises equivalently with DM or a history of myocardial infarction (MI) and the two are profoundly synergistic (**Fig. 1**).[3] In addition, DM (especially type 2 DM), is associated with clustered risk factors for cardiovascular disease (CVD). Among adults with DM there is a prevalence of 75% to 85% of hypertension, 70% to 80% for elevated low-density lipoprotein (LDL), and 60% to 70% for obesity.[4] CAD is the main cause of death in both type 1 and type 2 DM,[5] and DM is associated with a twofold to fourfold increased mortality risk from heart disease. More than 70% of people older than 65 years with DM will die from some form of heart disease or stroke.[2] Furthermore, in patients with DM there is an increased mortality after MI, and worse overall long-term prognosis with CAD.[6,7]

In the United States, approximately one-third of all percutaneous coronary intervention (PCI) procedures are performed on patients with DM and approximately 25% of patients undergoing coronary artery bypass graft (CABG) surgery have DM[5]; the outcomes of these procedures is less effective than in those without DM. DM modifies the response to arterial injury, with profound clinical consequences in terms of risk for restenosis[8] and stent thrombosis.[9] Although there has been considerable improvement in the management of patients with CAD, coronary event rates remain

[a] Department of Cardiology, Rambam Medical Center, Technion, Israel Institute of Technology, P.O.B 9602, Haifa 31096, Israel; [b] Cardiovascular Division, Department of Medicine, Institute for Medical Science and Engineering, Massachusetts Institute of Technology, Brigham and Women's Hospital, Harvard Medical School, 75 Francis Street, Boston, MA 02115, USA
* Corresponding author.
E-mail address: daronson@tx.technion.ac.il

Cardiol Clin 32 (2014) 439–455
http://dx.doi.org/10.1016/j.ccl.2014.04.001
0733-8651/14/$ – see front matter © 2014 Elsevier Inc. All rights reserved.

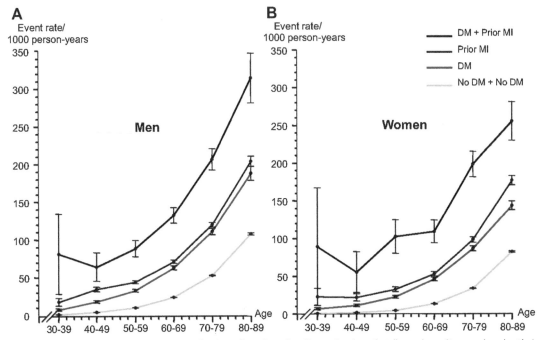

Fig. 1. Event rates for the composite endpoint of MI (nonfatal), stroke (nonfatal), and cardiovascular death in men (*A*) and women (*B*), stratified by age in relation to DM and a prior MI. (*From* Schramm TK, Gislason GH, Kober L, et al. Diabetes patients requiring glucose-lowering therapy and nondiabetics with a prior myocardial infarction carry the same cardiovascular risk: a population study of 3.3 million people. Circulation 2008;117:1945–54; with permission.)

heightened among patients with DM.[2,10–12] Therefore, optimal medical therapy (OMT) and appropriate selection of myocardial revascularization strategy are critical for patients with DM. This review summarizes the current evidence regarding the effectiveness of various medical therapies and revascularization strategies in patients with DM.

GLYCEMIC CONTROL AND CARDIOVASCULAR OUTCOMES

DM is a fascinating disease in that although it has been known since antiquity, the disease we refer to can be dated only to the era after the widespread use of insulin. Before the introduction of insulin replacement, DM was an almost universally fatal disease that primarily struck children. The DM of today, with all of its chronic manifestations, is the associated consequence of life-saving and life-prolonging effects of insulin and naturally many have wondered how "tight" control of blood sugar with precise insulin dosing would affect cardiovascular risk. The results have been sobering; in general, tight glycemic control is associated with an increased risk for hypoglycemia, but minimal to no benefit on mortality. The Action to Control Cardiovascular Risk in Diabetes (ACCORD) trial was designed to test whether treatment

targeting nearly normal glycemic control reduces the risk of cardiovascular events in type 2 DM. More than 10,000 patients were randomized to either a standard treatment strategy that targeted HbA1c levels between 7% and 8% or an intensive strategy that sought to attain a hemoglobin (Hb) A1c lower than 6.0%. The median HbA1c with the standard strategy was 7.5%; the intensive strategy achieved a median HbA1c of 6.4%.[13] Yet, the intensive strategy was associated with 22% increase in all-cause mortality and the study was stopped after a median follow-up of 3.4 years.

The Action in Diabetes and Vascular Disease: A Preterax and Diamicron Modified Release Controlled Evaluation (ADVANCE) trial randomized 11,140 participants to a strategy of intensive glycemic control (with primary therapy being the sulfonylurea gliclazide and additional medications as needed to achieve a target HbA1c of <6.5%) or to standard therapy, with the glycemic target set according to "local guidelines." The median HbA1c levels achieved in the intensive and standard arms were 6.3% and 7.0%, respectively. Intensive treatment produced a relative reduction of 10% in the primary composite outcome of major macrovascular and microvascular events (hazard ratio [HR] 0.90; 95% confidence interval [CI] 0.82–0.98; *P* = .01), primarily as a consequence of a reduction in nephropathy (a microvascular complication). However, when major macrovascular events were considered separately (MI, stroke, and cardiovascular death), there was no observed significant reduction (HR 0.94; 95% CI 0.84–1.06; $P = .32$).[13]

The Veterans Affairs Diabetes Trial (VADT) randomized 1791 participants with type 2 DM uncontrolled on insulin or maximal-dose oral agents (median entry HbA1c, 9.4%) to intensive glycemic control (goal HbA1c, <6.0%) or standard glycemic control, with a planned HbA1c separation of at least 1.5%.[14] Over a 5.6-year follow-up period, there was no significant difference in the primary outcome of a composite of MI, stroke, cardiovascular death, revascularization, hospitalization for heart failure, and amputation for ischemia.

A large retrospective cohort study from the UK General Practice Research Database showed a U-shaped pattern of risk association between HbA1c and all-cause mortality and progression to large-vessel disease events among patients with type 2 DM.[15] An HbA1c of approximately 7.5% was associated with the lowest risk and an increase or decrease from this mean HbA1c value was associated with a heightened risk of adverse outcomes (**Fig. 2**).

The most compelling message from these studies is that near-normal glycemic control for a median of 3.5 to 5.0 years does not reduce cardiovascular events within that period.[16] The contribution of glucose lowering to the reduction of macrovascular events in the ADVANCE and ACCORD trials appears to be minimal. It may very well be that even 90 years after insulin's introduction as a therapeutic modality, we are still

unclear on the drivers of cardiovascular morbidity as a chronic manifestation of DM.

For the prevention of macrovascular disease, the general goal of HbA1c lower than 7% appears reasonable (American College of Cardiology/American Heart Association, Class IIb recommendation; Level of Evidence: A).[17] For selected individual patients, lower HbA1c goals may be reasonable in an attempt to reduce microvascular complications (low risk of hypoglycemia, short duration of diabetes, long life expectancy, and no significant CVD). Yet, it also has become clear that the potential risks of intensive glycemic control may outweigh its benefits in patients with a long duration of diabetes, known history of severe hypoglycemia, advanced atherosclerosis, and advanced age/frailty. Here, less stringent HbA1c goals may be appropriate (7.5%–8.0% or possibly even slightly higher).[17,18]

Antidiabetic Drug Safety

Until recently, insulin and then oral agents based on metformin and sulfonylureas dominated the therapy of DM. There are now several additional classes of drugs approved for diabetes management: α-glucosidase inhibitors, thiazolidinediones, meglitinides, glucagonlike peptide analogues, amylin analogues, dipeptidyl peptidase IV inhibitors, and sodium-glucose cotransporter 2 inhibitors.[19] Most oral diabetes medications reduce HbA1c levels by a similar amount, by approximately 1 absolute percentage point.[20] Glycated hemoglobin, however, may not be a valid surrogate for assessing either the cardiovascular risks or benefits of diabetes therapy,[21] and the long-term

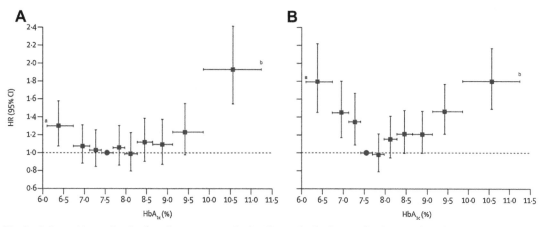

Fig. 2. Adjusted hazard ratios for all-cause mortality by HbA1c deciles in people given oral combination and insulin-based therapies. Vertical error bars show 95% CIs, horizontal bars show HbA1c range. The red squares are the hazard ratios. Red circle = reference decile. [a] Truncated at lower quartile. [b] Truncated at upper quartile. Metformin plus sulphonylureas (A); and insulin-based regimens (B). (*From* Currie CJ, Peters JR, Tynan A, et al. Survival as a function of HbA(1c) in people with type 2 diabetes: a retrospective cohort study. Lancet 2010;375:481–9; with permission.)

safety of these newer drugs with respect to CVD (the leading cause of illness and death among patients with diabetes) remains poorly characterized. In addition, antidiabetic agents may have multiple, additional potential effects on risk factors for CAD and on cardiac function (**Table 1**).

Concerns have been raised that some antidiabetes agents may impart greater cardiovascular risk. The University Group Diabetes Project study suggested increased CV risk in patients treated with tolbutamide, a first-generation sulfonylurea. These results have been widely criticized based on study design flaws.[22] A meta-analysis of clinical trials of rosiglitazone (Avandia), a thiazolidinedione, pointed to an increased risk of MI,[23] although the Rosiglitazone Evaluated for Cardiac Outcomes and Regulation of Glycaemia in Diabetes (RECORD) study did show an increased risk of major adverse cardiovascular events.[24]

The initial concern with rosiglitazone led the Food and Drug Administration (FDA) to issue an updated Guidance for Industry in 2008 requiring preapproval and post approval studies for all new antidiabetic drugs to rule out excess cardiovascular risk. In a postmarketing trial, the 2-sided 95% CI for the estimated increased risk (risk ratio) should be less than 1.3.[25]

The Bypass Angioplasty Revascularization Investigation 2 Diabetes (BARI 2D) trial assessed therapeutic strategies rather than any specific drug. No safety concerns were seen for the insulin-sensitizing group, in which more than 60% received thiazolidinediones, predominantly rosiglitazone (55%).[26] Notwithstanding, given that other options are now available, the use of rosiglitazone is not recommended.[27] Newer antidiabetic agents, such as, agonists of the glucagonlike peptide-1 (GLP1) receptor or dipeptidyl peptidase 4 (DPP4) inhibitors, which prevent the breakdown of endogenous GLP1, have shown beneficial effects in patients undergoing angioplasty and CABG in small studies.[28,29] However, in the Saxagliptin Assessment of Vascular Outcomes Recorded in Patients with Diabetes Mellitus (SAVOR), the DPP4 inhibitor saxagliptin did not change the primary composite end point of cardiovascular death, myocardial infarction, or ischemic stroke, when added to the standard of care in patients at high risk for cardiovascular events.[30] Although saxagliptin clearly met the FDA guidance for cardiovascular safety, therapy with the drug was associated with an unexpected increased risk of hospitalization for heart failure (especially in patients with high baseline brain natriuretic

Table 1
Effect of antidiabetic agents on the cardiovascular system

Therapeutic Classes	Effects on CVD Risk Factors	Other Direct and Indirect Effects on the Heart
Biguanides (Metformin)	Reduction in macrovascular end points[110] Improved lipid profile	—
Sulfonylureas	Weight gain	Hypoglycemia Impaired ischemic preconditioning[111]
Prandial glucose regulators (meglitinides)	Weight gain	Hypoglycemia
Thiazolidinediones/ Glitazones	Increased LDL levels[20,112] Reduced restenosis after coronary stenting[113,114]	Heart failure[115,116] Excess ischemic cardiovascular risk with rosiglitazone (?)[23,24]
Alpha-glucosidase inhibitors	Reduced inflammatory markers[112] Possible decrease in risk of cardiovascular disease event[117]	—
DPP4 inhibitors (gliptins)	—	Heart failure[30,116]
Amylin analogues (Pramlintide)	Weight loss	—
Incretin mimetics (GLP-1 analogues)	Weight loss	—
Insulin	Weight gain[118]	Hypoglycemia

Abbreviations: CVD, cardiovascular disease; DPP4, dipeptidyl peptidase 4; GLP, glucagonlike peptide; LDL, low-density lipoprotein.
  Data from Refs.[20,32,112,116,119]

peptide levels) and a higher frequency of hypoglycemia.[30] Similarly, in the Examination of Cardiovascular Outcomes with Alogliptin versus Standard of Care (EXAMINE) trial, the DPP4 inhibitor alogliptin was neutral with regard to major cardiovascular events in patients with type 2 diabetes and CVD or high cardiovascular risk, but met the FDA guidance for cardiovascular safety.[31] Currently, there is no sufficient evidence to definitively support one drug or combination of drugs over another for long-term clinical outcomes of mortality and macrovascular and microvascular complications of diabetes.[20,32]

Hypoglycemia and Mortality

Iatrogenic hypoglycemia is the limiting factor in the glycemic management of DM, and classically arises from the interplay of mild-to-moderate absolute or even relative therapeutic hyperinsulinemia and compromised physiologic and behavioral defenses against falling plasma glucose concentrations.[33] Hypoglycemia is a substantial, independent cause of excess morbidity and mortality. In the ACCORD trial, severe hypoglycemia was associated with increased mortality by twofold and fourfold in the intensive and conventional groups, respectively. However, hypoglycemia was not identified as the cause for this excess mortality in the intensive group.[34]

In the ADVANCE trial, severe hypoglycemia was associated with excess cardiovascular events and total mortality.[35] However, neither a close temporal relationship nor a dose-response relationship was observed between hypoglycemic events and subsequent cardiovascular or fatal events. Therefore, hypoglycemia might be a marker for patient-related disorders or complications, which could predispose patients to an excess risk of coronary heart disease.[34,35]

Plausible mechanisms by which hypoglycemia might cause cardiovascular events or lead to death from CVD include sympathoadrenal activation, abnormal cardiac repolarization, increased thrombogenesis, inflammation, and vasoconstriction leading to cardiac ischemia or fatal arrhythmia during recognized or unrecognized episodes of hypoglycemia.[36,37] Although the relationship in hospitalized patients with acute MI between hypoglycemia and cardiovascular outcomes is complex,[38] there was a clear J-shaped relationship between glucose values and adverse outcomes, including increased mortality.[39,40] In this context, hypoglycemia has been shown to lower myocardial blood flow reserve[41] and increase experimental infarct size.[42] Although it is reasonable to suspect that iatrogenic hypoglycemia contributes

directly to the excess mortality during intensive glycemic therapy, especially during acute ischemia, the association may represent increased vulnerability of people who are prone to hypoglycemia to other serious health outcomes due to the coexistence of other risk factors[35,38] or hypoglycemia may be a marker for more critical illness.[43] Notwithstanding, these data provide compelling reasons to minimize the risk of hypoglycemia in patients with diabetes and CAD.

The use of insulin infusions to control hyperglycemia or to provide metabolic support in face of stress is falling off, as severe hypoglycemia (<2.2 mmol/L [40 mg/dL]) occurs frequently (5%–17%)[44,45] and is associated with higher mortality.[46] There is no additional benefit from the lowering of blood glucose levels below the range of approximately 140 to 180 mg/dL.[47–49] For most critically ill patients, the American Diabetes Association recommends initiating insulin therapy for treatment of persistent hyperglycemia, starting at a threshold of no greater than 180 mg/dL (10.0 mmol/L), and aiming for glucose range of 140 to 180 mg/dL (7.8–10.0 mmol/L).[47] Similar recommendations were provided by the American College of Physicians[48] and the American Heart Association (**Fig. 3**).[49]

MANAGEMENT OF HYPERLIPIDEMIA IN PATIENTS WITH DM

Hydroxymethyl glutaryl coenzyme A reductase inhibitors (statins) are the cornerstone of lipid-associated cardiovascular-risk reduction, with established benefits in reducing clinical events in patients with diabetes shown in a multitude of trials. The Cholesterol Treatment Trialists' (CTT) Collaboration analysis of data from 18,686 individuals with diabetes (1466 with type 1 and 17,220 with type 2) in the context of 14 randomized trials of statin therapy, showed that statin therapy reduced the 5-year incidence of major vascular events by about a fifth per 1.0 mmol/L reduction in LDL cholesterol (LDL-C), with similar proportional reductions in major coronary events, stroke, and the need for coronary revascularization.[50]

For *primary prevention*, patients with DM ages 40 to 75 years with an LDL-C of 70 to189 mg/dL and without clinical CVD, are one of the major statin benefit groups. Among the 4 randomized controlled trials focused exclusively on primary prevention, the highest rate of cardiovascular events occurred in the Collaborative Atorvastatin Diabetes Study (CARDS),[51] which exclusively enrolled a primary prevention population with diabetes. The CTT meta-analyses also supports

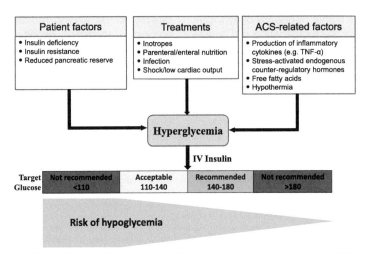

Fig. 3. Management of hyperglycemia in patients with acute coronary syndromes. ACS, acute coronary syndromes; IV, intravenous; TNF, tumor necrosis factor. (*Adapted from* Aronson D, Edelman ER. Role of CABG in the management of obstructive coronary arterial disease in patients with diabetes mellitus. Curr Opin Pharmacol 2012;12:134–41; with permission.)

the use of statins to reduce the risk of CVD in individuals with type 1 or 2 diabetes (**Fig. 4**).[50,52] Thus, a high level of evidence supports the use of moderate-intensity statin therapy in all primary-prevention–eligible adults ages 40 to 75 years with DM (**Table 2**). The estimated 10-year cardiovascular risk also can be used to guide the intensity of statin therapy; such that when the estimated 10-year CVD risk is 7.5% or higher, a high-intensity statin can be used. The percent reduction in LDL-C can be used as an indication of response and adherence to therapy, but is not in itself a treatment goal.[53] For *secondary prevention*, high-intensity statin therapy should be initiated for adults 75 years or younger who are not receiving statin therapy or the intensity should be increased in those receiving a low- or moderate-intensity statin.[53] Combination therapy does not provide additional cardiovascular benefit above statin therapy alone and is not generally recommended.[54]

STATIN USE AND RISK OF DIABETES

There has recently emerged a concern that statin use may be associated with the development of DM. A collaborative meta-analysis of 13 randomized placebo-controlled trials with more than 90,000 participants found a small, 9% increased risk for incident diabetes after 4 years of statin treatment, particularly in older people.[55] For 255 patients (95% CI 150–852) treated for 4 years with a statin, 1 additional patient would develop diabetes. Another meta-analysis showed that intensive-dose statin therapy is associated with a

somewhat higher risk than moderate-dose therapy.[56] In higher-risk secondary prevention patients with established CAD, the diabetes risk associated with statin therapy is low in absolute terms when compared with the reduction in cardiovascular events. Based on these studies, the FDA added a warning regarding diabetes risk to the labeling of statins.[57]

In the randomized placebo-controlled Justification for Use of statins in Prevention: an Intervention Trial Evaluating Rosuvastatin (JUPITER) trial, there was a modest risk of developing diabetes on statin therapy that was limited to patients who had preexisting biochemical evidence of impaired fasting glucose or multiple components of metabolic syndrome.[58] However, even in the setting of this primary prevention trial, the cardiovascular and mortality benefits of statin therapy exceeded the diabetes hazard in the trial population as a whole, as well as among those at higher risk for developing diabetes.

Overall, the risk of DM is approximately 1 excess case per 1000 individuals treated with a moderate-intensity statin for 1 year and approximately 3 excess cases per 1000 individuals treated with a high-intensity statin for 1 year.[53] Individuals receiving statin therapy should be evaluated for new-onset DM. Those who develop DM during statin therapy should continue statin therapy to reduce their risk of CVD events.[53] To date, a potential mechanism to explain the findings of a higher incidence of DM with statin therapy compared with placebo, and intensive-dose therapy compared with moderate-dose therapy, has not been clearly identified.

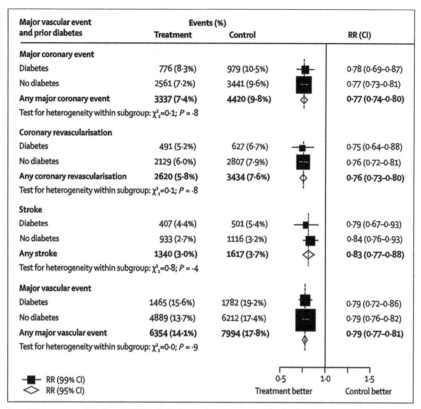

Fig. 4. Cholesterol Treatment Trialists' (CTT) Collaboration meta-analysis showing proportional effects of statins on major vascular events per mmol/L reduction in LDL cholesterol in participants presenting with or without diabetes. (*From* Cholesterol Treatment Trialists Collaborators, Kearney PM, Blackwell L, Collins R, et al. Efficacy of cholesterol-lowering therapy in 18,686 people with diabetes in 14 randomised trials of statins: a meta-analysis. Lancet 2008;371:117–25; with permission.)

Table 2
Recommendations for treatment of blood cholesterol to reduce atherosclerotic cardiovascular risk in adults with diabetes—statin treatment

Recommendations	NHLBI Grade	ACC/AHA COR	ACC/AHA LOE
Moderate-intensity statin[a] therapy should be initiated or continued for adults 40 to 75 y of age with diabetes mellitus.	A (Strong)	I	A
High-intensity statin[b] therapy is reasonable for adults 40 to 75 y of age with diabetes mellitus with a ≥7.5% estimated 10-year CVD risk unless contraindicated.	E (Expert Opinion)	IIa	B
In adults with diabetes mellitus, who are <40 or >75 y of age, it is reasonable to evaluate the potential for CVD benefits and for adverse effects, for drug-drug interactions, and to consider patient preferences when deciding to initiate, continue, or intensify statin therapy.	E (Expert Opinion)	IIa	C

Abbreviations: ACC/AHA, American College of Cardiology/American Heart Association; COR, Class of Recommendation; CVD, cardiovascular disease; LOE, level of evidence; NHLBI, National Heart, Lung, and Blood Institute.
[a] Daily dose lowers low-density lipoprotein cholesterol (LDL-C) on average, by approximately 30% to less than 50% (eg, atorvastatin 10 mg, rosuvastatin 10 mg, simvastatin 20–40 mg and pravastatin 40 mg).
[b] Daily dose lowers LDL-C on average, by approximately ≥50% (eg, atorvastatin 40–80 mg or rosuvastatin 20–40 mg).
Adapted from Stone NJ, Robinson J, Lichtenstein AH, et al. 2013 ACC/AHA Guideline on the treatment of blood cholesterol to reduce atherosclerotic cardiovascular risk in adults: a report of the American College of Cardiology/American Heart Association Task Force on Practice Guidelines. Circulation 2013; with permission.

CORONARY REVASCULARIZATION IN PATIENTS WITH DM

Revascularization Versus Medical Therapy

Patients with DM and CAD are at high risk of cardiovascular events regardless of symptoms.[59] Whether such patients with stable CAD should undergo prompt revascularization is an important clinical question, with broad implications for risk stratification and treatment.[60] As such, the BARI 2D trial tested the hypothesis that in patients with DM and stable CAD, prompt revascularization with either CABG or PCI would reduce long-term rates of death and cardiovascular events as compared with OMT alone. BARI 2D randomized patients with demonstrated ischemia who were asymptomatic or who had mild to moderate symptoms, and documented CAD by angiography. The appropriate method of revascularization for each patient (PCI or CABG) was determined a priori by the responsible physician, resulting in a population of patients with a much greater atherosclerotic burden in the CABG stratum. The 5-year survival rate was 88.3% among patients in the revascularization group and not statistically different in the medical-therapy group (87.8%). Similarly, the major cardiovascular event rate did not differ significantly between the revascularization and the OMT groups. As compared with OMT, patients who underwent CABG (but not PCI) had significantly fewer major cardiac events, mainly a reduction in nonfatal MIs.[26]

The benefits of revascularization in terms of freedom from angina were documented mostly during the year after the intervention, and most importantly were noticeably greater in patients undergoing CABG than PCI (**Fig. 5**).[26,61] Similarly, in COURAGE (Clinical Outcomes Utilizing Revascularization and Aggressive Drug Evaluation), the addition of early PCI to optimal medical therapy did not significantly reduce the risk of death or MI regardless of DM status.[62]

Use of Drug-Eluting Stents in Patients with DM

Although the magnitude of restenosis reduction achieved with drug-eluting stents (DESs) is impressive, it is important to recognize that these trials mandated an angiographic follow-up. Revascularization was therefore driven not only by clinical necessity but also by the angiographic appearance of narrowing within the treated segment even in patients who did not have documented ischemia.[63] In real-world practice, the benefit of DESs in patients with DM appears to be less impressive.[64] For example, in the Swedish Coronary Angiography and Angioplasty Registry, the numbers needed to treat a diabetic patient with DES to avoid 1 additional restenosis per year with bare metal stent (BMS) ranged from 21 to 47 lesions in patients treated with 1 stent and 11 to 27 in patients with multiple stents.[65] DES significantly reduced restenosis to half the rate seen with BMS. However, there was no difference in the combined outcome of death or MIs in diabetic patients treated with DES or BMS with up to 4 years of follow-up.[65]

Recent studies evaluated the comparative effectiveness of second-generation DES among diabetic patients.[60] A post hoc subgroup analysis from 4 pooled randomized trials with 27.6% diabetic patients compared the Xience V everolimus eluting stent (EES) with a first-generation DES, Taxus PES (paclitaxel-eluting stent, Express and Liberté)[66] In these 1869 patients with diabetes, there were no differences in clinical outcomes after 2 years between the first- and newer-generation DESs.[66]

Data regarding the latest-generation Resolute zotarolimus-eluting stent (ZES; with controlled drug release over a longer time period) was analyzed using pooled patient-level data from the 5130 patients (1535 with DM). Target-vessel failure (TVF) was defined as a composite of cardiac death, target vessel myocardial infarction, and ischemia-driven target vessel revascularization. The rate of TVF in a prespecified analysis of patients with diabetes at 12 months was 7.8%, considerably less than the predefined DES performance goal of 14.5% ($P<.001$).[67] After 2 years, the cumulative incidence of target lesion failure (TLF) in patients with noninsulin-treated diabetes was comparable to that of patients without diabetes (8.0% vs 7.1%). The higher-risk insulin-treated DM demonstrated a significantly higher TLF (13.7%). Rates of stent thrombosis (ST) were not significantly different between patients with and without diabetes (1.2% vs 0.8%). Based on this analysis, the FDA approved the Resolute ZES with specific labeling indication for patients with DM.

Although both of the newer-generation DESs (ie, the Resolute ZES and the Xience V) have improved outcomes compared with first-generation DES, there is still an opportunity to improve the treatment of CAD in patients DM, particularly those treated with insulin. Overall, the results emphasize the lack of mechanistic understanding with regard to the antiproliferative drugs eluted by the stent and adverse events after PCI.[60]

Stent Thrombosis After DES Implantation

The possibility of increased rates of ST after DES has been a matter of concern and can be particularly pertinent to diabetic patients. ST is classified

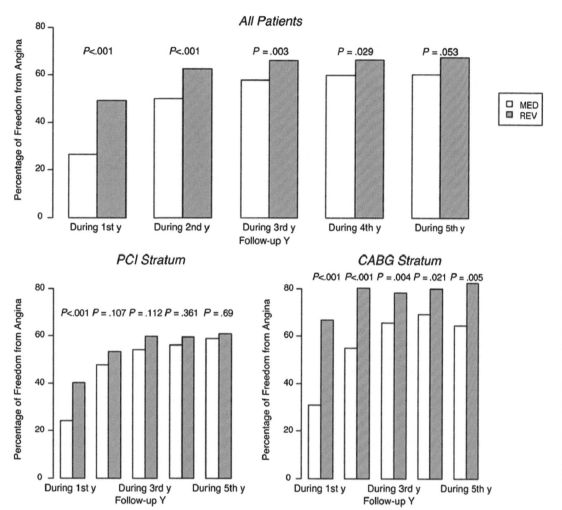

Fig. 5. Annual occurrence of freedom from angina in 1434 patients with angina at entry in BARI 2D. In the PCI stratum, the increase in freedom from angina was documented only at the first year of the follow-up. In the CABG stratum, the freedom from angina was increased during the 5-year follow-up. (*From* Dagenais GR, Lu J, Faxon DP, et al. Effects of optimal medical treatment with or without coronary revascularization on angina and subsequent revascularizations in patients with type 2 diabetes mellitus and stable ischemic heart disease. Circulation 2011;123:1492–500; with permission.)

based on the time of the adverse event relative to the index procedure. Early ST refers to the first 30 days after stent implantation and is further stratified into acute (<24 hours) and subacute (24 hours–30 days). Late ST defines the time interval between 1 month and 1 year after stent implantation; very late ST includes any event beyond 1 year.[68] After DES implantation, very late ST occurs at a relatively constant rate over time up to at least 5 years after stent implantation.[69]

ST is a multifactorial problem related to patient, lesion, and procedural factors and to the coagulation system and response to antiplatelet therapy.[68] Delayed healing and impaired endothelialization (ie, incomplete endothelial coverage of stent struts associated with persistence of fibrin deposits) is a

common features of most cases of late and very late ST, which either alone or in combination with chronic inflammation and hypersensitivity reactions, and outward remodeling promote ST.[70] All of these pathologic processes are amplified in DM and it therefore is not surprising that several studies demonstrated higher ST rates in diabetic patients, particularly in insulin-treated patients.[9,69,71,72]

In the Acute Catheterization and Urgent Intervention Triage Strategy (ACUITY) trial, insulin-requiring DM was a significant independent predictor of definite or probable ST occurring within 30 days (odds ratio, 2.35).[73] In the Trial to Assess Improvement in Therapeutic Outcomes by Optimizing Platelet Inhibition With Prasugrel–Thrombolysis in Myocardial Infarction 38 (TRITON-TIMI 38), patients with DM and acute coronary syndrome (n = 3146) had twice the rate of stent thrombosis than those without DM (2.8% vs 1.4%, P<.0001), with highest rates among subjects treated with insulin (3.7%, P<.0001).[74] In the Harmonizing Outcomes With Revascularization and Stents in Acute Myocardial Infarction (HORIZONS-AMI) trial, insulin-treated DM was an independent predictor of acute, subacute, late, and very late ST.[75]

In a large 2-institutional cohort study of 8146 patients who underwent PCI with a sirolimus-eluting stent (SES) (n = 3823) or a PES (n = 4323) and were followed for 4 years after stent implantation, DM was an independent predictor of overall, early, and late-definite ST.[76] Similarly, in the Swedish Coronary Angiography and Angioplasty Registry of almost 74,000 DES and BMS, insulin-treated DM was an independent predictor of ST (relative risk [RR] 1.77).[77] Finally, in the e-Cypher registry (n = 15,157), insulin-dependent DM was an independent predictor of ST at 1 year (2.8-fold risk increase).[71]

The increased risk of diabetic patients for ST might be related to the more diffuse nature of atherosclerosis, accompanied by longer lesion lengths, smaller vessel size, and greater plaque burden, which might impose less optimal procedural results. Additionally, the detrimental effects of DM on endothelial function[78] and platelet function[79] may also promote the development of ST. However, further studies are needed to elucidate the mechanisms leading to increased ST risk among diabetic patients.

CABG Versus PCI in Multivessel CAD

The Bypass Angioplasty Revascularization Investigation (BARI) study compared multivessel angioplasty with CABG in patients with medically treated DM and found a near doubling of mortality at 5 years with PCI (35% vs 19%, P = .003).[80] The survival benefit of CABG in patients with diabetes persisted at 10 years (Percutaneous transluminal coronary angioplasty [PTCA] 45.5% vs CABG 57.8%, P = .025).[81] In an analysis based on pooled individual patient data from 10 randomized trials comparing CABG with PCI (median follow-up of 5.9 years), mortality among patients with DM was 30% lower in the CABG group than in the PCI group.[82] These large differences in mortality underscore the importance of appropriate decisions regarding the mode of revascularization in DM.

However, many cardiologists dismissed the results of these earlier randomized studies as outdated because of the advent of DES technology.[83] Two contemporary trials comparing PCI with DES to CABG in patients with DM attempted to address this renewed controversy. The prespecified DM-subgroup analysis (n = 452) of SYNTAX (SYNergy Between PCI With TAXus and Cardiac Surgery)[84] showed that the 5-year composite Major Adverse Cardiac and Cerebrovascular event (MACCE) rate was significantly higher in patients with DM after PCI compared with CABG (PCI: 46.5% vs CABG: 29.0%; P<.001) mainly due to an increased risk of repeat revascularization (PCI: 35.3% vs CABG: 14.6%; P<.001).[85] However, the difference between PCI and CABG is larger for patients with DM than for those without.

The CARDia (Coronary Artery Revascularization in Diabetes) trial enrolled patients with DM (n = 510) with either multivessel CAD or complex single-vessel CAD (ostial or proximal left anterior descending artery disease) in whom coronary revascularization was recommended on clinical grounds.[86] The primary end point was a composite of death, MI, and stroke, with a major secondary end point of the composite of the primary outcome and repeat revascularization using a noninferiority design. SESs were used in 69% of patients in the PCI arm. The study could not demonstrate noninferiority of PCI for the primary end point (10.5% with CABG compared with 13.0% with PCI).

The long-term Future Revascularization Evaluation in Patients with Diabetes Mellitus: Optimal Management of Multivessel Disease (FREEDOM) trial enrolled 1900 patients with diabetes and multivessel CAD (about as many patients with diabetes as in all previous trials combined) who were randomly assigned to undergo either CABG or PCI with drug-eluting stents (primarily first-generation PES or SES).[87] After 5 years of follow-up, the 947 patients assigned to undergo CABG had significantly lower mortality (10.9% vs 16.3%) and fewer myocardial infarctions (6.0% vs 13.9%) than the 953 patients assigned to undergo PCI. However, patients in the CABG group had significantly more strokes (5.2% vs 2.4%), mostly those that occurred within 30 days after revascularization. In the CABG group, the primary composite outcome of death, MI, or stroke over 5 years was reduced by 7.9%, or a relative decrease of 30%, as compared with PCI (18.7% vs 26.6%, P = .005).[87] There was no interaction between SYNTAX score and outcomes among the overall population, suggesting that the increased event rate among patients randomized to PCI was not related to the anatomic complexity of disease at the time of revascularization.

Ongoing randomized studies of second-generation DES address important questions about revascularization strategies in patients with severe CAD and DM. Currently, however, the results of the FREEDOM and other trials suggest that the comparative effectiveness of CABG and PCI on hard outcomes remains similar whether PCI is performed without stents, with bare-metal stents, or with drug-eluting stents,[83] albeit at the price of an increased risk of nonfatal stroke.

Explaining the Mortality Benefit of CABG

The protective effects of CABG may be related to the increased restenosis rates following angioplasty in DM and incomplete revascularization associated with multivessel angioplasty.[88,89] In the BARI study population, 3.1 grafts were placed per patient undergoing CABG, whereas the mean number of successfully treated lesions in the PTCA group was 2.0.[80] Together with the greater degree of baseline atherosclerosis and the high restenosis rate among diabetic patients, it is likely that a higher proportion of the myocardium remains unprotected and unrevascularized in patients with DM, and a greater proportion of the myocardium becomes ischemic during an acute spontaneous myocardial infarction. The impact of incomplete revascularization may be even more severe because after PCI, progression of diffuse disease in diabetic patients forms new lesions that may cause ischemia and/or symptoms.

The amount of jeopardized myocardium decreases initially following revascularization and increases subsequently with target lesion restenosis, graft failure, or the development of new narrowings in native vessels. Follow-up angiographic analysis of the BARI patients at years 1 and 5 revealed that the total percentage of jeopardized myocardium, defined as the overall percentage of the coronary perfusion territory compromised by stenoses of greater than or equal to 50%, was higher in diabetic patients.[90] The mean percentage increase in total jeopardized myocardium was significantly greater in diabetic compared with nondiabetic patients at 1-year protocol-directed angiography (42% vs 24%, $P = .05$) and on the first clinically performed (unscheduled) angiogram within 30 months (63% vs 50%, $P = .01$) but not at 5-year protocol-directed angiography (34% vs 26%, $P = .33$). In contrast, among patients with CABG, DM was not associated with an increase in jeopardized myocardium at any angiographic follow-up interval. In this context, DM does not seem to affect the patency of internal thoracic artery (ITA) grafts, or the accelerated atherosclerotic process that characterizes vein grafts.[91,92] The lower rate of nonfatal MI with surgical revascularization observed in BARI 2D[26] is consistent with the hypothesis that bypass grafts to the mid coronary vessel treat the culprit lesion and prophylaxes against new proximal disease, progression of proximal narrowing, or plaque rupture occurring proximal to a patent graft insertion. Proximal coronary arterial stents, bare metal and drug-eluting, cannot protect against new disease, however.[93]

Graft Selection and Patency in Patients with DM

DM does not appear to adversely affect patency of ITA grafts.[91,94] Nonrandomized analyses indicate that bilateral internal thoracic artery (BITA) grafting appears to be particularly important in the diabetic population.[95] However, the use of BITA results in greater sternal wound complications in patients with DM (especially insulin-treated).[96,97] Harvesting skeletonized ITA may reduce the risk of sternal wound complications associated with BITA by minimizing the risk of devascularization of the sternum as compared with removal with an attached muscle pedicle.[95,98] Therefore, some surgeons believe that DM is not a contraindication for skeletonized BITA.[99] Notwithstanding, presently, it is unclear whether selective referral of patients with DM for skeletonized BITA grafting despite higher risks of sternal infection is justified.[100]

The radial artery (RA) conduits obtained from patients with DM has greater tendency to spasm compared with RAs from patients without DM, and exhibits impaired endothelial function.[101] In a randomized trial comparing angiographic RA graft patency versus saphenous vein graft (SVG) patency at 1 year after CABG, there was a significant interaction between graft type and DM; RA grafts had lower patency rate than SVGs in patients with DM and the reverse was true in patients without DM.[102]

APPROACH TO CORONARY REVASCULARIZATION IN PATIENTS WITH DM

Although revascularization therapies mechanically address specific local lesions, they all have limited longevity. As discussed, DM is a systemic disease with a vast array of metabolic effects that often escalate with time. It goes without saying then that the optimal therapy for vascular disease in diabetes is optimization of control of diabetes, and there is significant overlap in that drugs and approaches that control DM also regulate atherosclerotic disease and CVD. Yet, almost a century after insulin transformed DM we still do not fully comprehend the breadth and depth of this disease and, as such, there is both promise of new therapies yet to be appreciated and the challenge of balancing the harm and benefit of tight glucose control. Careful medical therapy is an excellent first-line strategy for coronary disease in patients with DM who are asymptomatic[103] or with mild symptoms (CCS Class I or II) and less-severe CAD (single-vessel or 2-vessel CAD not involving the proximal left anterior descending artery).[26,104] For these patients, it is unlikely that an initial revascularization strategy is better than medical therapy and may even be worse.[105] Revascularization can reduce anginal symptoms[61] and may be applied later if medical therapy does not adequately control symptoms (see **Fig. 5**). In patients who require intervention after optimization of medical therapy, there is a significantly higher risk of repeat revascularizations with PCI. DES, albeit, is superior to BMS in ischemia-driven repeat revascularization

procedures (target lesion revascularization)[100,106] and is a reasonable approach in these patients (see **Fig. 5**). But there remains consistently higher repeat revascularization rates after PCI compared with surgical revascularization in patients with DM.[86,107,108] The surgical approach has better survival, fewer recurrent infarctions, and greater freedom from reintervention for patients with treated DM, moderate to severe symptoms and multivessel CAD,[107,109] or significant involvement of the proximal left anterior descending or left main coronary artery (**Fig. 6**).[26,104,109]

Ultimately, no single treatment approach can be applied to all patients given the confluence of

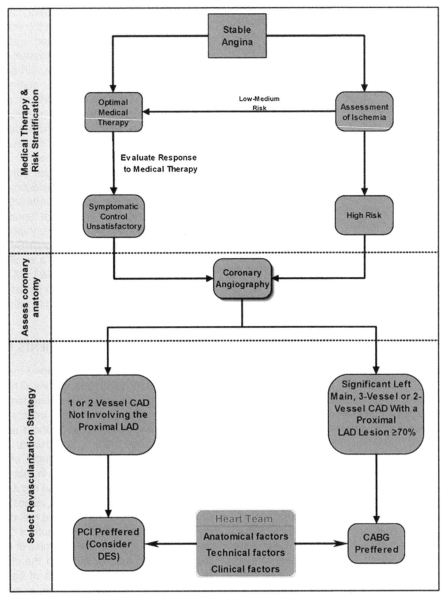

Fig. 6. Revascularization strategy in patients with DM and stable angina.

chronic obstructive atherosclerosis and the profound divergent metabolic derangements of DM. Decisions regarding potential revascularization must take into account multiple factors, and as such require a multidisciplinary team approach ("heart team"). The heart team approach guarantees that all therapeutic options (ie, OMT, PCI, and CABG) are transparently discussed, and the individual patient preferences are considered in the decision-making process.[109]

REFERENCES

1. Danaei G, Finucane MM, Lu Y, et al. National, regional, and global trends in fasting plasma glucose and diabetes prevalence since 1980: systematic analysis of health examination surveys and epidemiological studies with 370 country-years and 2.7 million participants. Lancet 2011; 378:31–40.

2. Go AS, Mozaffarian D, Roger VL, et al. Heart disease and stroke statistics—2014 update: a report from the American Heart Association. Circulation 2014;129:e28–292.

3. Schramm TK, Gislason GH, Kober L, et al. Diabetes patients requiring glucose-lowering therapy and nondiabetics with a prior myocardial infarction carry the same cardiovascular risk: a population study of 3.3 million people. Circulation 2008;117: 1945–54.

4. Preis SR, Pencina MJ, Hwang SJ, et al. Trends in cardiovascular disease risk factors in individuals with and without diabetes mellitus in the Framingham Heart Study. Circulation 2009;120:212–20.

5. Berry C, Tardif JC, Bourassa MG. Coronary heart disease in patients with diabetes: part II: recent advances in coronary revascularization. J Am Coll Cardiol 2007;49:643–56.

6. Aronson D, Rayfield EJ, Chesebro JH. Mechanisms determining course and outcome of diabetic patients who have had acute myocardial infarction. Ann Intern Med 1997;126:296–306.

7. Donahoe SM, Stewart GC, McCabe CH, et al. Diabetes and mortality following acute coronary syndromes. JAMA 2007;298:765–75.

8. Aronson D, Bloomgarden Z, Rayfield EJ. Potential mechanisms promoting restenosis in diabetic patients. J Am Coll Cardiol 1996;27:528–35.

9. Iakovou I, Schmidt T, Bonizzoni E, et al. Incidence, predictors, and outcome of thrombosis after successful implantation of drug-eluting stents. JAMA 2005;293:2126–30.

10. Haffner SM, Lehto S, Ronnemaa T, et al. Mortality from coronary heart disease in subjects with type 2 diabetes and in nondiabetic subjects with and without prior myocardial infarction. N Engl J Med 1998;339:229–34.

11. Gerstein HC, Miller ME, Byington RP, et al. Effects of intensive glucose lowering in type 2 diabetes. N Engl J Med 2008;358:2545–59.

12. Preis SR, Hwang SJ, Coady S, et al. Trends in all-cause and cardiovascular disease mortality among women and men with and without diabetes mellitus in the Framingham Heart Study, 1950 to 2005. Circulation 2009;119:1728–35.

13. Advance Collaborative Group, Patel A, MacMahon S, Chalmers J, et al. Intensive blood glucose control and vascular outcomes in patients with type 2 diabetes. N Engl J Med 2008;358: 2560–72.

14. Duckworth W, Abraira C, Moritz T, et al. Glucose control and vascular complications in veterans with type 2 diabetes. N Engl J Med 2009;360: 129–39.

15. Currie CJ, Peters JR, Tynan A, et al. Survival as a function of HbA(1c) in people with type 2 diabetes: a retrospective cohort study. Lancet 2010;375: 481–9.

16. Dluhy RG, McMahon GT. Intensive glycemic control in the ACCORD and ADVANCE trials. N Engl J Med 2008;358:2630–3.

17. Skyler JS, Bergenstal R, Bonow RO, et al. Intensive glycemic control and the prevention of cardiovascular events: implications of the ACCORD, ADVANCE, and VA diabetes trials: a position statement of the American Diabetes Association and a scientific statement of the American College of Cardiology Foundation and the American Heart Association. Circulation 2009;119:351–7.

18. Sue Kirkman M, Briscoe VJ, Clark N, et al. Diabetes in older adults: a consensus report. J Am Geriatr Soc 2012;60:2342–56.

19. Inzucchi SE, Bergenstal RM, Buse JB, et al. Management of hyperglycemia in type 2 diabetes: a patient-centered approach: position statement of the American Diabetes Association (ADA) and the European Association for the Study of Diabetes (EASD). Diabetes Care 2012;35:1364–79.

20. Bennett WL, Maruthur NM, Singh S, et al. Comparative effectiveness and safety of medications for type 2 diabetes: an update including new drugs and 2-drug combinations. Ann Intern Med 2011; 154:602–13.

21. Hiatt WR, Kaul S, Smith RJ. The cardiovascular safety of diabetes drugs—insights from the rosiglitazone experience. N Engl J Med 2013;369: 1285–7.

22. Meinert CL, Knatterud GL, Prout TE, et al. A study of the effects of hypoglycemic agents on vascular complications in patients with adult-onset diabetes. II. Mortality results. Diabetes 1970;19(Suppl):789–830.

23. Nissen SE, Wolski K. Effect of rosiglitazone on the risk of myocardial infarction and death from cardiovascular causes. N Engl J Med 2007;356:2457–71.

24. Home PD, Pocock SJ, Beck-Nielsen H, et al. Rosiglitazone evaluated for cardiovascular outcomes in oral agent combination therapy for type 2 diabetes (RECORD): a multicentre, randomised, open-label trial. Lancet 2009;373:2125–35.

25. Food and Drug Administration. Guidance for industry: diabetes mellitus—evaluating cardiovascular risk in new antidiabetic therapies to treat type 2 diabetes. 2008. Available at: www.fda.gov/downloads/Drugs/GuidanceComplianceRegulatoryInformation/Guidances/ucm071627.pdf. Accessed May 19, 2014.

26. Frye RL, August P, Brooks MM, et al. A randomized trial of therapies for type 2 diabetes and coronary artery disease. N Engl J Med 2009;360:2503–15.

27. Nathan DM, Buse JB, Davidson MB, et al. Medical management of hyperglycemia in type 2 diabetes: a consensus algorithm for the initiation and adjustment of therapy: a consensus statement of the American Diabetes Association and the European Association for the Study of Diabetes. Diabetes Care 2009;32:193–203.

28. Nikolaidis LA, Mankad S, Sokos GG, et al. Effects of glucagon-like peptide-1 in patients with acute myocardial infarction and left ventricular dysfunction after successful reperfusion. Circulation 2004; 109:962–5.

29. Sokos GG, Bolukoglu H, German J, et al. Effect of glucagon-like peptide-1 (GLP-1) on glycemic control and left ventricular function in patients undergoing coronary artery bypass grafting. Am J Cardiol 2007;100:824–9.

30. Scirica BM, Bhatt DL, Braunwald E, et al. Saxagliptin and cardiovascular outcomes in patients with type 2 diabetes mellitus. N Engl J Med 2013;369:1317–26.

31. White WB, Cannon CP, Heller SR, et al. Alogliptin after acute coronary syndrome in patients with type 2 diabetes. N Engl J Med 2013;369:1327–35.

32. Bianchi C, Miccoli R, Daniele G, et al. Is there evidence that oral hypoglycemic agents reduce cardiovascular morbidity/mortality? Yes. Diabetes Care 2009;32(Suppl 2):S342–8.

33. Cryer PE. Severe hypoglycemia predicts mortality in diabetes. Diabetes Care 2012;35:1814–6.

34. Bonds DE, Miller ME, Bergenstal RM, et al. The association between symptomatic, severe hypoglycaemia and mortality in type 2 diabetes: retrospective epidemiological analysis of the ACCORD study. BMJ 2010;340:b4909.

35. Zoungas S, Patel A, Chalmers J, et al. Severe hypoglycemia and risks of vascular events and death. N Engl J Med 2010;363:1410–8.

36. Frier BM, Schernthaner G, Heller SR. Hypoglycemia and cardiovascular risks. Diabetes Care 2011;34(Suppl 2):S132–7.

37. Desouza C, Salazar H, Cheong B, et al. Association of hypoglycemia and cardiac ischemia: a study based on continuous monitoring. Diabetes Care 2003;26:1485–9.

38. Yakubovich N, Gerstein HC. Serious cardiovascular outcomes in diabetes: the role of hypoglycemia. Circulation 2011;123:342–8.

39. Pinto DS, Skolnick AH, Kirtane AJ, et al. U-shaped relationship of blood glucose with adverse outcomes among patients with ST-segment elevation myocardial infarction. J Am Coll Cardiol 2005;46: 178–80.

40. Kosiborod M, Rathore SS, Inzucchi SE, et al. Admission glucose and mortality in elderly patients hospitalized with acute myocardial infarction: implications for patients with and without recognized diabetes. Circulation 2005;111:3078–86.

41. Rana O, Byrne CD, Kerr D, et al. Acute hypoglycemia decreases myocardial blood flow reserve in patients with type 1 diabetes mellitus and in healthy humans. Circulation 2011;124:1548–56.

42. Libby P, Maroko PR, Braunwald E. The effect of hypoglycemia on myocardial ischemic injury during acute experimental coronary artery occlusion. Circulation 1975;51:621–6.

43. Kosiborod M, Inzucchi SE, Goyal A, et al. Relationship between spontaneous and iatrogenic hypoglycemia and mortality in patients hospitalized with acute myocardial infarction. JAMA 2009;301: 1556–64.

44. Gandhi GY, Nuttall GA, Abel MD, et al. Intensive intraoperative insulin therapy versus conventional glucose management during cardiac surgery: a randomized trial. Ann Intern Med 2007; 146:233–43.

45. Griesdale DE, de Souza RJ, van Dam RM, et al. Intensive insulin therapy and mortality among critically ill patients: a meta-analysis including NICE-SUGAR study data. CMAJ 2009;180:821–7 [discussion: 799–800].

46. D'Ancona G, Bertuzzi F, Sacchi L, et al. Iatrogenic hypoglycemia secondary to tight glucose control is an independent determinant for mortality and cardiac morbidity. Eur J Cardiothorac Surg 2011;40: 360–6.

47. Moghissi ES, Korytkowski MT, DiNardo M, et al. American Association of Clinical Endocrinologists and American Diabetes Association consensus statement on inpatient glycemic control. Diabetes Care 2009;32:1119–31.

48. Qaseem A, Humphrey LL, Chou R, et al. Use of intensive insulin therapy for the management of glycemic control in hospitalized patients: a clinical practice guideline from the American College of Physicians. Ann Intern Med 2011;154:260–7.

49. Deedwania P, Kosiborod M, Barrett E, et al. Hyperglycemia and acute coronary syndrome: a scientific statement from the American Heart Association Diabetes Committee of the Council on Nutrition,

Physical Activity, and Metabolism. Circulation 2008;117:1610–9.

50. Cholesterol Treatment Trialists Collaborators, Kearney PM, Blackwell L, Collins R, et al. Efficacy of cholesterol-lowering therapy in 18,686 people with diabetes in 14 randomised trials of statins: a meta-analysis. Lancet 2008;371:117–25.

51. Colhoun HM, Betteridge DJ, Durrington PN, et al. Primary prevention of cardiovascular disease with atorvastatin in type 2 diabetes in the Collaborative Atorvastatin Diabetes Study (CARDS): multicentre randomised placebo-controlled trial. Lancet 2004; 364:685–96.

52. Cholesterol Treatment Trialists Collaborators, Baigent C, Blackwell L, Emberson J, et al. Efficacy and safety of more intensive lowering of LDL cholesterol: a meta-analysis of data from 170,000 participants in 26 randomised trials. Lancet 2010; 376:1670–81.

53. Stone NJ, Robinson J, Lichtenstein AH, et al. 2013 ACC/AHA guideline on the treatment of blood cholesterol to reduce atherosclerotic cardiovascular risk in adults: a report of the American College of Cardiology/American Heart Association Task Force on Practice Guidelines. Circulation 2013. Available at: http://circ.ahajournals.org/content/early/2013/11/11/01.cir.0000437738.63853.7a.short. Accessed May 19, 2014.

54. American Diabetes Association. Standards of medical care in diabetes—2014. Diabetes Care 2014; 37(Suppl 1):S14–80.

55. Sattar N, Preiss D, Murray HM, et al. Statins and risk of incident diabetes: a collaborative meta-analysis of randomised statin trials. Lancet 2010;375:735–42.

56. Preiss D, Seshasai SR, Welsh P, et al. Risk of incident diabetes with intensive-dose compared with moderate-dose statin therapy: a meta-analysis. JAMA 2011;305:2556–64.

57. United States Food and Drug Administration. DA Drug Safety Communication: Important safety label changes to cholesterol lowering statin drugs. 2012. Available at: http://www.fda.gov/Drugs/DrugSafety/ucm293101.htm. Accessed May 19, 2014.

58. Ridker PM, Pradhan A, MacFadyen JG, et al. Cardiovascular benefits and diabetes risks of statin therapy in primary prevention: an analysis from the JUPITER trial. Lancet 2012;380:565–71.

59. Dagenais GR, Lu J, Faxon DP, et al. Prognostic impact of the presence and absence of angina on mortality and cardiovascular outcomes in patients with type 2 diabetes and stable coronary artery disease: results from the BARI 2D (Bypass Angioplasty Revascularization Investigation 2 Diabetes) trial. J Am Coll Cardiol 2013;61:702–11.

60. Armstrong EJ, Rutledge JC, Rogers JH. Coronary artery revascularization in patients with diabetes mellitus. Circulation 2013;128:1675–85.

61. Dagenais GR, Lu J, Faxon DP, et al. Effects of optimal medical treatment with or without coronary revascularization on angina and subsequent revascularizations in patients with type 2 diabetes mellitus and stable ischemic heart disease. Circulation 2011;123:1492–500.

62. Maron DJ, Boden WE, Spertus JA, et al. Impact of metabolic syndrome and diabetes on prognosis and outcomes with early percutaneous coronary intervention in the COURAGE (Clinical Outcomes Utilizing Revascularization and Aggressive Drug Evaluation) trial. J Am Coll Cardiol 2011;58:131–7.

63. King SB 3rd. Is surgery preferred for the diabetic with multivessel disease? Surgery is preferred for the diabetic with multivessel disease. Circulation 2005;112:1500–7 [discussion: 1514–5].

64. Legrand V. Therapy insight: diabetes and drug-eluting stents. Nat Clin Pract Cardiovasc Med 2007;4:143–50.

65. Stenestrand U, James SK, Lindback J, et al. Safety and efficacy of drug-eluting vs. bare metal stents in patients with diabetes mellitus: long-term of follow-up in the Swedish Coronary Angiography and Angioplasty Registry (SCAAR). Eur Heart J 2010;31(2):177–86.

66. Stone GW, Kedhi E, Kereiakes DJ, et al. Differential clinical responses to everolimus-eluting and Paclitaxel-eluting coronary stents in patients with and without diabetes mellitus. Circulation 2011; 124:893–900.

67. Silber S, Serruys PW, Leon MB, et al. Clinical outcome of patients with and without diabetes mellitus after percutaneous coronary intervention with the resolute zotarolimus-eluting stent: 2-year results from the prospectively pooled analysis of the international global RESOLUTE program. JACC Cardiovasc Interv 2013;6:357–68.

68. Windecker S, Meier B. Late coronary stent thrombosis. Circulation 2007;116:1952–65.

69. Kimura T, Morimoto T, Nakagawa Y, et al. Very late stent thrombosis and late target lesion revascularization after sirolimus-eluting stent implantation: five-year outcome of the j-Cypher Registry. Circulation 2012;125:584–91.

70. Pfisterer ME. Late stent thrombosis after drug-eluting stent implantation for acute myocardial infarction: a new red flag is raised. Circulation 2008;118:1117–9.

71. Urban P, Gershlick AH, Guagliumi G, et al. Safety of coronary sirolimus-eluting stents in daily clinical practice: one-year follow-up of the e-Cypher registry. Circulation 2006;113:1434–41.

72. Machecourt J, Danchin N, Lablanche JM, et al. Risk factors for stent thrombosis after implantation of sirolimus-eluting stents in diabetic and nondiabetic patients: the EVASTENT Matched-Cohort Registry. J Am Coll Cardiol 2007;50:501–8.

73. Aoki J, Lansky AJ, Mehran R, et al. Early stent thrombosis in patients with acute coronary syndromes treated with drug-eluting and bare metal stents: the Acute Catheterization and Urgent Intervention Triage Strategy trial. Circulation 2009;119: 687–98.

74. Wiviott SD, Braunwald E, Angiolillo DJ, et al. Greater clinical benefit of more intensive oral antiplatelet therapy with prasugrel in patients with diabetes mellitus in the trial to assess improvement in therapeutic outcomes by optimizing platelet inhibition with prasugrel-Thrombolysis in Myocardial Infarction 38. Circulation 2008;118:1626–36.

75. Dangas GD, Caixeta A, Mehran R, et al. Frequency and predictors of stent thrombosis after percutaneous coronary intervention in acute myocardial infarction. Circulation 2011;123:1745–56.

76. Wenaweser P, Daemen J, Zwahlen M, et al. Incidence and correlates of drug-eluting stent thrombosis in routine clinical practice. 4-year results from a large 2-institutional cohort study. J Am Coll Cardiol 2008;52:1134–40.

77. Lagerqvist B, Carlsson J, Frobert O, et al. Stent thrombosis in Sweden: a report from the Swedish coronary angiography and angioplasty registry. Circ Cardiovasc Interv 2009;2:401–8.

78. Rask-Madsen C, King GL. Mechanisms of disease: endothelial dysfunction in insulin resistance and diabetes. Nat Clin Pract Endocrinol Metab 2007; 3:46–56.

79. Colwell JA, Nesto RW. The platelet in diabetes: focus on prevention of ischemic events. Diabetes Care 2003;26:2181–8.

80. Influence of diabetes on 5-year mortality and morbidity in a randomized trial comparing CABG and PTCA in patients with multivessel disease: the Bypass Angioplasty Revascularization Investigation (BARI) [see comments]. Circulation 1997; 96:1761–9.

81. BARI Investigators. The final 10-year follow-up results from the BARI randomized trial. J Am Coll Cardiol 2007;49:1600–6.

82. Hlatky MA, Boothroyd DB, Bravata DM, et al. Coronary artery bypass surgery compared with percutaneous coronary interventions for multivessel disease: a collaborative analysis of individual patient data from ten randomised trials. Lancet 2009;373:1190–7.

83. Hlatky MA. Compelling evidence for coronary-bypass surgery in patients with diabetes. N Engl J Med 2012;367:2437–8.

84. Mohr FW, Morice MC, Kappetein AP, et al. Coronary artery bypass graft surgery versus percutaneous coronary intervention in patients with three-vessel disease and left main coronary disease: 5-year follow-up of the randomised, clinical SYNTAX trial. Lancet 2013;381:629–38.

85. Kappetein AP, Head SJ, Morice MC, et al. Treatment of complex coronary artery disease in patients with diabetes: 5-year results comparing outcomes of bypass surgery and percutaneous coronary intervention in the SYNTAX trial. Eur J Cardiothorac Surg 2013;43:1006–13.

86. Kapur A, Hall R, Malik I, et al. Randomized comparison of percutaneous coronary intervention with coronary artery bypass grafting in diabetic patients: 1-year results of the CARDia (Coronary Artery Revascularization in Diabetes) trial. J Am Coll Cardiol 2010;55:432–40.

87. Farkouh ME, Domanski M, Sleeper LA, et al. Strategies for multivessel revascularization in patients with diabetes. N Engl J Med 2012;367:2375–84.

88. Gum P, O'Keefe JJ, Borkon A, et al. Bypass surgery versus coronary angioplasty for revascularization of treated diabetic patients. Circulation 1997; 96:II7–10.

89. Detre KM, Lombardero MS, Brooks MM, et al. The effect of previous coronary-artery bypass surgery on the prognosis of patients with diabetes who have acute myocardial infarction. Bypass Angioplasty Revascularization Investigation Investigators. N Engl J Med 2000;342:989–97.

90. Kip KE, Alderman EL, Bourassa MG, et al. Differential influence of diabetes mellitus on increased jeopardized myocardium after initial angioplasty or bypass surgery: bypass angioplasty revascularization investigation. Circulation 2002;105:1914–20.

91. Schwartz L, Kip KE, Frye RL, et al. Coronary bypass graft patency in patients with diabetes in the Bypass Angioplasty Revascularization Investigation (BARI). Circulation 2002;106:2652–8.

92. Hoogwerf BJ, Waness A, Cressman M, et al. Effects of aggressive cholesterol lowering and low-dose anticoagulation on clinical and angiographic outcomes in patients with diabetes: the Post Coronary Artery Bypass Graft Trial. Diabetes 1999;48: 1289–94.

93. Aronson D, Edelman ER. Role of CABG in the management of obstructive coronary arterial disease in patients with diabetes mellitus. Curr Opin Pharmacol 2012;12:134–41.

94. Hwang HY, Choi JS, Kim KB. Diabetes does not affect long-term results after total arterial off-pump coronary revascularization. Ann Thorac Surg 2010;90:1180–6.

95. Kinoshita T, Asai T, Nishimura O, et al. Off-pump bilateral versus single skeletonized internal thoracic artery grafting in patients with diabetes. Ann Thorac Surg 2010;90:1173–9.

96. Pevni D, Uretzky G, Mohr A, et al. Routine use of bilateral skeletonized internal thoracic artery grafting: long-term results. Circulation 2008;118:705–12.

97. Nakano J, Okabayashi H, Hanyu M, et al. Risk factors for wound infection after off-pump

coronary artery bypass grafting: should bilateral internal thoracic arteries be harvested in patients with diabetes? J Thorac Cardiovasc Surg 2008; 135:540–5.

98. Saso S, James D, Vecht JA, et al. Effect of skeletonization of the internal thoracic artery for coronary revascularization on the incidence of sternal wound infection. Ann Thorac Surg 2010;89:661–70.

99. Kinoshita T, Asai T, Suzuki T, et al. Off-pump bilateral versus single skeletonized internal thoracic artery grafting in high-risk patients. Circulation 2011; 124:S130–4.

100. Roffi M, Angiolillo DJ, Kappetein AP. Current concepts on coronary revascularization in diabetic patients. Eur Heart J 2011;32:2748–57.

101. Choudhary BP, Antoniades C, Brading AF, et al. Diabetes mellitus as a predictor for radial artery vasoreactivity in patients undergoing coronary artery bypass grafting. J Am Coll Cardiol 2007;50: 1047–53.

102. Goldman S, Sethi GK, Holman W, et al. Radial artery grafts vs saphenous vein grafts in coronary artery bypass surgery: a randomized trial. JAMA 2011;305:167–74.

103. Young LH, Wackers FJ, Chyun DA, et al. Cardiac outcomes after screening for asymptomatic coronary artery disease in patients with type 2 diabetes: the DIAD study: a randomized controlled trial. JAMA 2009;301:1547–55.

104. Chaitman BR, Hardison RM, Adler D, et al. The bypass angioplasty revascularization investigation 2 diabetes randomized trial of different treatment strategies in type 2 diabetes mellitus with stable ischemic heart disease: impact of treatment strategy on cardiac mortality and myocardial infarction. Circulation 2009;120:2529–40.

105. Patel MR, Dehmer GJ, Hirshfeld JW, et al. ACCF/ SCAI/STS/AATS/AHA/ASNC 2009 Appropriateness Criteria for coronary revascularization: a report by the American College of Cardiology Foundation Appropriateness Criteria Task Force, Society for Cardiovascular Angiography and Interventions, Society of Thoracic Surgeons, American Association for Thoracic Surgery, American Heart Association, and the American Society of Nuclear Cardiology endorsed by the American Society of Echocardiography, the Heart Failure Society of America, and the Society of Cardiovascular Computed Tomography. J Am Coll Cardiol 2009; 53:530–53.

106. Aronson D, Edelman ER. Revascularization for coronary artery disease in diabetes mellitus: angioplasty, stents and coronary artery bypass grafting. Rev Endocr Metab Disord 2010;11:75–86.

107. Banning AP, Westaby S, Morice MC, et al. Diabetic and nondiabetic patients with left main and/or 3-vessel coronary artery disease: comparison of outcomes with cardiac surgery and paclitaxel-eluting stents. J Am Coll Cardiol 2010;55:1067–75.

108. Onuma Y, Wykrzykowska JJ, Garg S, et al. 5-year follow-up of coronary revascularization in diabetic patients with multivessel coronary artery disease: insights from ARTS (Arterial Revascularization Therapy Study)-II and ARTS-I trials. JACC Cardiovasc Interv 2011;4:317–23.

109. Wijns W, Kolh P, Danchin N, et al. Guidelines on myocardial revascularization: the Task Force on Myocardial Revascularization of the European Society of Cardiology (ESC) and the European Association for Cardio-Thoracic Surgery (EACTS). Eur Heart J 2010;31:2501–55.

110. Kooy A, de Jager J, Lehert P, et al. Long-term effects of metformin on metabolism and microvascular and macrovascular disease in patients with type 2 diabetes mellitus. Arch Intern Med 2009;169:616–25.

111. Engler RL, Yellon DM. Sulfonylurea KATP blockade in type II diabetes and preconditioning in cardiovascular disease. Time for reconsideration [see comments]. Circulation 1996;94:2297–301.

112. Singh S, Bhat J, Wang PH. Cardiovascular effects of anti-diabetic medications in type 2 diabetes mellitus. Curr Cardiol Rep 2013;15:327.

113. Marx N, Wohrle J, Nusser T, et al. Pioglitazone reduces neointima volume after coronary stent implantation: a randomized, placebo-controlled, double-blind trial in nondiabetic patients. Circulation 2005;112:2792–8.

114. Takagi T, Akasaka T, Yamamuro A, et al. Troglitazone reduces neointimal tissue proliferation after coronary stent implantation in patients with non-insulin dependent diabetes mellitus: a serial intravascular ultrasound study. J Am Coll Cardiol 2000;36:1529–35.

115. Nesto RW, Bell D, Bonow RO, et al. Thiazolidinedione use, fluid retention, and congestive heart failure: a consensus statement from the American Heart Association and American Diabetes Association. October 7, 2003. Circulation 2003;108:2941–8.

116. McMurray JJ, Gerstein HC, Holman RR, et al. Heart failure: a cardiovascular outcome in diabetes that can no longer be ignored. Lancet Diabetes Endocrinol 2014. http://dx.doi.org/10.1016/S2213-8587(14)70031-2. [Epub ahead of print].

117. Chiasson JL, Josse RG, Gomis R, et al. Acarbose treatment and the risk of cardiovascular disease and hypertension in patients with impaired glucose tolerance: the STOP-NIDDM trial. JAMA 2003;290: 486–94.

118. Fox CS. Weighty matters: balancing weight gain with cardiovascular risk among patients with type 1 diabetes mellitus on intensive insulin therapy. Circulation 2013;127:157–9.

119. Ismail-Beigi F. Clinical practice. Glycemic management of type 2 diabetes mellitus. N Engl J Med 2012;366:1319–27.

Revascularization Options
Coronary Artery Bypass Surgery and Percutaneous Coronary Intervention

A. Pieter Kappetein, MD, PhD[a],*,
Nicolas M. van Mieghem, MD[b], Stuart J. Head, PhD[a]

KEYWORDS

- Coronary artery bypass grafting • Percutaneous coronary intervention • Three-vessel disease
- Left main disease • SYNTAX score • Revascularization

KEY POINTS

- The SYNTAX score is an independent predictor of adverse events of patients undergoing percutaneous coronary intervention (PCI).
- Comorbidities play an important role in predicting the clinical outcome after coronary artery bypass grafting (CABG).
- Decision making regarding the best mode of revascularization (PCI or CABG) should take place in a multidisciplinary heart team discussion, with a noninterventional/clinical cardiologist, interventional cardiologist, and cardiovascular surgeon.

INTRODUCTION

Coronary artery disease (CAD) is the leading cause of death globally. Revascularization with coronary artery bypass grafting (CABG) and percutaneous coronary intervention (PCI) are options for patients presenting with angina pectoris on optimal medical therapy. However, the choice of the most appropriate revascularization modality is controversial in some patient groups. The first saphenous vein bypass from the ascending aorta to the anterior descending coronary artery was performed in the 1960s by Kolesov and Favaloro.[1] This was the start of CABG, whereas PCI was first performed in 1977 by Dr Grüntzig, who opened a coronary lesion in the left anterior descending artery with a distensible balloon. During the last decade both technologies have undergone major advances. PCI started with balloon angioplasty followed by bare metal stents (BMS) and later with drug eluting stents (DES). Together with antiplatelet and antithrombotic treatments, the outcome of PCI has improved by reducing adverse events, in particular repeat revascularization. CABG has also progressed with the use of more arterial grafts, improvements in cardiopulmonary bypass, myocardial protection, improved perioperative care, and optimizing medical treatment after surgery.[2] However, randomized studies have never been able to show that off-pump CABG techniques optimize outcome compared with on-pump techniques.[3,4]

In the United States approximately 3700 individuals per million adults undergo revascularization with PCI, whereas 1100 per million adults undergo

[a] Department of Cardiothoracic Surgery, Thoraxcenter Erasmus MC, PO Box 2040, Rotterdam 3000 CA, The Netherlands; [b] Department of Cardiology, Thoraxcenter Erasmus MC, PO Box 2040, Rotterdam 3000 CA, The Netherlands
* Corresponding author. Department of Thoracic Surgery, Erasmus Medical Center, Room BD 569, PO Box 2040, Rotterdam 3000 CA, The Netherlands.
E-mail address: a.kappetein@erasmusmc.nl

Cardiol Clin 32 (2014) 457–461
http://dx.doi.org/10.1016/j.ccl.2014.04.011
0733-8651/14/$ – see front matter © 2014 Elsevier Inc. All rights reserved.

CABG. The number of patients undergoing CABG is decreasing, whereas the number of PCI procedures has remained constant.[5]

Randomized trials have attempted to determine which of the techniques is superior. Special subgroups of patients, including those with unprotected left main disease, multivessel disease, diabetes mellitus, and left ventricular dysfunction have been studied.

CLINICAL TRIALS COMPARING CABG VERSUS PCI

Over the past 2 decades, almost 30 randomized controlled trials have investigated CABG versus PCI. At first, CABG was compared with balloon angioplasty, then with BMS, and most recently with DES. The Synergy Between Percutaneous Coronary Intervention With Taxus and Cardiac Surgery (SYNTAX) trial is one of the most important trials that randomized patients to CABG or PCI with DES.[6] The SYNTAX trial was an all-comers trial for patients with either left main disease or 3-vessel CAD. Participants deemed suitable for both CABG and PCI with paclitaxel-eluting stents by a heart team (surgeon and interventional cardiologist) were eligible for randomization. A total of 1800 patients were enrolled in the randomized arm and if patients could not be randomized they were enrolled in a CABG-ineligible PCI registry (n = 198) or PCI-ineligible CABG registry (n = 1077).[7] The primary end point of the study was major adverse cardiac and cerebrovascular events (MACCE) and the hypothesis was that PCI would be noninferior to CABG at 1 year. However, MACCE was significantly lower following CABG compared with PCI (12.4% vs 17.8%; $P = .002$) and the primary hypothesis was rejected. Patients in the CABG group had more strokes compared with patients undergoing PCI, whereas patients in the PCI group had a higher rate of repeat revascularization.[6] After 5 years of follow-up MACCE were 26.9% in the CABG group and 37.3% in the PCI group ($P<.0001$). Compared with CABG, PCI had significantly higher rates of myocardial infarction (9.7% vs 3.8%; $P<.0001$) and repeat revascularization (13.7% vs 25.9%; $P<.0001$). Rates of all-cause death (11.4% in the CABG group vs 13.9% in the PCI group; $P = .10$) and stroke (3.7% vs 2.4%; $P = .09$) were not significantly different between groups.[8]

An important tool derived from the SYNTAX study was the SYNTAX score, an anatomic scoring system, based on the coronary angiogram, which quantifies lesion complexity. The SYNTAX score was created with preexisting classifications, which included the American Heart Association (AHA) classification of coronary artery tree segments modified for the Arterial Revascularization Therapy Study (ARTS), the Leaman score, the American College of Cardiology (ACC)/AHA lesion classification system, the total occlusion classification system, the Duke and International Classification for Patient Safety (ICPS) classification system for bifurcation lesions, and a consensus opinion from experts.[9] The SYNTAX score was designed to quantify the complexity of left main or 3-vessel disease. Using the online calculator (http://www.syntaxscore.com) it is possible to determine each patient's SYNTAX score (**Fig. 1**). The SYNTAX score proved to be an independent predictor of MACCE in patients undergoing PCI but not CABG. The 5-year results of the SYNTAX study showed that, in patients with intermediate (22–32) or high ($\geq$33) SYNTAX scores, MACCE was significantly increased with PCI (intermediate score, 25.8% of the CABG group vs 36.0% of the PCI group, $P = .008$; high score, 26.8% vs 44.0%, $P<.0001$). However, the drawback to this score is that it does not take into consideration the comorbidities of the patient. For this reason, the SYNTAX II score has been developed as a decision-making tool that combines the SYNTAX score with various clinical factors.

The Future Revascularization Evaluation in Patients with Diabetes Mellitus: Optimal Management of Multivessel Disease (FREEDOM) trial compared PCI with CABG in patients with diabetes and multivessel coronary disease and the composite primary 5-year end point of death, stroke, or myocardial infarction occurred less frequently in the CABG group than in the PCI group (18.7% vs 26.6%; $P = .005$). Stroke rates were significantly higher in the CABG group than in the PCI group (5.2% vs 2.4%; $P = .03$).[10] The results of the diabetic population of the SYNTAX study also favored CABG in most patients: 5-year rates were significantly higher for PCI versus CABG for MACCE (PCI 46.5% vs CABG 29.0%; $P<.001$) and repeat revascularization (PCI 35.3% vs CABG 14.6%; $P<.001$).

The decision to undertake CABG or PCI should be made collaboratively (the so-called heart team approach) by cardiac surgeons and cardiologists[11] from an assessment of an individual patient's coronary disease pattern, comorbidities, and risk of complications.

MULTIVESSEL DISEASE

Most (70%) coronary revascularizations concern patients with multivessel disease. After the start of CABG it became clear that the treatment was successful in relieving angina. It was more difficult

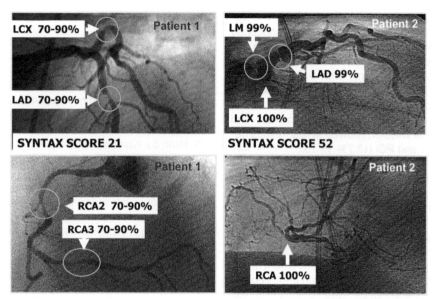

Fig. 1. Example of two patients both with three vessel disease but one with a low SYNTAX score (21) and one with a high SYNTAX score (52).

to prove that use of CABG achieved improved survival compared with medical therapy. Trials comparing CABG versus medical therapy were often underpowered. A meta-analysis comprising 7 trials showed that at 10 years 41% of medically treated patients had undergone CABG surgery.[12] There was an increased life expectancy of patients who underwent CABG compared with medical therapy at 5 years (89.8% vs 84.2%) and at 10 years (73.6% vs 69.5%). Survival was predominantly better in patients with extensive CAD, confirming the hypothesis that the benefits of CABG are higher when more myocardium is at risk. Current guidelines recommend CABG with a class IA recommendation for patients with multivessel disease.[13]

A subgroup analysis of the SYNTAX trial showed that in patients with 3-vessel disease and a low SYNTAX score, MACCE rates were similar between PCI and CABG at 5-year follow-up (CABG 26.8% vs PCI 33.3%; $P = .21$). In those with 3-vessel disease and intermediate (23–32) or high ($\geq$33) SYNTAX scores, the rate of MACCE was significantly increased in favor of CABG (23–32, CABG 22.6% vs PCI 37.9%, $P<.001$; $\geq$33, CABG 24.1% vs PCI 41.9%, $P<.001$). In patients with 3-vessel disease and a SYNTAX score greater than or equal to 33, mortality (CABG 8.8% vs PCI 17.8%; $P = .015$) and MI (1.9% vs 8.7%; $P = .008$) were significantly higher in the PCI arm.[14]

Trials comparing PCI with medical therapy also showed that PCI reduces angina.[15] In the Clinical Outcomes Utilizing Revascularization and Aggressive Drug Evaluation (COURAGE) trial patients

were randomized to PCI and optimal medical therapy or optimal medical therapy alone.[16] After almost 5 years of follow-up there was no difference between PCI and the optimal medical therapy group in the composite end point of mortality and myocardial infarction. However, angina relief was greater with PCI.

In the Fractional Flow Reserve versus Angiography for Multivessel Evaluation 2 (FAME 2) trial, patients with stable angina who underwent PCI guided by a fractional flow reserve to treat a functionally significant coronary lesion were less likely to need an urgent reintervention than those treated with medical therapy alone.[17] However, the trial did not show any reduction in mortality or myocardial infarction with PCI.

Recent trials have consistently shown a favorable effect of PCI compared with optimal medical therapy in terms of relief of angina. PCI consequently has a class IIb recommendation with a level B evidence level compared with optimal medical therapy in the ACC/AHA guidelines and a IIa recommendation in the European guidelines.[13,18]

LEFT MAIN DISEASE

The left main coronary artery supplies at least 70% of the left ventricular myocardium with blood. Patients treated medically for left main coronary artery disease have a decreased life expectancy and CABG has become the standard therapy for left main disease because there is an increased survival benefit compared with medical treatment. The significant reduction of restenosis rates associated with DES has augmented interest in treating patients with left main disease with PCI. The SYNTAX trial involved 705 patients with unprotected left main disease, most with distal left main lesions.[6] Because it is a subgroup analysis caution is needed in interpreting the results,[19] but the primary end point of 1-year MACCE showed similar results between CABG and PCI (13.7% vs 15.8%; $P = .44$). The 5-year results for the left main cohort showed no difference in MACCE between CABG and PCI with low and intermediate SYNTAX scores. However, in patients with high SYNTAX scores MACCE rates were significantly worse for PCI compared with surgery (46.5% vs 29.7%; $P = .003$). These results suggest that both treatments are valid options for patients with left main disease. The extent of disease should be accounted for when choosing between surgery and PCI because patients with high SYNTAX scores seem to benefit more from surgery compared with the lower terciles.[20] The hypothesis that can be generated from the SYNTAX study that PCI is noninferior to CABG in patients with left main disease needs to be evaluated in a study with an appropriate sample size calculation. The Evaluation of Xience Prime or Xience V versus Coronary Artery Bypass Surgery for Effectiveness of Left Main Revascularization (EXCEL) study has recently completed enrollment and will report the composite end point of all-cause mortality, myocardial infarction, and stroke at a median follow-up of 3 years.[21]

SUMMARY

CABG is superior to PCI in terms of a reduction in mortality in certain patient subgroups and an improvement in the overall composite end points of angina, recurrent MI, and repeat revascularization procedures; this is especially apparent in patients with complex coronary lesions (high or intermediate SYNTAX scores). However, CABG is associated with a higher perioperative stroke risk compared with PCI. For patients with less complex disease (low SYNTAX scores) or left main coronary disease (low or intermediate SYNTAX scores), PCI is an acceptable alternative to CABG. This finding suggests that lesion complexity defined by the SYNTAX score is an essential consideration for stenting, whereas patient comorbidity is an essential consideration for CABG surgery. However, all patients with complex multivessel coronary artery disease should be reviewed and discussed by a heart team including a cardiac surgeon and interventional cardiologist to reach consensus on optimum treatment.

REFERENCES

1. Head SJ, Kieser TM, Falk V, et al. Coronary artery bypass grafting: part 1–the evolution over the first 50 years. Eur Heart J 2013;34(37):2862–72.
2. Head SJ, Börgermann J, Osnabrugge RL, et al. Coronary artery bypass grafting: part 2–optimizing outcomes and future prospects. Eur Heart J 2013; 34(37):2873–86.
3. Head SJ, Kappetein AP. Off-pump or on-pump coronary-artery bypass grafting. N Engl J Med 2012; 367(6):577–8.
4. Lamy A, Devereaux PJ, Prabhakaran D, et al. Off-pump or on-pump coronary-artery bypass grafting at 30 days. N Engl J Med 2012;366(16):1489–97.
5. Osnabrugge RL, Head SJ, Bogers AJ, et al. Multivessel coronary artery disease: quantifying how recent trials should influence clinical practice. Expert Rev Cardiovasc Ther 2013;11(7):903–18.
6. Serruys PW, Morice MC, Kappetein AP, et al. Percutaneous coronary intervention versus coronary-artery bypass grafting for severe coronary artery disease. N Engl J Med 2009;360(10):961–72.
7. Head SJ, Holmes DR, Mack MJ, et al. Risk profile and 3-year outcomes from the SYNTAX percutaneous coronary intervention and coronary artery bypass grafting nested registries. JACC Cardiovasc Interv 2012;5(6):618–25.
8. Mohr FW, Morice MC, Kappetein AP, et al. Coronary artery bypass graft surgery versus percutaneous coronary intervention in patients with three-vessel disease and left main coronary disease: 5-year follow-up of the randomised, clinical SYNTAX trial. Lancet 2013;381(9867):629–38.
9. Head SJ, Farooq V, Serruys PW, et al. The SYNTAX score and its clinical implications. Heart 2014; 100(2):169–77.
10. Farkouh ME, Domanski M, Sleeper LA, et al. Strategies for multivessel revascularization in patients with diabetes. N Engl J Med 2012;367(25): 2375–84.
11. Head SJ, Kaul S, Mack MJ, et al. The rationale for heart team decision-making for patients with stable, complex coronary artery disease. Eur Heart J 2013; 34(32):2510–8.
12. Yusuf S, Zucker D, Passamani E, et al. Effect of coronary artery bypass graft surgery on survival: overview of 10-year results from randomised trials by the Coronary Artery Bypass Graft Surgery Trialists Collaboration. Lancet 1994;344(8922): 563–70.
13. Kolh P, Wijns W, Danchin N, et al. Guidelines on myocardial revascularization. Eur J Cardiothorac Surg 2010;38(Suppl):S1–52.
14. Kappetein AP, Feldman TE, Mack MJ, et al. Comparison of coronary bypass surgery with drug-eluting stenting for the treatment of left main and/or

three-vessel disease: 3-year follow-up of the SYNTAX trial. Eur Heart J 2011;32(17):2125–34.

15. Katritsis DG, Ioannidis JP. Percutaneous coronary intervention versus conservative therapy in nonacute coronary artery disease: a meta-analysis. Circulation 2005;111:2906–12.

16. Boden WE, O'Rourke RA, Teo KK, et al. Optimal medical therapy with or without PCI for stable coronary disease. N Engl J Med 2007;356(15):1503–16.

17. De Bruyne B, Pijls NH, Kalesan B, et al. Fractional flow reserve-guided PCI versus medical therapy in stable coronary disease. N Engl J Med 2012; 367(11):991–1001.

18. Fihn SD, Gardin JM, Abrams J, et al. 2012 ACCF/ AHA/ACP/AATS/PCNA/SCAI/STS guideline for the diagnosis and management of patients with stable ischemic heart disease: a report of the American College of Cardiology Foundation/American Heart Association Task Force on Practice Guidelines, and the American College of Physicians, American Association for Thoracic Surgery, Preventive Cardiovascular Nurses Association, Society for Cardiovascular Angiography and Interventions, and Society of Thoracic Surgeons. Circulation 2012;126(25):e354–471.

19. Head SJ, Kaul S, Tijssen JG, et al. Subgroup analyses in trial reports comparing percutaneous coronary intervention with coronary artery bypass surgery. JAMA 2013;310(19):2097–8.

20. Morice MC, Serruys PW, Kappetein AP, et al. Five-year outcomes in patients with left main disease treated with either percutaneous coronary intervention or coronary artery bypass grafting in the SYNTAX trial. Circulation 2014. [Epub ahead of print].

21. Kappetein AP. Editorial comment: is there enough evidence that proves clinical equipoise between stenting and coronary surgery for patients with left main coronary artery disease? Eur J Cardiothorac Surg 2010;38(4):428–30.

Cardiac Syndrome X:
Update 2014

Shilpa Agrawal, BS[a], Puja K. Mehta, MD[b],*, C. Noel Bairey Merz, MD[b]

KEYWORDS

- Cardiac syndrome X • Angina • Ischemia • Microvascular endothelial dysfunction
- Myocardial hypersensitivity

KEY POINTS

- Up to 20% to 30% of patients presenting with chest discomfort characteristic of angina show no obstructive coronary artery disease (CAD), defined as 50% or more stenosis in at least 1 major coronary artery, on angiography.
- The lifetime cost of health care for a woman with chest pain and no obstructive CAD is estimated at approximately $1 million as a result of challenges in diagnosis and treatment.
- To diagnose cardiac syndrome X, noncardiac causes, large vessel coronary disorders, and coronary microvascular dysfunction with associated myocardial disease must be ruled out.
- The proposed theories for the underlying pathogenesis of cardiac syndrome X include coronary microvascular dysfunction and associated ischemia, abnormal cardiac pain sensitivity, or a combination of both.
- Treatment strategies include anti-ischemic medications, analgesic medications, nonpharmacologic procedures, and lifestyle modifications.

INTRODUCTION

Cardiovascular (CV) disease is the leading cause of death worldwide, and coronary artery disease (CAD) is the most common type of CV disease.[1] Yet, up to 20% to 30% of patients presenting with chest discomfort characteristic of angina show no signs of obstructive CAD, defined as 50% or more stenosis in at least 1 major coronary artery, on angiography.[2] These patients are often given noncardiac diagnoses such as gastrointestinal or psychiatric disorders.[3] However, evidence of electrocardiographic (ECG) and metabolic abnormalities during stress induced by right atrial pacing in a subset of these patients led to the designation of a new disorder by Harvey Kemp in 1973[4] named cardiac syndrome X (CSX).

CSX can be defined broadly as anginalike chest discomfort, with normal epicardial coronary arteries on angiography. A proposed more strict definition of CSX entails the following criteria:

1. Exercise-induced, anginalike chest discomfort
2. ST segment depression during angina

This work was supported by contracts from the National Heart, Lung, and Blood Institute, N01-HV-68161, N01-HV-68162, N01-HV-68163, N01-HV-68164, grants K23HL105787, U0164829, U01 HL649141, U01 HL649241, T32HL69751, R01 HL090957, 1R03AG032631 from the National Institute on Aging, GCRC grant MO1-RR00425 from the National Center for Research Resources and grants from the Gustavus and Louis Pfeiffer Research Foundation, Danville, NJ, The Women's Guild of Cedars-Sinai Medical Center, Los Angeles, CA, The Ladies Hospital Aid Society of Western Pennsylvania, Pittsburgh, PA, and QMED, Laurence Harbor, NJ, the Edythe L. Broad Women's Heart Research Fellowship, Cedars-Sinai Medical Center, Los Angeles, California, and the Barbra Streisand Women's Cardiovascular Research and Education Program, Cedars-Sinai Medical Center, Los Angeles, and the Linda Joy Pollin Women's Heart Health Program, Cedars-Sinai Medical Center, Los Angeles.
Disclosures: None of the authors has any relevant conflicts of interest to disclose.
[a] David Geffen School of Medicine, University of California, Los Angeles, Los Angeles, CA 90095, USA;
[b] Department of Medicine, Cedars-Sinai Medical Center, Barbra Streisand Women's Heart Center, Cedars-Sinai Heart Institute, 127 South San Vicente Boulevard, Los Angeles, CA 90048, USA
* Corresponding author. 127 South San Vicente Boulevard, Suite A3212, Los Angeles, CA 90048.
E-mail address: puja.mehta@cshs.org

0733-8651/14/$ – see front matter © 2014 Elsevier Inc. All rights reserved.

3. Normal epicardial coronary arteries at angiography[2]
4. No spontaneous or inducible epicardial coronary artery spasm on egonovine or acetylcholine provocation
5. Absence of cardiac or systemic diseases associated with microvascular dysfunction, such as hypertrophic cardiomyopathy or diabetes[5]

There are several groups of patients who have anginalike chest pain and normal coronary arteries at angiography but fail to meet one of these criteria. Examples of these patients include those with angina predominantly at rest, those with diabetes or hypertension, or those with lack of ST depression on ECG during angina. It remains unclear whether the pathogenesis of angina in these patients is the same as in patients who fall under the strict definition of CSX. Throughout the scientific literature, the broad and strict definitions of CSX are used variably, reflecting the mystery that has historically surrounded the syndrome.[6]

EPIDEMIOLOGY

What is known is that CSX is relatively more prevalent in women. In a study of 32,856 patients presenting for their first cardiac catheterization with suspected ischemic heart disease,[7] 23.3% of women versus 7.1% of men were found to have normal coronaries after angiography. Another study[8] found that among 886 patients who were referred for chest pain and subsequently underwent angiography, a diagnosis of normal coronary arteries was more than 5 times more common in women than men (41% vs 8%). Furthermore, women who were perimenopausal or postmenopausal were found to have an increased risk of angina with no obstructive CAD.[5] A study of 99 patients with CSX[9] showed that the mean age of diagnosis was 48.5 years and that 61.5% of women were postmenopausal.

Individuals with CSX have a higher likelihood of presenting with features of the metabolic syndrome (eg, hypertension, dyslipidemia, and insulin resistance) than the general population (30% vs 8%, respectively). In addition, these patients have been shown to have a greater amount of endothelium-dependent and endothelium-independent impairment of cutaneous microvascular function compared with healthy controls.[10]

PROGNOSIS

For many years, it was believed that CSX had a benign prognosis. One study[9] followed 99 patients with CSX for an average of 7 years and showed no significant decline in ventricular function. In another study of 1491 patients with anginal symptoms and normal coronary arteries (no major epicardial artery with >25% stenosis),[11] myocardial infarction–free survival rates were 99% at 5 years and 98% at 10 years. In 486 patients with angina and no obstructive CAD (no major epicardial artery with ≥75% stenosis), myocardial infarction–free survival rates were 97% at 5 years and 90% at 10 years. A study[12] of 7-year survival in patients with symptoms suggestive of CAD but showing a normal or near-normal coronary arteriogram (<50% stenosis in ≥1 epicardial arteries) showed survival rates of 96% and 92%, respectively, in these 2 subpopulations.

However, recent evidence has challenged the assumption that anginalike pain without obstructive CAD is a benign condition. In the WISE (Women's Ischemia Syndrome Evaluation) study,[13] 5-year annualized event rates for CV events were 16.0% in 222 symptomatic women with nonobstructive CAD (stenosis in any coronary artery of 1%–49%), 7.9% in 318 symptomatic women with normal coronary arteries (0% stenosis in all coronary arteries), and 2.4% in 5932 asymptomatic women. CV events included myocardial infarction, hospitalization for heart failure, stroke, cardiac mortality, and all-cause mortality. Recent reports from Europe and Canada[14,15] replicate this adverse prognosis. In addition, some subsets of patients tend to have poorer prognoses than others. In 1 study,[16] 13 of 22 symptomatic patients with normal coronary angiograms and endothelial dysfunction assessed through acetylcholine-mediated dilatation developed CAD when followed for greater than 10 years. In contrast, 20 of 20 symptomatic patients with normal coronary angiograms and no endothelial dysfunction showed resolution of chest pain 6 to 36 months after angiography. Impaired coronary vasomotor response to acetylcholine has also been independently linked to earlier CV events regardless of CAD severity.[17]

Furthermore, CSX remains a major diagnostic and therapeutic challenge causing significant deterioration in a patient's functioning and quality of life. Diagnosis of CSX requires an extensive workup to rule out other potential causes of chest pain and can be expensive. Treatment with conventional antianginal medications is often not successful, which results in patients being limited in their daily activities, seeking emergency care for their chest pain, and needing to take time off or abandon their work because of persistent symptoms. Prolonged and recurrent chest pain also necessitates repeated coronary arteriographies as well as regular outpatient visits. The lifetime cost of health care for a woman with nonobstructive chest pain is estimated at approximately $1 million.[5]

DIAGNOSIS
Clinical Features

History
In approximately 50% of CSX cases, patients present with a history of exercise-induced chest pain, which is followed by 15 to 20 minutes of dull, persistent chest discomfort. Short-acting nitrates are often inadequate in relieving this pain.[18] Some patients also experience chest pain at rest in addition to the chest pain during exertion. Patients often describe the chest pain as retrosternal and radiating to the left arm. These episodes of chest pain occur frequently, with 1 study[9] showing that 31% of patients reported greater than 7 episodes per week and 30% of patients reported greater than 1 episode per day.

ECG
By definition, patients with CSX have ST segment depression induced by exercise ECG testing. However, evidence from Holter monitoring show that patients also have transient ST depression during their daily activities. In 1 study in which patients with CSX underwent 48 hours of Holter monitoring,[19] 63% of patients had transient ST segment depression. Transient ST depression is believed to occur in only 2% of healthy individuals. However, ST segment depression did not correlate with episodes of angina. In 50% of ST segment depression episodes, patients did not experience chest pain, and in 75% of anginal episodes, patients did not have ST segment depression.

Coronary angiography
Similar to the presence of ST depression, by definition, patients with CSX show no obstructive CAD on angiography. The traditional definition of obstructive CAD is stenosis of 50% or more of the diameter of the left main coronary artery or stenosis of 70% or more of the diameter of a coronary vessel greater than 2 mm in diameter. However, most studies require no stenosis of 50% or more in any coronary vessel for a patient to be classified in CSX.[20]

Among patients with angina and normal coronary angiography, 1 study[21] showed that approximately 75% of patients show ST segment depression during exercise treadmill testing. Among the 25% who do not show exercise-induced ST segment depression, 50% have detectable ST segment depression during their daily activities with Holter monitoring. A controversy in this field is whether patients with transient ST segment depression during Holter monitoring but not during exercise treadmill testing should be included in the definition of CSX.

Differential Diagnosis
The diagnosis of CSX in patients with recurrent chest pain and absence of any angiographic lesion greater than 50% in any coronary vessel is primarily a diagnosis of exclusion (**Fig. 1**).[22–26] First, chest pain of noncardiac origin (eg, gastrointestinal, musculoskeletal, pulmonary, or psychiatric) must be ruled out. If the chest pain is of cardiac origin, imaging modalities such as echocardiogram can be used to rule out structural and inflammatory disorders, such as pericarditis. If a diagnosis of coronary dysfunction is likely, the distinction between large and small vessel dysfunction is important. The primary large vessel coronary dysfunction, vasospastic angina, presents with angina at rest, reversible ischemic ECG changes (usually ST elevation rather than depression), and spontaneous/induced coronary spasm on angiography.[22,27] Various agents can be used for spasm provocation testing, including ergonovine and acetylcholine, but standardized guidelines on when to test for spasm are lacking.[28] Catheter-induced coronary spasm can occur on routine angiography, especially during engagement of the right coronary artery. This spasm is believed to occur as a result of mechanical irritation of the vessel, and factors such as the size of the catheter and catheter manipulation predispose to catheter-induced spasm. The clinical significance of asymptomatic catheter-induced spasm is unclear, but if a patient complains of chest pain during catheter-induced spasm, then, a diagnosis of vasospastic angina can be made and treatment initiated. When catheter-induced spasm occurs, the arterial pressure wave form can decrease and become ventricularized or dampened; in this setting, it is important to rule out significant ostial atherosclerosis. Intracoronary nitroglycerin or other epicardial vasodilators are routinely given in the setting of catheter-induced spasm.

With signs and symptoms of ischemia and no obstructive CAD, coronary microvascular dysfunction (CMD) should also be considered as a cause for chest pain. CMD can be associated with several myocardial diseases, as listed in **Fig. 1**. Whether this dysfunction is involved in the pathogenesis or is a consequence of these diseases is debatable, but the presence of myocardial diseases should be ruled out before making a diagnosis of CSX.[26] CSX must be distinguished from 2 other CMD disorders not associated with

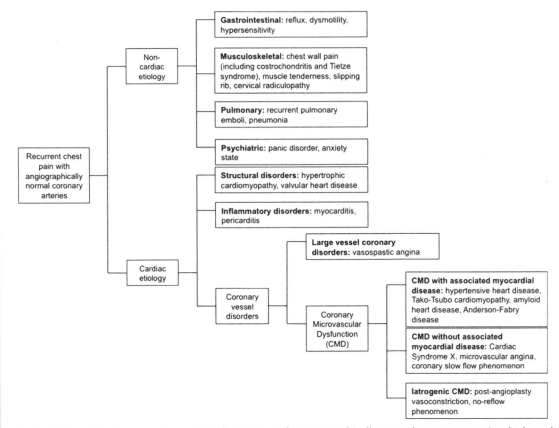

Fig. 1. Differential diagnosis of recurrent chest pain with angiographically normal coronary arteries. (*Adapted from* Refs.[22–26])

myocardial disease: microvascular angina and coronary slow flow phenomenon. In microvascular angina, CMD is present as indicated by impaired coronary vasodilator capacity. However, unlike in individuals with CSX, these patients do not show evidence of stress-induced ischemia. These patients primarily experience angina with rest rather than exertion and do not show ST depression during exercise ECG testing.[22] Coronary slow flow phenomenon, sometimes referred to as syndrome Y, is characterized by delayed distal vessel contrast flow on angiography. In contrast to CSX, clinical features include a higher prevalence in men and rest or mixed-pattern angina rather than angina on exertion.[29]

PATHOGENESIS OVERVIEW

The pathogenesis of CSX remains unclear, but several theories have been proposed. The 2 major hypotheses are (1) CMD, in which symptoms are believed to result from myocardial ischemia secondary to abnormal coronary microvasculature function, and (2) abnormal cardiac pain sensitivity, in which symptoms are believed to be a result of altered pain perception of myocardial

hypersensitivity. These processes could be acting synergistically, or different subpopulations of patients with CSX may have different underlying causes.[6]

CMD
Normal Coronary Microvascular Function

The coronary arterial system is composed of 3 types of vessels. The most proximal vessels are the large epicardial coronary arteries, ranging in diameter size from 500 μm to 2 to 5 mm. The function of these vessels is to store blood from the heart as flow changes. The prearterioles are distal to the epicardial coronary arteries, and these prearterioles are 100 to 500 μm in diameter. Their function is to maintain pressure with changes in blood flow. The most distal vessels are the intramural arterioles, which have a diameter of less than 100 μm. Their function is to match blood supply to tissue oxygen demand.[16] The coronary microcirculation is composed of the coronary arteries, which are too small to be visualized by angiography (<500 μm) but are important in regulating blood flow to match oxygen demand, growth, inflammation, coagulation, and permeability.[30]

Normally, when the heart tissue increases its oxygen consumption in response to increased work, for example, the intramural arterioles dilate in response to the release of metabolites from the myocardium. This dilation results in a decrease in pressure, triggering a dilation of the prearterioles and epicardial coronary arteries, increasing blood flow, and therefore, matching the increased oxygen demand of the tissue.[16]

Assessment of Coronary Microvascular Function

Because the vessels involved in the microcirculation are too small to be visualized by angiography, coronary blood flow measurements at baseline compared with maximal hyperemic stimuli are used to evaluate the function of the microcirculatory vessels. Hyperemic stimuli can be endothelium-independent or endothelium-dependent, and therefore, dysfunction of both types of stimuli must be assessed. Adenosine is used as the gold standard to invoke an endothelium-independent hyperemic response in vessels less than 150 μm by stimulating the adenosine A_2 receptors on smooth muscle cells. Acetylcholine is commonly used to assess endothelial-dependent dilation of the microvasculature.[30] A newer, less invasive diagnostic method is the use of cardiac magnetic resonance imaging to assess myocardial perfusion reserve index (MPRI) in response to adenosine. A recent study[31] showed that women with previously confirmed CMD had lower MPRI values globally and in subendocardial and subepicardial regions compared with controls.

Impaired Coronary Microvascular Function

It is believed that patients with CSX have impaired relaxation or increased sensitivity to vasoconstriction in the intramural arterioles and prearterioles. This situation results in impaired myocardial blood supply and episodes of ischemia, causing chest pain.[2] According to the traditional definition of CMD, coronary volumetric blood flow increases by less than 2.5 times baseline blood flow with maximal hyperemic stimuli.[30]

Studies in favor of the CMD theory underlying the pathogenesis of CSX have shown that patients with CSX have impaired vasodilation in response to endothelium-dependent and endothelium-independent hyperemic stimuli, greater ischemic metabolite production after pacing-induced tachycardia, decreased phosphocreatine/adenosine triphosphate (ATP) ratio after exercise, more heterogeneous blood flow, and greater thallium scan defects compared with healthy controls (**Table 1**).[32–40] Studies opposing the ischemic genesis hypothesis for CSX have shown that patients with CSX lack cardiac wall motion abnormalities during both hyperemic stimuli-mediated vasodilation and right atrial pacing, lack production of ischemic metabolites during right atrial pacing, and do not show significant change in myocardial blood flow with hyperemic stimuli when compared with control individuals (**Table 2**).[41–46]

Maseri and colleagues[47] proposed a hypothesis that explains these seemingly contradictory studies. These investigators described a population of patients with CSX with many abnormally constricted prearteriolar vessels who showed reduced coronary flow reserve and myocardial ischemia. They also described another population of patients with a limited and patchy distribution of abnormally constricted prearteriolar vessels. These vessels may stimulate the local release of adenosine, which, if intense and prolonged, could cause anginal pain. This pain could occur in the absence of signs of ischemia and reduction in total coronary flow reserve because of compensation by nonconstricted vessels. Furthermore, a patchy distribution of myocardial ischemia may be adequate to produce ST depression on ECG but may not result in detectable contractile dysfunction, because of the presence of normal surrounding tissue, and may not result in detection of ischemic metabolites, because of dilution with blood flow from normal tissue.[48]

Other possible reasons for the contradictory studies include methodological limitations and patient selection factors. None of the invasive or noninvasive techniques used in the assessment of coronary blood flow can accurately measure absolute flow. Furthermore, because the definition of CSX remains debatable, different studies have recruited patients with different inclusion criteria, making comparison between studies difficult.[2]

Risk Factors

Risk factors for CMD, and hence, potentially CSX, have not yet been fully elucidated. Traditional risk factors for atherosclerosis account for less than 20% of the variability seen in coronary reactivity to hyperemic stimuli.[49] Other potential risk factors include nitric oxide (NO) metabolism disorders, dysregulation of inflammatory cytokines, estrogen, or adrenergic pathways, and disruption in the expression and production of local vasoactive substances.[50]

ENHANCED PAIN SENSITIVITY
Origin of the Enhanced Pain Sensitivity Theory

The pain sensitivity theory was first proposed by Shapiro and colleagues,[51] when they observed

Table 1
Evidence supporting CMD in CSX

Authors and Year	Assessment Method	Key Findings
Lanza et al,[37] 2008	Dobutamine, adenosine-mediated dilatation	At peak dobutamine stress test, reversible perfusion defects found in 56% of patients with CSX but in none of the control individuals ($P = .004$) Coronary flow rate to adenosine lower in patients with CSX than in control individuals ($P = .0004$)[37]
Panting et al,[39] 2002	Adenosine-mediated dilatation	Although myocardial perfusion index in response to adenosine increased in both the subepicardium and subendocardium in normal controls, it did not change significantly in the subendocardium for patients with CSX ($P = .11$) Adenosine provoked chest pain in 95% of patients with CSX but only 40% of normal controls ($P<.001$)[39]
Buffon et al,[34] 2000	Metabolite production	Lipid hydroperoxides and conjugated dienes, 2 markers of ischemia-reperfusion oxidative stress, increased in the great cardiac vein in patients with CSX ($P<.01$) but did not change in normal controls after pacing-induced tachycardia[34]
Buchthal et al,[33] 2000	Phosphocreatine/ATP ratio after exercise	7/35 women with CSX had decreases in the phosphocreatine/ATP ratio during isometric handgrip exercise that were more than 2 standard deviations less than the mean value in controls, providing evidence of an abnormal metabolic response to exercise consistent with myocardial ischemia[33]
Bottcher et al,[32] 1999	Dipyridamole-mediated dilatation	Hyperemic response to intravenous dipyridamole less in CSX group compared with normal controls ($P<.05$)[32]
Chauhan et al,[35] 1997	Papaverine, acetylcholine-mediated dilatation	Mean increase in coronary blood flow to endothelium-independent vasodilator papaverine and endothelium-depending vasodilator acetylcholine was less in patients with CSX than normal controls ($P<.001$)[35]
Meeder et al,[38] 1995	Heterogeneity of perfusion using positron emission tomography	Mean perfusion and its coefficient of variation, as a measure of perfusion heterogeneity, were higher in patients with CSX compared with normal controls, indicating patchy distribution of hyperactive small coronary vessels with compensatory release of adenosine[38]
Galassi et al,[36] 1993	Dipyridamole-mediated dilatation	Baseline and postintravenous dipyridamole myocardial blood flow more heterogeneous in patients with CSX than in healthy controls ($P<.01$)[36]
Tweddel et al,[40] 1992	Thallium scan	98/100 patients with angina and normal coronary arteriograms had thallium scan defects that suggest microvascular angina[40]

Data from Refs.[32–40]

that patients with CSX experienced chest pain during cardiac catheterization. This chest pain was similar to the recurrent episodes that were experienced before catheterization and was stimulated when the venous catheter was moved within the proximal 3 to 5 cm of the superior vena cava and the entire right atrium. Furthermore, injection of saline into the right atrium also provoked the pain. In contrast, none of the patients with CAD or mitral valve disease experienced pain during movement of the catheter. Shapiro and colleagues[51] proposed that the mechanism

Table 2
Evidence against CMD in CSX

Authors and Year	Assessment Method	Key Findings
Panza et al,[44] 1997	Dobutamine-mediated dilatation	Like normal controls, patients with CSX showed a quantitatively normal myocardial contractile response without development of wall motion abnormalities in response to dobutamine[44]
Rosano et al,[45] 1996	Blood pH and lactate levels during right atrial pacing	Patients with CAD showed a greater decrease of coronary sinus pH, oxygen saturation, and lactate extraction ratio compared with patients with CSX ($P<.01$, $P<.05$, and $P<.01$ respectively)[45]
Rosen et al,[46] 1994	Dipyridamole-mediated dilatation	Myocardial blood flow in patients with CSX and control individuals at rest was 1.05 and 1.00, respectively, and after dipyridamole administration was 2.73 and 3.00, respectively (P = not significant)[46]
Camici et al,[41] 1992	Dipyridamole-mediated dilatation	Among patients with chest pain and angiographically normal coronary arteries, one-third had reduced coronary vasodilatory reserve after dipyridamole administration. 12/14 patients with reduced reserve had exercise ST segment depression, but 16/29 patients with normal reserve also had ST depression, suggesting the role of factors other than reduced coronary reserve and ischemia in the genesis of ST depression[41]
Camici et al,[42] 1991	Analysis of metabolites during rapid atrial pacing	No net lactate release in patients with CSX during atrial pacing Patients with CSX carried out the same external work with a smaller increase in blood flow, oxygen consumption, and energy expenditure than normal controls During atrial pacing, patients with CSX continued to rely on fatty acid substrates for oxidative metabolism[42]
Nihoyannopoulos et al,[43] 1991	Stress two-dimensional echocardiogram during right atrial pacing	In patients with CSX, no regional wall motion abnormalities seen on two-dimensional imaging of any myocardial segment Percent systolic wall thickening increased over values at rest in each myocardial segment during right atrial pacing[43]

Data from Refs.[41–46]

underlying chest pain in CSX may be hyperawareness of changes in right atrial pressure and volume during exertion. Additional studies with larger patient populations confirmed these observations and found that patients with CSX also had a low tolerance to pain induced by adenosine.[52,53]

Psychological and Behavioral Factors

Several groups have proposed that patients with CSX have an exaggerated response to pain. Studies have shown that certain behavioral characteristics such as hypochondriasis, anxiety, and panic disorders are common in patients with CSX. Wielgosz and colleagues[54] found that among 217 patients, a high hypochondriasis score (assessed by the Minnesota Multiphasic Personality Inventory) was the strongest determinant of continued pain in patients with no coronary artery stenosis. In women experiencing chest pain, a history of anxiety disorders is associated with a lower probability of CAD on angiography.[55] Panic disorder is believed to affect 1% to 2% of the US population but approximately one-third of patients with unexplained chest pain and angiographically normal coronary arteries.[56]

It remains unclear whether increased pain sensitivity or increased pain perception plays a role in this theory. A study was conducted by Pasceri and colleagues,[57] in which patients with CSX and control individuals underwent false and true pacing. The investigators found that patients with CSX had both increased cardiac pain sensitivity and higher likelihood of reporting pain with the expectation of pain but absence of stimulus (false pacing).

PATHOGENESIS SUMMARY

CMD and enhanced pain sensitivity may be independent causes manifesting in different subsets of patients with CSX. Alternatively, Crea and Lanza[6] have proposed a combined theory in which repeated episodes of transient ischemia may functionally alter cardiac afferent nerve endings to a hypersensitive state. Novel techniques and additional studies are necessary to further elucidate the pathogenesis of CSX.

TREATMENT OVERVIEW

Management of patients with CSX remains a significant challenge because of the limited effectiveness of conventional antianginal therapies. The difficulties in management may be caused by our incomplete understanding of the pathophysiology underlying CSX and hence the inability to target the underlying pathophysiology.[58] Current therapies include anti-ischemic and analgesic pharmacologic treatments, nonpharmacologic procedures, and lifestyle modifications (**Box 1**).

ANTI-ISCHEMIC PHARMACOLOGIC TREATMENTS
Nitrates

The therapeutic effect of nitrates results from the release of NO from nitrite, the activation of guanylyl cyclase, and the relaxation of blood vessels.[59] Although the effectiveness of nitrates in CSX has not been evaluated in large randomized clinical trials, observational studies have shown that nitrates have limited efficacy in alleviating chest pain. In an observational study of 99 patients with CSX, both sublingual nitrates as well as oral nitrates with calcium antagonists relieved episodes of chest pain in 42% of patients.[9] Furthermore, Russo and colleagues[60] reported that although patients with CAD had significantly improved exercise stress test results with the administration of short-

---

Box 1
Overview of treatment strategies for CSX

Anti-ischemic pharmacologic treatments
  Nitrates
  β-Blockers
  Calcium channel antagonists
  Ranolazine
  Angiotensin-converting enzyme inhibitors
  Statins
Analgesic pharmacologic treatments
  Xanthine derivatives
  Tricyclic antidepressants
Nonpharmacologic treatments
  Cognitive-behavioral therapy
  Enhanced external counterpulsation
  Neurostimulation
    Transcutaneous electrical stimulation
    Spinal cord stimulation
  Stellate ganglionectomy
Lifestyle modifications
  Exercise
  Weight loss
  Smoking cessation
  Dietary changes (Mediterranean diet)

---

acting nitrates, patients with microvascular angina did not. These findings supported the hypothesis that the dilator effect of nitrates on small coronary vessels is poor. Despite their unpredictable effectiveness, nitrates have historically been the mainstay of CSX therapy.[61]

β-Adrenergic Receptor Blockers

β-Adrenergic receptor blockers (β-blockers) work as an antianginal therapy by blocking catecholamine-induced increases in heart rate, blood pressure, and myocardial contractility, thereby reducing myocardial oxygen consumption.[62] They have been shown to improve anginal symptoms, functional capacity, and exercise testing in up to 75% of patients with CSX.[63] Propranolol has been shown to significantly reduce the average number of ischemic episodes per 24 hours compared with placebo, and atenolol has been shown to significantly improve symptoms, exercise performance, and diastolic function in patients with CSX when compared with placebo.[64,65]

Compared with traditional β-blockers, the third-generation β-blockers nebivolol and carvedilol have additional endothelium-dependent vasodilating properties and may be more effective than traditional β-blockers.[66] In patients with CSX, nebivolol has been shown to significantly increase circulating endothelial function parameters, such as plasma asymmetric dimethylarginine (ADMA), L-arginine, and NO levels, and improve exercise stress test parameters, such as exercise duration to 1-mm ST depression and total exercise duration, compared with metoprolol.[67] Kaski and colleagues[68] showed that after administration of a single dose of carvedilol, 10 of 15 patients with CSX did not have angina at peak exercise and 5 of 15 patients had ST shifts of less than 1 mm (P<.01 compared with placebo). Overall, β-blockers may represent the first line of treatment of patients with CSX.[64]

Calcium Channel Antagonists

Calcium channel antagonists block L-type calcium channels, thereby reducing intracellular calcium concentrations. This process results in negative chronotropic and inotropic effects as well as a decrease in peripheral vascular resistance.[69] The efficacy of calcium channel antagonists for treating CSX remains unclear. Verapamil and nifedipine have been shown to decrease the frequency of anginal episodes and prolong exercise duration compared with placebo.[70] However, administration of intravenous diltiazem did not increase coronary flow reserve in patients with angina, normal coronary arteries, and reduced coronary flow reserve.[71] Furthermore, β-blockers have been shown to be more effective than calcium channel antagonists. Propranolol was shown to be more effective than verapamil and atenolol was more effective than amlodipine in reducing frequency of anginal episodes.[72]

Ranolazine

The functional molecular mechanisms of ranolazine, a newer antianginal medication, have been debated, but the consensus is that ranolazine inhibits the late inward sodium channel, thereby preventing high intracellular sodium concentrations from disrupting myocardial function.[69] Chaitman and colleagues[73,74] have reported in patients with chronic severe angina that ranolazine used as monotherapy increases exercise performance, and when combined with standard doses or atenolol, amlodipine, or diltiazem, provides additional antianginal relief. Furthermore, ranolazine has been shown to modulate neuronal voltage-gated sodium channels involved in neuropathic pain,

and therefore, may be especially beneficial as an antianginal therapy for patients with CSX.[75] Mehta and colleagues[76] showed that in women with angina, evidence of ischemia, and no obstructive CAD, 4-week treatment with ranolazine improves physical functioning, angina stability, and quality of life as measured by Seattle Angina Questionnaire scores.

Angiotensin-Converting Enzyme Inhibitors

Angiotensin-converting enzyme inhibitors (ACE-I) have 2 main mechanisms of action. First, they decrease production of angiotensin II, which has vasoconstrictive properties, and therefore are used in blood pressure management. Second, they decrease degradation of endothelial bradykinin, which stimulates the production of NO and other vasodilators and is antiapoptotic.[77] Therefore, they are hypothesized to be beneficial for treating patients with CSX. ACE-I have been shown to improve exercise tolerance, improve endothelial function, improve coronary flow rates, and decrease angina in patients with CSX. Studies have shown that both cilazapril and enalapril increase total exercise duration, prolong time to 1 mm of ST segment depression, and decrease magnitude of ST segment depression compared with placebo.[78,79] Chen and colleagues[80] showed that enalapril improved endothelial function by reducing von Willebrand factor and ADMA levels and increasing NO and L-arginine/ADMA ratio levels. Pauly and colleagues[81] showed that quinapril improved anginal episode frequency as well as increased coronary flow rate. The women who presented with the lowest baseline coronary flow rate benefited the most from quinapril.

Statins

Similar to ACE-I, statins have 2 main mechanisms of action. They are used primarily to lower cholesterol because of their ability to inhibit 3-hydroxy-3-methyl-glutaryl–coenzyme A reductase. However, they also improve endothelium-dependent vasomotion and hence may be beneficial in patients with CSX.[82] Studies have shown that patients with CSX receiving pravastatin or simvastatin show significant improvement in both exercise-induced ischemia as well as in brachial artery flow-mediated dilatation within 4 months.[83,84] Statins combined with calcium channel blockers have also proved beneficial. Zhang and colleagues[85] showed that patients who were treated with fluvastatin and diltiazem for 90 days showed improved coronary flow reserve and prolonged time to 1 mm ST segment depression as well as a significant increase in NO levels and a reduction in endothelin 1 when compared with patients treated with either medication alone.

ANALGESIC PHARMACOLOGIC TREATMENTS
Xanthine Derivatives

As mentioned earlier, enhanced pain sensitivity has been proposed as one of the pathophysiologic mechanisms underlying the pain experienced by patients with CSX. Therefore, it has been proposed[86] that xanthine derivatives, which are adenosine receptor blockers, can modulate the anginal pain in CSX. In a double-blind crossover study, patients with CSX who were given oral aminophylline for 3 weeks reported fewer episodes of chest pain when they were taking the medication than when they were taking placebo pills. Furthermore, after 3 weeks of aminophylline, patients had a higher exercise-induced chest pain threshold. However, frequency of ST depression measured by Holter monitoring and peak exercise ST depression did not change with the medication.[86] Improved exercise capacity with aminophylline has also been documented in other studies.[87,88] Despite the proven efficacy of xanthine derivatives when taken over a span of several weeks, Lanza and colleagues[89] showed that they may not have any acute benefit. These investigators showed that 1 intravenous infusion of bamiphylline had little effect on anginal pain during exercise testing in patients with CSX.

Tricyclic Antidepressants

In addition to their antidepressive effects, tricyclic antidepressants show analgesic activity because of their balanced reuptake inhibition of the neurotransmitters serotonin and noradrenaline.[90] In a study of patients with chest pain and normal angiograms,[91] patients experienced a 52% decrease in episodes of chest pain during the imipramine-treatment phase. In addition, patients experienced significant improvement in sensitivity to cardiac pain during right ventricular electrical stimulation or intracoronary infusion of adenosine compared with baseline. Cox and colleagues[92] also showed that imipramine treatment decreased anginal frequency. However, they also reported the failure of imipramine to improve quality of life, likely because of the side effects of treatment, including dry mouth, dizziness, nausea, and constipation.

NONPHARMACOLOGIC TREATMENT
Cognitive-Behavioral Therapy

Cognitive-behavioral therapy (CBT) consists of opportunities for patients to discuss their experiences of pain and its management, receive counseling and education about cardiac disease and angina, learn stress management and relaxation techniques, regain exposure to activities avoided because of pain, and engage in light physical exercise.[93,94] In women with chest pain despite normal angiography, 8 weeks of CBT can help reduce patients' anxiety, depression, and disability as well as increase exercise tolerance.[94] Furthermore, CBT can reduce yearly hospital admissions among patients with CSX, likely because educating patients and demystifying angina put patients at greater ease. One study[93] showed that 8 weeks of CBT decreased total hospital admissions from 2.40 to 1.78 per patient per year and decreased total hospital bed day occupancy from 15.48 to 10.34 days per patient per year. CBT should be considered in the management of CSX, especially when patients have continued pain despite pharmacologic treatment.

Enhanced External Counterpulsation

Enhanced external counterpulsation consists of treatment sessions in which cuffs are wrapped around a patient's legs and inflated and deflated in sequence with the cardiac cycle. During early diastole, the cuff is inflated sequentially from the lower legs to the upper thighs, thereby propelling blood to the heart. During end-diastole, the cuff is deflated, reducing vascular resistance. This technique is believed to provide anginal relief through several mechanisms:

1. Increased transmyocardial pressure gradients during the treatment sessions may open collaterals in the heart.
2. When the coronary and peripheral arterial beds are exposed to increased blood flow and shear forces, the endothelium increases production of NO and prostacyclin.
3. Increased blood flow may regulate paracrine substances involved in vascular remodeling and reactivity.[95]

Kronhaus and Lawson[96] have shown that enhanced external counterpulsation is beneficial in patients with CSX. In their study, they showed that enhanced external counterpulsation treatment in 30 patients with CSX resulted in an improvement in angina and regional ischemia. After 12 months, 87% of these patients maintained their improvement in angina.

Neurostimulation

Neural modulation can be performed either through transcutaneous electrical nerve stimulation (TENS) or spinal cord stimulation. It has been proposed that an autonomic imbalance with increased sympathetic activity and decreased parasympathetic activity may cause both endothelial dysfunction and increased pain sensitivity in patients with CSX.[97,98] Neurostimulation is believed to enhance parasympathetic activity and reduce spinothalamic tract cell activity, thereby potentially being an effective therapy for patients with CSX.[99]

de Vries and colleagues[99] performed a study in which patients who presented with anginal pain, normal coronary arteries, and benefit from a 2-week trial of TENS were treated with continued TENS for 5 years. If patients developed side effects, they had the option of switching to spinal cord stimulation. After 5 years of neurostimulation, patients reported a 57% reduction in pain and a 30% improvement in exercise capacity. Furthermore, Lanza and colleagues[100] reported that patients with angina and normal coronary arteries who underwent spinal cord stimulation showed an improvement in the Seattle Angina Questionnaire, reduction in angina severity and duration, and improvement in ischemic burden as measured by Holter monitoring.

Stellate Ganglionectomy

Sympathetic blockade is a technique used to block sympathetic fibers. One type of sympathetic blockade is the stellate (cervicothoracic) blockade. This blockade involves the stellate ganglion, which is formed from the fusion between the lower cervical and first thoracic ganglia, and provides part of the sympathetic innervation to the head, neck, arm, and heart. The heart lacks sensory nerves, and therefore, the sympathetic nervous system transmits the sensation of angina to the brain. Blocking the stellate ganglion, and hence sympathetic transmission, is believed to provide relief from angina.[101] Blockade is usually performed with an anesthetic and is transient. To achieve long-term blockade, a ganglionectomy can be performed.[102] Case reports of successful treatment with stellate ganglionectomy have been reported in conditions with augmentation of sympathetic activity, including congenital long QT syndrome, ventricular tachycardia storm, and palmar hyperhidrosis.[103–105] Furthermore, it has been shown[101] as a safe and effective procedure for pain conditions, including chronic refractory angina. Stellate ganglionectomy could be a viable option for patients with CSX, but further research is necessary.

LIFESTYLE MODIFICATIONS

The only lifestyle modification that has been evaluated in patients with CSX is exercise. Eriksson and colleagues[106] showed that exercise training for 8 weeks resulted in an increased exercise capacity with later onset of anginal pain. Exercise training also increased endothelium-dependent blood flow. However, training did not improve cardiac hypersensitivity to low-dose adenosine infusion. Another study[107] showed that the tolerated exertion during 6 minutes of walking and the health-related qualify of life measured by both the Stress and Crisis Inventory and the Sickness Impact Profile improved when patients with CSX underwent 8 weeks of physical training.

Along with these results, the INTERHEART study,[108] a global case-control study involving 27,098 participants from 52 countries, showed that not only does physical activity decrease the risk of a future myocardial infarction but that physical activity is more protective in women than in men. Physical activity can be performed by patients on their own or as part of a cardiac rehabilitation program. Cardiac rehabilitation programs are group-based or home-based CV exercise programs that focus on improving aerobic conditioning, functional capacity, muscular strength, endurance, and flexibility.[109] Asbury and colleagues[109] showed that women with CSX who underwent an 8-week cardiac rehabilitation program showed improved exercise tolerance, quality of life, symptom severity, and psychological morbidity not found among control CSX women.

Other lifestyle modifications that can be encouraged include weight loss, smoking cessation, and a Mediterranean diet. Both weight loss and smoking cessation have been shown to improve endothelial function and therefore may be beneficial in women with CSX.[110,111] The current American diet consists of highly processed, calorie-dense, and nutrient-depleted foods, which trigger oxidative stress, causing inflammation and damage to the endothelium. The Mediterranean diet, which is rich in minimally processed, high-fiber, plant-based foods such as vegetables and fruits, whole grains, legumes, and nuts, reduces oxidative stress, inflammation, and damage to the endothelium.[112]

TREATMENT CONCLUSION

In patients with CSX, a combination therapeutic approach, including anti-ischemic and analgesic pharmacologic treatment and lifestyle modifications, is often necessary. Nonpharmacologic therapies can be added as necessary. Studies have shown the effectiveness of individual therapies, but further work is needed in evaluating the best combination of treatments, and guidelines are necessary for the order in which treatments should be administered.

SUMMARY

CSX, the condition of angina, normal coronary arteries, and ST segment depression on ECG, was once characterized as benign. However, it is now recognized as a condition that carries significant morbidity and increases the risk for CV events. Diagnosis of the syndrome is challenging and expensive. The pathogenesis is not fully understood, which makes treatment difficult. Many pharmacologic and nonpharmacologic treatments have been shown to be at least partially effective, but guidelines are lacking on the best course of treatment.

REFERENCES

1. Wachira JK, Stys TP. Cardiovascular disease and bridging the diagnostic gap. S D Med 2013; 66(9):366–9.
2. Melikian N, De Bruyne B, Fearon WF, et al. The pathophysiology and clinical course of the normal coronary angina syndrome (cardiac syndrome X). Prog Cardiovasc Dis 2008;50(4):294–310.
3. Phan A, Shufelt C, Merz CN. Persistent chest pain and no obstructive coronary artery disease. JAMA 2009;301(14):1468–74.
4. Kemp HG Jr. Left ventricular function in patients with the anginal syndrome and normal coronary arteriograms. Am J Cardiol 1973;32(3):375–6.
5. Parsyan A, Pilote L. Cardiac syndrome X: mystery continues. Can J Cardiol 2012;28(Suppl 2):S3–6.
6. Crea F, Lanza GA. Angina pectoris and normal coronary arteries: cardiac syndrome X. Heart 2004; 90(4):457–63.
7. Humphries KH, Pu A, Gao M, et al. Angina with "normal" coronary arteries: sex differences in outcomes. Am Heart J 2008;155(2):375–81.
8. Sullivan AK, Holdright DR, Wright CA, et al. Chest pain in women: clinical, investigative, and prognostic features. BMJ 1994;308(6933):883–6.
9. Kaski JC, Rosano GM, Collins P, et al. Cardiac syndrome X: clinical characteristics and left ventricular function. Long-term follow-up study. J Am Coll Cardiol 1995;25(4):807–14.
10. Jadhav ST, Ferrell WR, Petrie JR, et al. Microvascular function, metabolic syndrome, and novel risk factor status in women with cardiac syndrome X. Am J Cardiol 2006;97(12):1727–31.
11. Papanicolaou MN, Califf RM, Hlatky MA, et al. Prognostic implications of angiographically normal and insignificantly narrowed coronary arteries. Am J Cardiol 1986;58(13):1181–7.
12. Kemp HG, Kronmal RA, Vlietstra RE, et al. Seven year survival of patients with normal or near normal coronary arteriograms: a CASS registry study. J Am Coll Cardiol 1986;7(3):479–83.
13. Gulati M, Cooper-DeHoff RM, McClure C, et al. Adverse cardiovascular outcomes in women with nonobstructive coronary artery disease: a report from the Women's Ischemia Syndrome Evaluation Study and the St James Women Take Heart Project. Arch Intern Med 2009;169(9):843–50.
14. Jespersen L, Hvelplund A, Abildstrom SZ, et al. Stable angina pectoris with no obstructive coronary artery disease is associated with increased risks of major adverse cardiovascular events. Eur Heart J 2012;33(6):734–44.
15. Sedlak TL, Lee M, Izadnegahdar M, et al. Sex differences in clinical outcomes in patients with stable angina and no obstructive coronary artery disease. Am Heart J 2013;166(1):38–44.
16. Camici PG, Crea F. Coronary microvascular dysfunction. N Engl J Med 2007;356(8):830–40.
17. von Mering GO, Arant CB, Wessel TR, et al. Abnormal coronary vasomotion as a prognostic indicator of cardiovascular events in women: results from the National Heart, Lung, and Blood Institute-Sponsored Women's Ischemia Syndrome Evaluation (WISE). Circulation 2004;109(6):722–5.
18. Singh M, Singh S, Arora R, et al. Cardiac syndrome X: current concepts. Int J Cardiol 2010; 142(2):113–9.
19. Kaski JC, Crea F, Nihoyannopoulos P, et al. Transient myocardial ischemia during daily life in patients with syndrome X. Am J Cardiol 1986; 58(13):1242–7.
20. Patel MR, Peterson ED, Dai D, et al. Low diagnostic yield of elective coronary angiography. N Engl J Med 2010;362(10):886–95.
21. Lanza GA, Manzoli A, Pasceri V, et al. Ischemic-like ST-segment changes during Holter monitoring in patients with angina pectoris and normal coronary arteries but negative exercise testing. Am J Cardiol 1997;79(1):1–6.
22. Di Fiore DP, Beltrame JF. Chest pain in patients with 'normal angiography': could it be cardiac? Int J Evid Based Healthc 2013;11(1):56–68.
23. Fass R, Achem SR. Noncardiac chest pain: diagnostic evaluation. Dis Esophagus 2012; 25(2):89–101.
24. McConaghy JR, Oza RS. Outpatient diagnosis of acute chest pain in adults. Am Fam Physician 2013;87(3):177–82.
25. Stochkendahl MJ, Christensen HW. Chest pain in focal musculoskeletal disorders. Med Clin North Am 2010;94(2):259–73.
26. Beltrame JF, Crea F, Camici P. Advances in coronary microvascular dysfunction. Heart Lung Circ 2009;18(1):19–27.
27. Beltrame JF, Sasayama S, Maseri A. Racial heterogeneity in coronary artery vasomotor reactivity: differences between Japanese and Caucasian patients. J Am Coll Cardiol 1999;33(6):1442–52.

28. Zaya M, Mehta PK, Merz CN. Provocative testing for coronary reactivity and spasm. J Am Coll Cardiol 2014;63(2):103–9.

29. Beltrame JF. Defining the coronary slow flow phenomenon. Circ J 2012;76(4):818–20.

30. Kothawade K, Bairey Merz CN. Microvascular coronary dysfunction in women: pathophysiology, diagnosis, and management. Curr Probl Cardiol 2011;36(8):291–318.

31. Shufelt CL, Thomson LE, Goykhman P, et al. Cardiac magnetic resonance imaging myocardial perfusion reserve index assessment in women with microvascular coronary dysfunction and reference controls. Cardiovasc Diagn Ther 2013;3(3):153–60.

32. Bottcher M, Botker HE, Sonne H, et al. Endothelium-dependent and -independent perfusion reserve and the effect of L-arginine on myocardial perfusion in patients with syndrome X. Circulation 1999;99(14):1795–801.

33. Buchthal SD, den Hollander JA, Merz CN, et al. Abnormal myocardial phosphorus-31 nuclear magnetic resonance spectroscopy in women with chest pain but normal coronary angiograms. N Engl J Med 2000;342(12):829–35.

34. Buffon A, Rigattieri S, Santini SA, et al. Myocardial ischemia-reperfusion damage after pacing-induced tachycardia in patients with cardiac syndrome X. Am J Physiol Heart Circ Physiol 2000;279(6):H2627–33.

35. Chauhan A, Mullins PA, Taylor G, et al. Both endothelium-dependent and endothelium-independent function is impaired in patients with angina pectoris and normal coronary angiograms. Eur Heart J 1997;18(1):60–8.

36. Galassi AR, Crea F, Araujo LI, et al. Comparison of regional myocardial blood flow in syndrome X and one-vessel coronary artery disease. Am J Cardiol 1993;72(2):134–9.

37. Lanza GA, Buffon A, Sestito A, et al. Relation between stress-induced myocardial perfusion defects on cardiovascular magnetic resonance and coronary microvascular dysfunction in patients with cardiac syndrome X. J Am Coll Cardiol 2008;51(4):466–72.

38. Meeder JG, Blanksma PK, Crijns HJ, et al. Mechanisms of angina pectoris in syndrome X assessed by myocardial perfusion dynamics and heart rate variability. Eur Heart J 1995;16(11):1571–7.

39. Panting JR, Gatehouse PD, Yang GZ, et al. Abnormal subendocardial perfusion in cardiac syndrome X detected by cardiovascular magnetic resonance imaging. N Engl J Med 2002;346(25):1948–53.

40. Tweddel AC, Martin W, Hutton I. Thallium scans in syndrome X. Br Heart J 1992;68(1):48–50.

41. Camici PG, Gistri R, Lorenzoni R, et al. Coronary reserve and exercise ECG in patients with chest pain and normal coronary angiograms. Circulation 1992;86(1):179–86.

42. Camici PG, Marraccini P, Lorenzoni R, et al. Coronary hemodynamics and myocardial metabolism in patients with syndrome X: response to pacing stress. J Am Coll Cardiol 1991;17(7):1461–70.

43. Nihoyannopoulos P, Kaski JC, Crake T, et al. Absence of myocardial dysfunction during stress in patients with syndrome X. J Am Coll Cardiol 1991;18(6):1463–70.

44. Panza JA, Laurienzo JM, Curiel RV, et al. Investigation of the mechanism of chest pain in patients with angiographically normal coronary arteries using transesophageal dobutamine stress echocardiography. J Am Coll Cardiol 1997;29(2):293–301.

45. Rosano GM, Kaski JC, Arie S, et al. Failure to demonstrate myocardial ischaemia in patients with angina and normal coronary arteries. Evaluation by continuous coronary sinus pH monitoring and lactate metabolism. Eur Heart J 1996;17(8):1175–80.

46. Rosen SD, Uren NG, Kaski JC, et al. Coronary vasodilator reserve, pain perception, and sex in patients with syndrome X. Circulation 1994;90(1):50–60.

47. Maseri A, Crea F, Kaski JC, et al. Mechanisms of angina pectoris in syndrome X. J Am Coll Cardiol 1991;17(2):499–506.

48. Lanza GA, Crea F. Primary coronary microvascular dysfunction: clinical presentation, pathophysiology, and management. Circulation 2010;121(21):2317–25.

49. Wessel TR, Arant CB, McGorray SP, et al. Coronary microvascular reactivity is only partially predicted by atherosclerosis risk factors or coronary artery disease in women evaluated for suspected ischemia: results from the NHLBI Women's Ischemia Syndrome Evaluation (WISE). Clin Cardiol 2007;30(2):69–74.

50. Crea F, Camici PG, Bairey Merz CN. Coronary microvascular dysfunction: an update. Eur Heart J 2014;35(17):1101–11.

51. Shapiro LM, Crake T, Poole-Wilson PA. Is altered cardiac sensation responsible for chest pain in patients with normal coronary arteries? Clinical observation during cardiac catheterisation. Br Med J (Clin Res Ed) 1988;296(6616):170–1.

52. Cannon RO 3rd, Quyyumi AA, Schenke WH, et al. Abnormal cardiac sensitivity in patients with chest pain and normal coronary arteries. J Am Coll Cardiol 1990;16(6):1359–66.

53. Lagerqvist B, Sylven C, Waldenstrom A. Lower threshold for adenosine-induced chest pain in patients with angina and normal coronary angiograms. Br Heart J 1992;68(3):282–5.

54. Wielgosz AT, Fletcher RH, McCants CB, et al. Un-improved chest pain in patients with minimal or no coronary disease: a behavioral phenomenon. Am Heart J 1984;108(1):67–72.

55. Rutledge T, Reis SE, Olson M, et al. History of anxiety disorders is associated with a decreased likelihood of angiographic coronary artery disease in women with chest pain: the WISE study. J Am Coll Cardiol 2001;37(3):780–5.

56. Beitman BD. Panic disorder in patients with angiographically normal coronary arteries. Am J Med 1992;92(5A):33S–40S.

57. Pasceri V, Lanza GA, Buffon A, et al. Role of abnormal pain sensitivity and behavioral factors in determining chest pain in syndrome X. J Am Coll Cardiol 1998;31(1):62–6.

58. Lim TK, Choy AJ, Khan F, et al. Therapeutic development in cardiac syndrome X: a need to target the underlying pathophysiology. Cardiovasc Ther 2009;27(1):49–58.

59. Nossaman VE, Nossaman BD, Kadowitz PJ. Nitrates and nitrites in the treatment of ischemic cardiac disease. Cardiol Rev 2010;18(4):190–7.

60. Russo G, Di Franco A, Lamendola P, et al. Lack of effect of nitrates on exercise stress test results in patients with microvascular angina. Cardiovasc Drugs Ther 2013;27(3):229–34.

61. Larsen W, Mandleco B. Chest pain with angiographic clear coronary arteries: a provider's approach to cardiac syndrome X. J Am Acad Nurse Pract 2009;21(7):371–6.

62. Frishman WH. β-Adrenergic blockade in cardiovascular disease. J Cardiovasc Pharmacol Ther 2013;18(4):310–9.

63. Cotrim C, Almeida AG, Carrageta M. Cardiac syndrome X, intraventricular gradients and, beta-blockers. Rev Port Cardiol 2010;29(2):193–203.

64. Bugiardini R, Borghi A, Biagetti L, et al. Comparison of verapamil versus propranolol therapy in syndrome X. Am J Cardiol 1989;63(5):286–90.

65. Leonardo F, Fragasso G, Rossetti E, et al. Comparison of trimetazidine with atenolol in patients with syndrome X: effects on diastolic function and exercise tolerance. Cardiologia 1999;44(12):1065–9.

66. Kalinowski L, Dobrucki LW, Szczepanska-Konkel M, et al. Third-generation beta-blockers stimulate nitric oxide release from endothelial cells through ATP efflux: a novel mechanism for antihypertensive action. Circulation 2003;107(21):2747–52.

67. Sen N, Tavil Y, Erdamar H, et al. Nebivolol therapy improves endothelial function and increases exercise tolerance in patients with cardiac syndrome X. Anadolu Kardiyol Derg 2009;9(5):371–9.

68. Kaski JC, Rodriguez-Plaza L, Brown J, et al. Efficacy of carvedilol (BM 14,190), a new beta-blocking drug with vasodilating properties, in exercise-induced ischemia. Am J Cardiol 1985;56(1):35–40.

69. Parker JD, Parker JO. Stable angina pectoris: the medical management of symptomatic myocardial ischemia. Can J Cardiol 2012;28(Suppl 2):S70–80.

70. Cannon RO 3rd, Watson RM, Rosing DR, et al. Efficacy of calcium channel blocker therapy for angina pectoris resulting from small-vessel coronary artery disease and abnormal vasodilator reserve. Am J Cardiol 1985;56(4):242–6.

71. Sutsch G, Oechslin E, Mayer I, et al. Effect of diltiazem on coronary flow reserve in patients with microvascular angina. Int J Cardiol 1995;52(2):135–43.

72. Lanza GA, Colonna G, Pasceri V, et al. Atenolol versus amlodipine versus isosorbide-5-mononitrate on anginal symptoms in syndrome X. Am J Cardiol 1999;84(7):854–6. A858.

73. Chaitman BR, Pepine CJ, Parker JO, et al. Effects of ranolazine with atenolol, amlodipine, or diltiazem on exercise tolerance and angina frequency in patients with severe chronic angina: a randomized controlled trial. JAMA 2004;291(3):309–16.

74. Chaitman BR, Skettino SL, Parker JO, et al. Antiischemic effects and long-term survival during ranolazine monotherapy in patients with chronic severe angina. J Am Coll Cardiol 2004;43(8):1375–82.

75. Gould HJ 3rd, Garrett C, Donahue RR, et al. Ranolazine attenuates behavioral signs of neuropathic pain. Behav Pharmacol 2009;20(8):755–8.

76. Mehta PK, Goykhman P, Thomson LE, et al. Ranolazine improves angina in women with evidence of myocardial ischemia but no obstructive coronary artery disease. JACC Cardiovasc Imaging 2011;4(5):514–22.

77. Ferrari R, Guardigli G, Ceconi C. Secondary prevention of CAD with ACE inhibitors: a struggle between life and death of the endothelium. Cardiovasc Drugs Ther 2010;24(4):331–9.

78. Kaski JC, Rosano G, Gavrielides S, et al. Effects of angiotensin-converting enzyme inhibition on exercise-induced angina and ST segment depression in patients with microvascular angina. J Am Coll Cardiol 1994;23(3):652–7.

79. Nalbantgil I, Onder R, Altintig A, et al. Therapeutic benefits of cilazapril in patients with syndrome X. Cardiology 1998;89(2):130–3.

80. Chen JW, Hsu NW, Wu TC, et al. Long-term angiotensin-converting enzyme inhibition reduces plasma asymmetric dimethylarginine and improves endothelial nitric oxide bioavailability and coronary microvascular function in patients with syndrome X. Am J Cardiol 2002;90(9):974–82.

81. Pauly DF, Johnson BD, Anderson RD, et al. In women with symptoms of cardiac ischemia, nonobstructive coronary arteries, and microvascular

dysfunction, angiotensin-converting enzyme inhibition is associated with improved microvascular function: A double-blind randomized study from the National Heart, Lung and Blood Institute Women's Ischemia Syndrome Evaluation (WISE). Am Heart J 2011;162(4):678–84.

82. Anderson TJ, Meredith IT, Yeung AC, et al. The effect of cholesterol-lowering and antioxidant therapy on endothelium-dependent coronary vasomotion. N Engl J Med 1995;332(8):488–93.

83. Kayikcioglu M, Payzin S, Yavuzgil O, et al. Benefits of statin treatment in cardiac syndrome-X1. Eur Heart J 2003;24(22):1999–2005.

84. Fabian E, Varga A, Picano E, et al. Effect of simvastatin on endothelial function in cardiac syndrome X patients. Am J Cardiol 2004;94(5):652–5.

85. Zhang X, Li Q, Zhao J, et al. Effects of combination of statin and calcium channel blocker in patients with cardiac syndrome X. Coron Artery Dis 2014; 25(1):40–4.

86. Elliott PM, Krzyzowska-Dickinson K, Calvino R, et al. Effect of oral aminophylline in patients with angina and normal coronary arteriograms (cardiac syndrome X). Heart 1997;77(6):523–6.

87. Emdin M, Picano E, Lattanzi F, et al. Improved exercise capacity with acute aminophylline administration in patients with syndrome X. J Am Coll Cardiol 1989;14(6):1450–3.

88. Yoshio H, Shimizu M, Kita Y, et al. Effects of short-term aminophylline administration on cardiac functional reserve in patients with syndrome X. J Am Coll Cardiol 1995;25(7):1547–51.

89. Lanza GA, Gaspardone A, Pasceri V, et al. Effects of bamiphylline on exercise testing in patients with syndrome X. G Ital Cardiol 1997;27(1):50–4.

90. Sindrup SH, Jensen TS. Efficacy of pharmacological treatments of neuropathic pain: an update and effect related to mechanism of drug action. Pain 1999;83(3):389–400.

91. Cannon RO 3rd, Quyyumi AA, Mincemoyer R, et al. Imipramine in patients with chest pain despite normal coronary angiograms. N Engl J Med 1994; 330(20):1411–7.

92. Cox ID, Hann CM, Kaski JC. Low dose imipramine improves chest pain but not quality of life in patients with angina and normal coronary angiograms. Eur Heart J 1998;19(2):250–4.

93. Moore RK, Groves DG, Bridson JD, et al. A brief cognitive-behavioral intervention reduces hospital admissions in refractory angina patients. J Pain Symptom Manage 2007;33(3):310–6.

94. Potts SG, Lewin R, Fox KA, et al. Group psychological treatment for chest pain with normal coronary arteries. QJM 1999;92(2):81–6.

95. Arora RR, Chou TM, Jain D, et al. The multicenter study of enhanced external counterpulsation (MUST-EECP): effect of EECP on exercise-induced myocardial ischemia and anginal episodes. J Am Coll Cardiol 1999;33(7):1833–40.

96. Kronhaus KD, Lawson WE. Enhanced external counterpulsation is an effective treatment for syndrome X. Int J Cardiol 2009;135(2):256–7.

97. Frobert O, Molgaard H, Botker HE, et al. Autonomic balance in patients with angina and a normal coronary angiogram. Eur Heart J 1995;16(10):1356–60.

98. Gulli G, Cemin R, Pancera P, et al. Evidence of parasympathetic impairment in some patients with cardiac syndrome X. Cardiovasc Res 2001; 52(2):208–16.

99. de Vries J, Dejongste MJ, Durenkamp A, et al. The sustained benefits of long-term neurostimulation in patients with refractory chest pain and normal coronary arteries. Eur J Pain 2007;11(3):360–5.

100. Lanza GA, Sestito A, Sandric S, et al. Spinal cord stimulation in patients with refractory anginal pain and normal coronary arteries. Ital Heart J 2001;2(1):25–30.

101. Moore R, Groves D, Hammond C, et al. Temporary sympathectomy in the treatment of chronic refractory angina. J Pain Symptom Manage 2005;30(2):183–91.

102. Wong CW, Wang CH, Wen MS, et al. Effective therapy with transthoracic video-assisted endoscopic coagulation of the left stellate ganglion and upper sympathetic trunk in congenital long-QT syndrome. Am Heart J 1996;132(5):1060–3.

103. Drott C. Results of endoscopic thoracic sympathectomy (ETS) on hyperhidrosis, facial blushing, angina pectoris, vascular disorders and pain syndromes of the hand and arm. Clin Auton Res 2003;13(Suppl 1):I26–30.

104. Methangkool E, Chua JH, Gopinath A, et al. Anesthetic considerations for thoracoscopic sympathetic ganglionectomy to treat ventricular tachycardia storm: a single-center experience. J Cardiothorac Vasc Anesth 2014;28(1):69–75.

105. Moss AJ, McDonald J. Unilateral cervicothoracic sympathetic ganglionectomy for the treatment of long QT interval syndrome. N Engl J Med 1971; 285(16):903–4.

106. Eriksson BE, Tyni-Lenne R, Svedenhag J, et al. Physical training in syndrome X: physical training counteracts deconditioning and pain in syndrome X. J Am Coll Cardiol 2000;36(5):1619–25.

107. Tyni-Lenne R, Stryjan S, Eriksson B, et al. Beneficial therapeutic effects of physical training and relaxation therapy in women with coronary syndrome X. Physiother Res Int 2002;7(1):35–43.

108. Anand SS, Islam S, Rosengren A, et al. Risk factors for myocardial infarction in women and men: insights from the INTERHEART study. Eur Heart J 2008;29(7):932–40.

109. Asbury EA, Slattery C, Grant A, et al. Cardiac rehabilitation for the treatment of women with chest pain and normal coronary arteries. Menopause 2008; 15(3):454–60.

110. Gokce N, Vita JA, McDonnell M, et al. Effect of medical and surgical weight loss on endothelial vasomotor function in obese patients. Am J Cardiol 2005;95(2):266–8.

111. Raitakari OT, Adams MR, McCredie RJ, et al. Arterial endothelial dysfunction related to passive smoking is potentially reversible in healthy young adults. Ann Intern Med 1999;130(7):578–81.

112. O'Keefe JH, Gheewala NM, O'Keefe JO. Dietary strategies for improving post-prandial glucose, lipids, inflammation, and cardiovascular health. J Am Coll Cardiol 2008;51(3):249–55.

Index

Note: Page numbers of article titles are in **boldface** type.

Cardiol Clin 32 (2014) 479–483

http://dx.doi.org/10.1016/S0733-8651(14)00051-4

0733-8651/14/$ – see front matter © 2014 Elsevier Inc. All rights reserved.

Moving?

Printed and bound by CPI Group (UK) Ltd, Croydon, CR0 4YY

03/10/2024

01040381-0016